T0210173

Fetal Growth

Editors

NATHAN R. BLUE
ROBERT M. SILVER

OBSTETRICS AND GYNECOLOGY CLINICS OF NORTH AMERICA

www.obgyn.theclinics.com

Consulting Editor
WILLIAM F. RAYBURN

June 2021 • Volume 48 • Number 2

ELSEVIER

1600 John F. Kennedy Boulevard • Suite 1800 • Philadelphia, Pennsylvania, 19103-2899

http://www.theclinics.com

OBSTETRICS AND GYNECOLOGY CLINICS OF NORTH AMERICA Volume 48, Number 2
June 2021 ISSN 0889-8545, ISBN-13: 978-0-323-84973-9

Editor: Kerry Holland
Developmental Editor: Lopez Hannah Almira

Obstetrics and Gynecology Clinics (ISSN 0889-8545) is published quarterly by Elsevier Inc., 360 Park Avenue South, New York, NY 10010-1710. Months of issue are March, June, September, and December. Periodicals postage paid at New York, NY, and additional mailing offices. Subscription price per year is $335.00 (US individuals), $944.00 (US institutions), $100.00 (US students), $404.00 (Canadian individuals), $991.00 (Canadian institutions), $100.00 (Canadian students), $459.00 (international individuals), $991.00 (international institutions), and $225.00 (international students). To receive student/resident rate, orders must be accompanied by name of affiliated institution, date of term, and the signature of program/residency coordinator on institution letterhead. Orders will be billed at individual rate until proof of status is received. Foreign air speed delivery is included in all *Clinics* subscription prices. All prices are subject to change without notice. POSTMASTER: Send address changes to *Obstetrics and Gynecology Clinics*, Elsevier Health Sciences Division, Subscription Customer Service, 3251 Riverport Lane, Maryland Heights, MO 63043. **Customer Service: Telephone: 1-800-654-2452 (U.S. and Canada); 314-447-8871 (outside U.S. and Canada). Fax: 314-447-8029. E-mail: journalscustomerservice-usa@elsevier.com (for print support); journalsonlinesupport-usa@elsevier.com (for online support).**

Reprints. For copies of 100 or more of articles in this publication, please contact the Commercial Reprints Department, Elsevier Inc., 360 Park Avenue South, New York, New York 10010-1710. Tel.: 212-633-3874; Fax: 212-633-3820; E-mail: reprints@elsevier.com

Obstetrics and Gynecology Clinics of North America is also published in Spanish by McGraw-Hill Interamericana Editores S.A., P.O. Box 5-237, 06500, Mexico; in Portuguese by Reichmann and Affonso Editores, Rio de Janeiro, Brazil; and in Greek by Paschalidis Medical Publications, Athens, Greece.

Obstetrics and Gynecology Clinics of North America is covered in MEDLINE/PubMed (Index Medicus), Excerpta Medica, Current Concepts/Clinical Medicine, Science Citation Index, BIOSIS, CINAHL, and ISI/BIOMED.

Contributors

CONSULTING EDITOR

WILLIAM F. RAYBURN, MD, MBA
Adjunct Professor, Department of Obstetrics and Gynecology, College of Graduate
Studies, Medical University of South Carolina, Charleston, South Carolina; Associate
Dean, Continuing Medical Education and Professional Development, Distinguished
Professor and Emeritus Chair, Department of Obstetrics and Gynecology, University of
New Mexico School of Medicine, Albuquerque, New Mexico

EDITORS

NATHAN R. BLUE, MD
Assistant Professor, Maternal-Fetal Medicine, University of Utah, Health Intermountain
Healthcare, Salt Lake City, Utah

ROBERT M. SILVER, MD
Professor and Chair, Maternal-Fetal Medicine, University of Utah, Health Salt Lake City,
Utah

AUTHORS

NICHOLAS BEHRENDT, MD
Assistant Professor of Obstetrics and Gynecology, Division of Maternal-Fetal Medicine,
University of Colorado, Children's Hospital Colorado, Colorado Fetal Care Center, Aurora,
Colorado, USA

NATHAN R. BLUE, MD
Assistant Professor, Maternal-Fetal Medicine, University of Utah Health, Intermountain
Healthcare, Salt Lake City, Utah, USA

CLAARTJE BRUIN, MD
Department of Obstetrics and Gynecology, Amsterdam University Medical Centers,
University of Amsterdam, Amsterdam, The Netherlands

STEFANIE E. DAMHUIS, MD
Department of Obstetrics and Gynaecology, University Medical Center Groningen, University
of Groningen, Groningen; Department of Obstetrics and Gynaecology, University Medical
Centers Amsterdam, University of Amsterdam, Amsterdam, the Netherlands

JERAD H. DUMOLT, PhD
Division of Reproductive Sciences, Department of Obstetrics and Gynecology, University
of Colorado Anschutz Medical Campus, Aurora, Colorado, USA

CAMILLE FUNG, MD
Associate Professor, Division of Neonatology, Department of Pediatrics, University of
Utah, Salt Lake City, Utah, USA

HENRY L. GALAN, MD
Professor of Obstetrics and Gynecology, Division of Maternal-Fetal Medicine, University of Colorado, Children's Hospital Colorado, Colorado Fetal Care Center, Aurora, Colorado, USA

WESSEL GANZEVOORT, MD, PhD
Department of Obstetrics and Gynaecology, University Medical Centers Amsterdam, University of Amsterdam, Amsterdam, the Netherlands

SANNE J. GORDIJN, MD, PhD
Department of Obstetrics and Gynaecology, University Medical Center Groningen, University of Groningen, Groningen, the Netherlands

KATHERINE L. GRANTZ, MD, MS
Investigator, Division of Intramural Population Health Research, Eunice Kennedy Shriver National Institute of Child Health and Human Development, National Institutes of Health, Bethesda, Maryland, USA

THOMAS JANSSON, MD, PhD
Division of Reproductive Sciences, Department of Obstetrics and Gynecology, University of Colorado Anschutz Medical Campus, Aurora, Colorado, USA

ALEXANDROS MORAITIS, MD
Department of Obstetrics and Gynaecology, University of Cambridge, Cambridge, United Kingdom

MICHELLE T. NGUYEN, MD
Clinical Instructor, Department of Obstetrics and Gynecology, Division of Maternal-Fetal Medicine, University of Southern California, Keck School of Medicine, Los Angeles, California, USA

JOSEPH G. OUZOUNIAN, MD, MBA
Daniel R. Mishell Jr. MD Endowed Professor and Chair, Department of Obstetrics and Gynecology, USC/Keck School of Medicine, Los Angeles, California, USA

JESSICA M. PAGE, MD, MSCI
Assistant Professor, Maternal-Fetal Medicine, Intermountain Healthcare, University of Utah Health, Murray, Utah, USA

ARIS T. PAPAGEORGHIOU, MD
Nuffield Department of Women's and Reproductive Health, University of Oxford, Oxford, United Kingdom

THERESA L. POWELL, PhD
Division of Reproductive Sciences, Department of Obstetrics and Gynecology, University of Colorado Anschutz Medical Campus, Department of Pediatrics, Section of Neonatology, University of Colorado Anschutz Medical Campus, Aurora, Colorado, USA

CHRISTINA M. SCIFRES, MD
Associate Professor, Department of Obstetrics and Gynecology, Indiana University School of Medicine , Indianapolis, Indiana, USA

ALICE SELF, MD
Nuffield Department of Women's and Reproductive Health, University of Oxford, Oxford, United Kingdom

ROBERT M. SILVER, MD
Professor and Chair, Maternal-Fetal Medicine, University of Utah Health, Salt Lake City, Utah, USA

GORDON C.S. SMITH, DSc
Professor, Department of Obstetrics and Gynaecology, University of Cambridge, Cambridge, United Kingdom

KATIE STEPHENS, MBChB
Department of Obstetrics and Gynaecology, University of Cambridge, Cambridge, United Kingdom

ERIN ZINKHAN, MD
Adjunct Assistant Professor, Division of Neonatology, Department of Pediatrics, University of Utah, Salt Lake City, Utah, USA

Contents

> Placental regulation of fetal growth involves the integration of multiple signaling pathways that modulate an array of placental functions, including nutrient transport. As a result, the flux of oxygen and nutrients to the fetus is altered, leading to changes in placental and fetal growth. Placental insulin/insulinlike growth factor-1 and mechanistic target of rapamycin signaling and amino acid transport capacity are inhibited in fetal growth restriction and activated in fetal overgrowth, implicating these placental functions in driving fetal growth. With novel approaches to specifically target the placenta, clinical interventions to modulate placental function in high-risk pregnancies can be developed.

> Abnormal fetal growth (growth restriction and overgrowth) is associated with perinatal morbidity, mortality, and lifelong risks to health. To describe abnormal growth, "small for gestational age" and "large for gestational age" are commonly used terms. However, both are statistical definitions of fetal size below or above a certain threshold related to a reference population, rather than referring to an abnormal condition. Fetuses can be constitutionally small or large and thus healthy, whereas fetuses with seemingly normal size can be growth restricted or overgrown. Although golden standards to detect abnormal growth are lacking, understanding of both pathologic conditions has improved significantly.

> Three modern cohort studies have an advantage over historical fetal growth references because they included diverse populations. Despite similar inclusion criteria, estimated fetal weight percentiles for gestational age varied among studies, which result in different proportions of fetuses as being classified below or above a cutoff point. A universal reference would make comparison of fetal growth simpler for clinical use and for

comparison across populations but may misclassify small-for-gestational-age or large-for-gestational-age fetuses. It is important to know how a growth reference performs in a local population in relation to fetal morbidity and mortality when implementing in clinical practice.

Fetal growth restriction (FGR) is a common clinical manifestation of placental insufficiency. As such, FGR is a risk factor for stillbirth. This association has been demonstrated in numerous studies but is prone to overestimation because of the possibility of prolonged in utero retention before the recognition of the fetal death. Stillbirth risk reduction by optimizing maternal medical conditions and exposures and appropriate antenatal testing and delivery timing are essential to pregnancies affected by FGR. It is important to evaluate stillbirths with FGR with fetal autopsy, placental pathology, genetic testing, and assessment of antiphospholipid antibodies and fetal-maternal hemorrhage.

Fetal growth restriction (FGR) describes a fetus' inability to attain adequate weight gain based on genetic potential and gestational age and is the second most common cause of perinatal morbidity and mortality after prematurity. Infants who have suffered fetal growth restriction are at the greatest risks for short- and long-term complications. This article specifically details the neurologic and cardiometabolic sequalae associated with fetal growth restriction, as well as the purported mechanisms that underlie their pathogenesis. We end with a brief discussion about further work that is needed to gain a more complete understanding of fetal growth restriction.

Large for gestational age birth weight is associated with adverse short- and long-term outcomes. Infants born with large for gestational age birth weight are at increased risk for neonatal intensive care unit admission, respiratory distress, neonatal metabolic abnormalities including hypoglycemia, birth trauma, and even stillbirth or neonatal death. The risk for many of these complications increases with higher birth weights. Individuals with large for gestational age birth weight also appear to be at subsequent increased risk for overweight/obesity, diabetes, cardiovascular disease, and even some childhood cancers. These data highlight the need for effective interventions to decrease risk across the lifespan.

Antenatal imaging is crucial in the management of high-risk pregnancies. Accurate dating relies on acquisition of reliable and reproducible ultrasound images and measurements. Quality image acquisition is necessary for assessing fetal growth and performing Doppler measurements to help diagnose pregnancy complications, stratify risk, and guide management. Further research is needed to ascertain whether current methods for estimating fetal weight can be improved with 3-dimensional ultrasound or magnetic resonance imaging; optimize dating with late initiation of prenatal care; minimize under-diagnosis of fetal growth restriction; and identify the best strategies to make ultrasound more available in low-income and middle-income countries.

Several risk factors for adverse pregnancy outcomes can be identified by a routine third trimester ultrasound scan. However, there is also potential for harm, anxiety, and additional health care costs through unnecessary intervention due to false positive results. The evidence base informing the balance of risks and benefits of universal screening is inadequate to fully inform decision making. However, data on the diagnostic effectiveness of universal ultrasound suggest that better methods are required to result in net benefit, with the exception of screening for presentation near term, where a clinical and economic case can be made for its implementation.

Impaired fetal growth owing to placental insufficiency is a major contributor to adverse perinatal outcomes. No intervention is available that improves outcomes by changing the pathophysiologic process. Monitoring in early-onset fetal growth restriction (FGR) focuses on optimizing the timing of iatrogenic preterm delivery using cardiotocography and Doppler ultrasound. In late-onset FGR, identifying the fetus at risk for immediate hypoxia and who benefits from expedited delivery is challenging. It is likely that studies in the next decade will provide evidence how to best integrate different monitoring variables and other prognosticators in risk models that are aimed to optimize individual treatment strategies.

Macrosomia results from abnormal fetal growth and can lead to serious consequences for the mother and fetus. In cases of suspected macrosomia, patients must be counseled carefully regarding a delivery plan, and Cesarean section should be considered when indicated. Techniques to assess for suspected macrosomia include clinical measurements, ultrasound, and MRI.

Multifetal gestation pregnancies present a clinical challenge due to unique complications including growth issues, prematurity, maternal risk, and pathologic processes, such as selective intrauterine growth restriction (sIUGR), twin-to-twin transfusion syndrome (TTTS), and twin anemia-polycythemia sequence. If sIUGR is found, then management may involve some combination of increased surveillance, fetal procedures, and/or delivery. The combination of sIUGR with TTTS or other comorbidities increases the risk of pregnancy complications. Multifetal pregnancy reduction is an option when a problem is confined to a single fetus or when weighing the risks and benefits of a multifetal gestation in comparison to a singleton pregnancy.

Fetal growth restriction (FGR) is a common obstetric complication that predisposes to mortality across the lifespan. Women with a prior pregnancy affected by FGR have a 20% to 30% risk of recurrence, but effective preventive strategies are lacking. Pharmacologic interventions to prevent FGR are lacking. Low-dose aspirin may be somewhat effective, but low-molecular-weight heparin and sildenafil are not. Surveillance in a subsequent pregnancy may consist of serial ultrasonography with timing and frequency determined by the clinical severity in the index pregnancy. Once FGR is diagnosed, the principal management strategy consists of close surveillance and carefully timed delivery.

OBSTETRICS AND GYNECOLOGY CLINICS

SERIES OF RELATED INTEREST

Clinics in Perinatology
www.perinatology.theclinics.com

THE CLINICS ARE AVAILABLE ONLINE!
Access your subscription at:
www.theclinics.com

Foreword

Understanding the Intricacies of Individual Fetal Growth

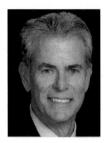

William F. Rayburn, MD, MBA
Consulting Editor

This quarterly issue of *Obstetrics and Gynecology Clinics of North America*, edited by Nathan Blue, MD and Robert Silver, MD, pertains to the intricacies of fetal growth. The eventual size of the newborn infant is a culmination of complex placental functions and fetal physiologic processes in adapting to maternal and environmental influences. This issue reviews the definition, prevalence, significance, risk factors, cause, and diagnosis and treatment of every fetus in which there is a deviation in normal growth in the form of either growth restriction or overgrowth. Each deviation can represent pressing and difficult clinical challenges. A smaller- or larger-than-expected fetal size or weight is usually related to constitutional factors. However, maternal factors (eg, hypertension, diabetes), maternal size (eg, obesity, undernutrition), maternal weight gain, or fetal abnormalities (eg, genetic, structural, infections, twins/triplets) require consideration.

The standard modality for fetal growth assessment is by 2-dimensional ultrasound evaluation. A small-for-gestational-age or large-for-gestational-age fetus/infant refers to growth either under or beyond a specific threshold for that gestation age. Using statistical approaches, any fetus/infant weighing <10th percentile or >90th percentile for gestational age is either small or large. Tables for estimating fetal weight between gestational ages 24 and 42 weeks have been drawn to show the 5th, 10th, 50th, 90th, and 95th percentile weights.

Fetal growth curves are nicely compared in this issue. Generating local tables, when possible, should be considered if the population is constitutionally more uniform and different from published tables. While racial and ethnic differences in fetal growth have been described, whether and how to incorporate them into clinical management are uncertain and remain an area of active investigation. Comparisons of published tables are made in this issue between the World Health Organization, the National

Obstet Gynecol Clin N Am 48 (2021) xiii–xv
https://doi.org/10.1016/j.ogc.2021.03.005
0889-8545/21/© 2021 Published by Elsevier Inc.

obgyn.theclinics.com

Institute of Child Health and Diseases, and the International Fetal and Newborn Growth Consortium for the 21st Century.

When repeated ultrasound examinations suggest impaired fetal growth, steps to be taken include reexamining gestational age determination, determining the cause and severity, counseling the parents, closely monitoring fetal growth and well-being, and determining the optimal time and route of delivery. Fetal growth restriction (FGR) resulting from intrinsic factors (aneuploidy, congenital malformation, infection) carries a guarded prognosis that often cannot be improved by any intervention. In contrast, FGR related to uteroplacental insufficiency has a more favorable prognosis, but the risk for an adverse outcome remains increased.

An initial approach is to confirm the diagnosis based on discrepancies between actual and expected sonographic biometric measurements for a given gestational age. No biometric measurement is highly sensitive and specific, although the abdominal circumference is especially important when assessing a larger- or smaller-than-expected size. An estimated fetal weight <10th percentile definition is clinically practical, but it alone does not distinguish between the constitutionally small fetus, that achieves its normal growth potential and is not at increased risk of adverse outcome, from the fetus whose restricted growth is at increased risk of perinatal morbidity and mortality.

Evaluation of the fetus with a growth discrepancy involves monitoring the fetal weight trajectories, managing any maternal comorbidities, and serially assessing fetal well-being. A detailed fetal anatomic survey is recommended, since anomalies are frequently associated with failure to maintain normal fetal growth. This issue focuses on umbilical artery diastolic flow and amniotic fluid volume. Although a significant decrease in the fetal weight percentile between 30 and 38 weeks may be of concern, the presence of a normal flow and volume is reassuring. Biophysical profiles weekly and delivery at 38 weeks seem to be reasonable, with preterm delivery for standard obstetric indications.

The timing and location of delivery are intended to maximize fetal maturity and growth while minimizing the risk of fetal and neonatal mortality and short-term and long-term morbidity. The presence of altered fetal growth is an important factor to consider in decision making about performance of delivery (eg, whether to use forceps or vacuum vs whether to proceed with cesarean delivery). Altered fetal growth, confirmed at birth, requires close monitoring of the newborn for hypoglycemia, respiratory problems, and minor congenital anomalies, which sometimes requires admission in a special care nursery. Furthermore, preconception counseling before any subsequent pregnancies should include an awareness of the tendency of a repeat smaller or larger fetus.

The intricacies of fetal growth depend on maternal, placental, and fetal factors that may manifest differently. These situations often involve a complexity of clinical scenarios that require continued vigilance and education of the parents-to-be. The international group of authors in this issue contributed their cutting-edge information.

Knowledge gleaned by the readers will assist in addressing the many questions resulting from altered fetal growth.

William F. Rayburn, MD, MBA
Department of Obstetrics and Gynecology
University of New Mexico School of Medicine
MSC 10 5580, 1 University of New Mexico
Albuquerque, NM 87131-0001, USA

E-mail address:
wrayburnmd@gmail.com

Preface

Fetal Growth in the Twenty-First Century: A Pressing Challenge for Clinicians and Researchers

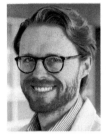 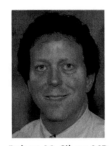

Nathan R. Blue, MD   Robert M. Silver, MD
Editors

Fetal growth is a culmination of complex fetal-placental-maternal processes that adapt to maternal and environmental factors. Deviations in normal growth occur in the form of fetal growth restriction (FGR) and fetal overgrowth and represent a pressing and difficult clinical challenge. The challenge is pressing because the global burden of morbidity from FGR and fetal overgrowth is considerable. It is difficult because of the limited available options for diagnosis and management; few are supported by robust evidence, and many more questions exist than answers. In 2021, expert clinicians remained vexed by rudimentary risk-stratification tools, inaccurate diagnostic modalities, and uncertainty about ideal delivery timing and mode. Finally, there are no therapeutic options available to families and pregnant people faced with a diagnosis of FGR or fetal overgrowth.

First among challenges to both researchers and clinicians is the lack of a gold standard against which screening and diagnostic approaches can be tested. For example, most small-for-gestational age (SGA) infants are healthy and do not suffer complications of pathologic smallness, making SGA a poor surrogate by which to define poor growth. The alternative is to use perinatal morbidity and mortality as the outcome to be predicted. While this represents an incremental improvement over an isolated size-for-age threshold, this approach is also limited in utility since there are many causal pathways to morbidity and mortality. Accordingly, prenatal diagnostic or risk-stratification strategies may never achieve useful specificity. This is merely one example of the many unresolved obstacles to progress in reducing morbidity and mortality from aberrant fetal growth.

We are indebted to our stellar group of international authors for their cutting-edge contributions to the ongoing efforts to address these difficult questions. Our hope is

Obstet Gynecol Clin N Am 48 (2021) xvii–xviii
https://doi.org/10.1016/j.ogc.2021.03.004
0889-8545/21/© 2021 Published by Elsevier Inc.

obgyn.theclinics.com

that this issue will serve as a useful reference by which clinicians can anchor and orient themselves to find a path forward when faced with the complex clinical scenarios that characterize daily obstetrics practice in 2021.

Nathan R. Blue, MD
Maternal-Fetal Medicine
University of Utah
Intermountain Healthcare
30 North 1900 East, 2A200
Salt Lake City, UT 84132, USA

Robert M. Silver, MD
Maternal-Fetal Medicine
University of Utah
30 North 1900 East, 2A200
Salt Lake City, UT 84132, USA

E-mail addresses:
nblue1297@gmail.com (N.R. Blue)
bob.silver@hsc.utah.edu (R.M. Silver)

Twitter: @Nateyblue (N.R. Blue)

Placental Function and the Development of Fetal Overgrowth and Fetal Growth Restriction

Jerad H. Dumolt, PhD[a],*, Theresa L. Powell, PhD[a,b,1],
Thomas Jansson, MD, PhD[a,2]

KEYWORDS

- Fetal development • Fetal growth restriction • Fetal overgrowth • Placental transport
- Maternal-fetal exchange • Syncytiotrophoblast

KEY POINTS

- Placental signaling and nutrient transport are determinants of fetal growth.
- In fetal growth restriction, placental insulin/insulinlike growth factor-1 (IGF-1) and mechanistic target of rapamycin (mTOR) signaling and nutrient transport are typically inhibited, which may contribute to the restricted fetal growth.
- Activation of placental insulin/IGF-1 and mTOR signaling and nutrient transporters and reduced placental adiponectin signaling may promote fetal overgrowth in some pregnancies complicated by maternal obesity and gestational diabetes mellitus.
- Therapeutic strategies designed to restore normal placental function and fetal growth in high-risk pregnancies are limited and have yielded conflicting results.
- Robust approaches to specifically target the placenta rather than the mother and the fetus and a better understanding of the placental molecular pathways driving fetal growth are required for the development of successful interventions to modulate placental function.

Funding: Supported by grants from NIH [grant numbers R01DK089989, HD089980, HD093950, HD065007, HD068370, HD078376, and T32HD007186].

[a] Division of Reproductive Sciences, Department of Obstetrics and Gynecology, University of Colorado Anschutz Medical Campus, Aurora, CO 80045, USA; [b] Department of Pediatrics, Section of Neonatology, University of Colorado Anschutz Medical Campus, Aurora, CO 80045, USA
[1] Present address: Research Complex 2, 12700 East 19th Avenue, Room 3100A, MS 8613, Aurora, CO 80045.
[2] Present address: Research Complex 2, 12700 East 19th Avenue, Room 3100C, MS 8613, Aurora, CO 80045.
* Corresponding author. Research Complex 2, 12700 East 19th Avenue, Room 3420B, Aurora, CO 80045.
E-mail address: jerad.dumolt@cuanschutz.edu

Obstet Gynecol Clin N Am 48 (2021) 247–266
https://doi.org/10.1016/j.ogc.2021.02.001
0889-8545/21/© 2021 Elsevier Inc. All rights reserved.

INTRODUCTION

The developing fetus undergoes a dynamic period of rapid growth that is responsive to changes in the in utero environment that may contribute to the development of fetal growth restriction (FGR) or fetal overgrowth resulting in the delivery of a large-for-gestational age (LGA) infant.[1] Pregnancies complicated by abnormal fetal growth have a major impact on public health because of the increased perinatal morbidity and mortality associated with FGR and LGA and because abnormal fetal growth is strongly associated with long-term health consequences for offspring, including the development of cardiovascular disease, metabolic dysfunction, and obesity later in life.[2–4] An array of conditions, including changes in maternal nutrient, endocrine, and metabolic status and impaired uteroplacental blood flow, are associated with altered fetal growth.[5] However, the precise mechanisms causing changes in the growth trajectory of the fetus remain to be fully established. Accumulating evidence suggests that changes in placental function may contribute to, or mediate, both FGR and fetal overgrowth.

Early clinical studies of fetal growth were instrumental in establishing a link between impaired uteroplacental blood flow and reduced fetal weight as a result of placental insufficiency.[6,7] Although impaired uteroplacental blood flow is an established risk factor for restricted fetal growth, placental insufficiency is more than reduced blood flow and may involve decreased transplacental nutrient transport capacity, altered activity in placental growth factor and inflammatory signaling pathways, and changes in the release of placental extracellular vesicles and their cargo. Placental cell signaling pathways, such as mechanistic target of rapamycin (mTOR), insulinlike growth factor (IGF), adipokine signaling, and nutrient transport are regulated by oxygen and nutrient levels as well as maternal metabolic hormones. Changes in placental function therefore link the availability of oxygen and nutrients for fetal growth to the fetal growth trajectory, in some cases resulting in FGR or, at the opposite end of the growth spectrum, LGA.[8,9]

This article discusses recent work showing compelling associations between changes in placental function and fetal growth. In particular, it focuses on distinct differences in transplacental nutrient transport, cellular signaling pathways, inflammatory markers, and extracellular vesicle regulatory functions that are unique to placentas of LGA and FGR infants. Furthermore, it discusses novel clinical interventions specifically targeting placental function as an avenue to rescue disordered fetal growth patterns. In addition, it speculates on future research and intervention priorities to prevent adverse infant outcomes in pregnancies complicated by altered placental function and fetal growth.

HUMAN PLACENTA

The human placenta is derived from the fetal trophectoderm, the outermost layer of the blastocyst. After implantation, the trophectoderm differentiates into mononuclear villous cytotrophoblasts that can further differentiate into either extravillous trophoblasts or they can fuse to form the multinucleated syncytiotrophoblast (STB). The extravillous trophoblasts proliferate and invade the myometrium to reach the spiral arteries, where they eventually replace smooth muscle cells of the arterial media with eosinophilic materials, resulting in decreased vasoreactivity, allowing the marked increase in uteroplacental blood flow throughout gestation that characterizes a normal pregnancy. During the first weeks after implantation, cytotrophoblasts rapidly proliferate to form the functional unit of the placenta, the trophoblast villous tree, which is lined with a continuous outer layer of STB. Following the onset of the uteroplacental circulation in late first trimester, the STB is directly exposed to maternal blood in the intervillous space, and serve as the primary barrier between maternal and fetal blood supply as well as the site of placental hormone production and maternal-fetal oxygen, nutrient, and ion transfer.[10,11]

Maternal-fetal exchange occurs across 2 largely continuous cell layers, the fetal capillary endothelium and STB, which separate maternal and fetal blood supplies. Fetal capillary endothelial cells allow largely unrestricted transfer of small molecules such as glucose, amino acids, and ions through intercellular junctions,[12] making STB the limiting factor for maternal-fetal solute exchange. In contrast, although the mechanisms involved remain to be fully established, transplacental transfer of lipids likely requires transport across both STB and fetal capillary endothelium.[13] The STB consists of 2 polarized plasma membranes, the apical or maternal-facing microvillous plasma membrane (MVM), and the fetal-facing basal plasma membrane (BM). The MVM and BM express an array of different transporter proteins critical for mediating vectorial maternal-to-fetal transfer of nutrients[14] and fetal-to-maternal transfer of waste products (**Fig. 1**).

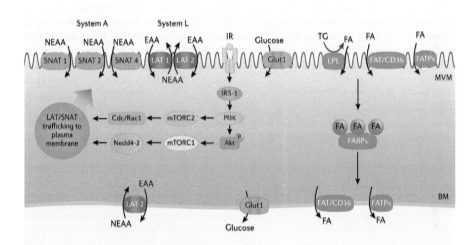

Fig. 1. Some key placental signaling pathways and nutrient transporters. The syncytiotrophoblast consists of 2 polarized plasma membranes, MVM and BM, that express an array of transport proteins that mediate maternal-to-fetal transfer of amino acids, glucose, and fatty acids. The uptake of nonessential and essential amino acids from maternal circulation across the MVM is mediated by system A (SNAT1, 2, 4) and system L (LAT1, 2) transport systems that are trafficked to the plasma membrane as a result of activation of insulin/IGF-1 and mTOR signaling. Glucose transporter-1 (GLUT-1) is highly expressed in the MVM and BM of the syncytiotrophoblast and is considered the primary glucose transporter in the human placenta at term. Maternal triglycerides are hydrolyzed into free fatty acids (FFAs) by membrane-bound lipases and transferred across the MVM by FAT/CD36 and fatty acid transport proteins (FATPs). Internalized FFAs are transferred to the BM by fatty acid binding proteins (FABPs) for export into fetal circulation. Akt, protein kinase B; Cdc/Rac1, cell division control protein/ras-related C3 botulinum toxin substrate 1; EAA, essential amino acids; FA, fatty acids; FAT/CD36, fatty acid translocase/cluster of differentiation 36;IR, insulin receptor; IRS-1, insulin receptor substrate 1; LAT, L-amino acid transporter; LPL, lipoprotein lipase; mTORC, mTOR complex; Nedd4-2, neuronal precursor cell-expressed, developmentally downregulated gene 4 isoform 2; NEAA, nonessential amino acids; SNAT, sodium-coupled neutral amino acid transporter; TG, triglycerides. (*Courtesy of* KIMEN Design4Research, with permission.)

PLACENTAL SIGNALING

Placental receptors for many metabolic hormones and growth factors, including receptors for insulin,[15] IGF-1,[16] and adiponectin,[17] are localized on the MVM of syncytiotrophoblast, mediating regulation of placental function by maternal circulating factors. The coordinated actions of insulin/IGF-1 and adiponectin through downstream mTOR signaling act to regulate mitochondrial function, protein synthesis, and the flux of glucose, amino acids, lipids, and folate across the placental barrier. Importantly, these signaling pathways are differentially regulated in pregnancies complicated by fetal overgrowth and FGR (**Fig. 2**).

Insulin/insulinlike growth factor-1 and mechanistic target of rapamycin Signaling

The insulin/IGF-1 signaling pathway is primarily composed of a system of ligands (IGF-1, IGF-2, and insulin), tyrosine kinase receptors (IGF-1 receptor and insulin receptor isoforms [INSR] A and B), and downstream activation of target proteins insulin receptor substrate 1 (IRS-1), protein kinase B (Akt), and mTOR. Activation of placental insulin/IGF-1 signaling is crucial for normal trophoblast function and fetal growth and development by promoting hormone synthesis, protein synthesis, and nutrient transfer, in part as a result of mTOR activation.[18,19] During pregnancy, IGF-1 availability in the maternal circulation and at the maternal-fetal interface is primarily regulated by IGF binding proteins such as IGFBP-1 synthesized by the decidua.[20] Phosphorylation of IGFBP-1 at serine residues

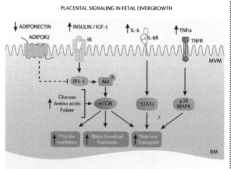
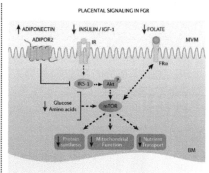

Fig. 2. Placental signaling in fetal overgrowth and FGR. The coordinated actions of placental insulin/IGF-1, mTOR, adiponectin, and inflammatory cytokine signaling pathways act to regulate mitochondrial function, protein synthesis, and the flux of glucose, amino acids, lipids, and folate across the placental barrier. Placental insulin/IGF-1 and mTOR signaling is activated in women with obesity delivering LGA infants likely because of increased circulating maternal insulin/IGF-1 levels and increased availably of nutrients. Moreover, low maternal levels of circulating adiponectin in pregnancies complicated by maternal obesity contribute to enhance placental insulin signaling because of decreased inhibition of insulin receptor substrate (IRS)-1. Levels of maternal circulating proinflammatory cytokines interleukin (IL)-6 and tumor necrosis factor (TNF)-α are increased in pregnancies with obesity and may contribute to fetal overgrowth by activating signal transducer and activator of transcription 3 (STAT3) and p38 mitogen-activated protein kinase (MAPK) signaling pathways. Conversely, lower levels of maternal circulating insulin/IGF-1 and folate, and increased adiponectin level, contribute to reduced placental insulin/IGF-1 and mTOR signaling in FGR pregnancies. Thus, differential regulation of placental signaling pathways and subsequent impact on placental function and nutrient transfer likely contribute to fetal overgrowth and FGR. ADIPOR2, adiponectin receptor 2; FRα, folate receptor-α; IL-6R, IL-6 receptor; TNFR, tumor necrosis factor-α receptor. (*Courtesy of* KIMEN Design4Research, with permission.)

(Ser101, 119, and 169) markedly increases IGFBP-1 binding affinity for IGF-1, effectively reducing IGF-1 availability and function.[21] FGR pregnancies are associated with reduced maternal serum IGF-1 concentrations and increased abundance[22] and phosphorylation[23,24] of IGFBP-1. In addition, decreased placental IGF-1 expression has been reported in human FGR,[25] which may contribute to the inhibition of placental insulin/IGF-1 signaling pathway in this pregnancy complication.[26–28] In contrast, placental insulin/IGF-1 signaling is enhanced in women with obesity[29] or gestational diabetes mellitus (GDM)[30] delivering a large infant. There are likely multiple factors underlying the activation of placental insulin/IGF-1 signaling in fetal overgrowth, including increased maternal IGF-1 level[22] and lower circulating levels of adiponectin in the mother,[31] as discussed later.

Activation of mTOR complex 1 (mTORC1) occurs by several mechanisms, including insulin/IGF-1 ligand binding and increased availability of ATP, amino acids, fatty acids, folate, and glucose, whereas mTOR complex 2 (mTORC2) primarily responds to insulin/phosphoinositide 3-kinase(Akt) signaling.[32] In the placenta, mTORC1 serves as a positive regulator of amino acid[33] and folate transport,[34] and mitochondrial biogenesis.[35] In contrast, mTORC2 promotes cell proliferation by phosphorylation of Akt, PKCα, and SGK1, which regulate cytoskeletal remodeling and cell migration.[32] Placental mTORC1 activity has been found to be closely related to fetal growth. A consistent decrease in placental mTORC1 activity has been reported in humans[27,36,37] and animal models[38,39] of FGR, whereas human GDM[40] and obesity[29] and rodent models of fetal overgrowth[41,42] are often associated with placental mTORC1 activation. Further, inhibition of mTOR in decidual cells increased the release of hyperphosphorylated IGFBP-1, which decreases IGF-1 bioavailability and is associated with restricted fetal growth.[43] Likewise, mTORC1 is inhibited by adenosine monophosphate-activated protein kinase (AMPK), a critical nutrient sensor that is activated when ATP levels are depleted.[44] Placental mTORC1 activity is positively correlated to infant birthweight, whereas placental AMPK activity shows an inverse relationship, suggesting that the placental mTORC1 signaling pathway constitutes an important link between placental nutrient status and fetal growth.[29]

Adiponectin Signaling

As in nonpregnant individuals, circulating levels of adiponectin are inversely correlated to body mass index (BMI) in pregnant women. Moreover, maternal serum adiponectin level is negatively associated with birth weight.[45] In agreement with these associations, low adiponectin level increases the risk of fetal overgrowth,[31,46–48] whereas maternal adiponectin level tends to be increased in FGR.[45] Adiponectin is the most abundant protein secreted from adipose tissue and has well-documented insulin-sensitizing effects in adipose, liver, and skeletal muscle tissues.[49] Adiponectin binds to adiponectin receptor (AdipoR) 1 and AdipoR2, which activate downstream AMPK, p38 mitogen-activated protein kinase (MAPK), and/or PPARα.[50] Surprisingly, adiponectin blunts insulin signaling in primary human trophoblast cells[51] by PPARα--mediated synthesis of ceramide, which phosphorylates IRS-1 at an inhibitory site.[52] These findings are consistent with the possibility that low circulating adiponectin level, a feature of maternal obesity and GDM, is mechanistically linked to activation of placental insulin/IGF-1/mTOR signaling, stimulating fetal growth. In support of this model, adiponectin supplementation prevented the adverse effects of maternal obesity on placental function and fetal growth in mice.[41] Moreover, normalization of maternal circulating adiponectin levels in obese pregnant mice largely prevented the development of cardiac[53] and metabolic disease[54] in adult progeny, implicating low maternal adiponectin levels as a mechanism underpinning fetal overgrowth and developmental programming of cardiovascular and metabolic disease.

INFLAMMATION

Pregnancy is characterized by a tightly regulated balance between proinflammatory and antiinflammatory cytokines necessary for implantation and placentation. Although results of studies exploring the effect of maternal obesity and GDM on maternal cytokine levels are inconsistent,[55] women with obesity,[56] GDM,[57] or preeclampsia[58] generally are thought to have increased levels of circulating proinflammatory cytokines, such as IL-6 and tumor necrosis factor (TNF)-α. Placental cytokine production, which is critical for the maintenance of pregnancy from implantation to parturition,[59] is altered in pregnancies complicated with obesity and GDM.[55] Maternal BMI is positively associated with activation of distinct placental inflammatory pathways, including p38 MAPK and signal transducer and activator of transcription 3 (STAT3) signaling without changes in classic inflammatory pathways or fetal cytokine profile.[60] These findings suggest that maternal and placental inflammation in maternal obesity and GDM may affect fetal development by altering placental function rather than direct fetal exposure to increased levels of proinflammatory cytokines.

The transcription of placental IL-6 and TNF-α messenger RNA (mRNA) is increased in maternal obesity,[61] which may promote placental lipid and amino acid transfer. In cultured primary human trophoblasts, IL-6 was shown to upregulate STAT3-dependent system A amino acid transport activity through increased sodium-coupled neutral amino acid transporter (SNAT) 2 expression,[62] whereas TNF-α stimulated system A amino acid transport through activation of p38 MAPK signaling.[63] In contrast, IL-1β downregulates insulin-stimulated system A transport but activates system L activity in primary trophoblasts.[64] Collectively, data from in vitro experiments show a mechanistic link between placental response to inflammation and altered nutrient transport. However, the cumulative effects of inflammation on placental nutrient transport are complex and may vary depending on the degree of inflammation and specific cytokine levels that are increased.

NUTRIENT TRANSPORT
Glucose

Glucose is the primary energy substrate for the placenta and the fetus. Fetoplacental glucose needs are met entirely by placental uptake from the maternal circulation via facilitated diffusion and in response to increased postprandial maternal glucose levels. Glucose transporter (GLUT)-1 is highly expressed in the MVM and BM of the STB; however, GLUT-1 localized in the BM is considered the primary glucose transporter in the human placenta at term.[65] BM GLUT-1 expression is associated with birthweight and is increased in pregnancies complicated by obesity and fetal overgrowth.[66] Similarly, GLUT-4 expression and translocation to the BM is upregulated by insulin, which may enhance glucose transport in response to postprandial hyperinsulinemia.[15] MVM and BM GLUT-1 protein expression and activity seem not to be affected in FGR[65]; however, reduced MVM GLUT-1 protein level, activity, and glucose transfer have been reported in preeclampsia.[67] Some FGR fetuses are hypoglycemic in utero, this may be caused by impaired uteroplacental blood flow, increased placental glucose consumption, or altered glycolytic pathways.[21,68]

Amino Acids

Placental uptake of amino acids is mediated by an array of distinct transporter systems. Of these, system A and system L are thought to be some of the most important, in part because these transporters are subjected to regulation. System A is a sodium-dependent transporter mediating the uptake of nonessential neutral amino acids into the cell. System A comprises 3 isoforms, which are all expressed in the human placenta: SNAT 1 (SLC38A1), SNAT 2 (SLC38A2), and SNAT 4 (SLC38A4).[69] The system L amino acid transporter is a heterodimer, consisting of a light chain, typically L-amino acid transporter (LAT) 1 (SLC7A5) or LAT2 (SLC7A8), and a heavy chain, 4F2hc/CD98 (SLC3A2). System L is a sodium-independent exchanger mediating cellular uptake of essential amino acids, including leucine, in exchange for nonessential system A substrates such as glycine. As a result, the coordinated activity of both system A and system L activity is required for placental transport of nonessential and essential amino acids across pregnancy.[70] Activation of trophoblast system A and system L amino acid transport occurs as a direct result of upstream mTORC1 and mTORC2 activation.[33] mTORC1 modulates SNAT2 and LAT1 trafficking by Nedd4-2-regulated ubiquitination in normal term pregnancies,[69] whereas mTORC2 regulates amino acid transporter trafficking through interactions with Cdc42 and Rac1, which are downregulated in FGR.[71] Placental amino acid transport capacity has been consistently shown to be reduced in human FGR.[37,72–77] The authors have reported that downregulation of key placental amino acid transport systems precedes the development of FGR in rodents[38,78] and nonhuman primates,[39,79,80] supporting the concept that downregulation of placental nutrient transport is a primary event that directly contributes to FGR, rather than a response to a changing fetal demand. In contrast, as previously discussed, activation of placental amino acid transport systems caused by upstream activation of mTOR signaling by increased maternal hormone levels (insulin/IGF, leptin), low adiponectin level, excess nutrients, and a mild proinflammatory activation may contribute to fetal overgrowth in pregnancies complicated by obesity.[29,42,52,62]

Lipids

Placental uptake of lipids from the maternal circulation is mediated by several membrane-bound transport proteins and lipases. Triglycerides (TGs) packaged in circulating lipoproteins (very-low-density lipoprotein, low-density lipoprotein [LDL], chylomicrons) are hydrolyzed into nonesterified fatty acids and glycerol by lipoprotein lipase (LPL) and endothelial lipase (EL) before entering the syncytiotrophoblast. Long-chain fatty acids are transported across the MVM by fatty acid transport proteins (FATPs) and fatty acid translocase/cluster of differentiation 36 (FAT/CD36).[81] Once internalized, free fatty acids are esterified with coenzyme A (CoA) producing acyl-CoAs that are trafficked by cytosolic fatty acid binding proteins for use in placental mitochondrial respiration, incorporated into lipid droplets for placental storage, or transferred to the BM for export.[82] Maternal obesity is generally thought to increase lipid transport, possibly contributing to greater fetal adipogenesis and birthweight.[61] Although the relationship between maternal obesity, placental lipid transport, and fetal growth remains incompletely understood, maternal obesity is associated with decreased placental total FATP1 and FATP4 mRNA and increased FATP6 and FAT/CD36 protein content.[83] FATP2 and FATP4 expression is greater on the BM compared with the MVM in the human placenta, with BM FATP2 expression positively correlated to maternal BMI.[84] In contrast, FAT/CD36 expression is higher in the MVM compared with the BM, but was not associated with maternal BMI.[84] Increased BM FATP2 expression may reflect increased transplacental lipid transfer; however, direct evidence showing an association between increased BM FATP expression and fetal overgrowth is currently lacking. Maternal obesity is also associated with reduced placental EL expression and increased placental storage of long-chain polyunsaturated fatty acids (LCPUFAs), which may limit transplacental transport of LCPUFA species in maternal obesity.[83]

Pregnancies complicated by FGR are also associated with changes in placental lipid transport mechanisms. Placental EL mRNA and MVM LPL activity have been reported to be decreased, but placental LPL gene expression is increased,[85,86] in FGR. The divergence between LPL activity and mRNA expression may reflect that regulation of LPL-mediated lipid transfer does not occur at the transcriptional level.[21] MVM FATP6 and CD36 protein levels are increased in FGR, and LCPUFAs seem to be preferentially routed to storage in placental TG, suggesting a possible defect in intracellular LCPUFA trafficking and export.[87] Further, fetal and placental weights and placental expression of genes related to fatty acid mobilization and TG content were not altered in mice deficient in FATP2 and FATP4.[88] Interestingly, protein expression of placental FATP1, FATP2, FATP4, FATP5, and FATP6 is increased across late gestation in a baboon model of FGR, suggesting a coordinated placental adaptation to facilitate fatty acid transport.[89] However, the potential overlap and redundancy of FATPs involved in placental fatty acid trafficking throughout gestation remains unresolved and warrants further investigation. The expression of LDL receptor (LDLr) mRNA and scavenger receptor class B type I (SR-B1) protein, which are membrane-bound proteins responsible for the uptake of LDL and high-density lipoprotein from maternal circulation, is reduced in FGR placentas. However, whether changes in placental cholesterol transport in FGR influence fetal development is not fully elicited.[90]

Folate

Folate has a well-characterized role in DNA replication, amino acid metabolism, and as a methyl donor. Folate deficiency during pregnancy is associated with FGR and congenital abnormalities such as neural tube defects. Interestingly, mTOR functions as a folate sensor in the trophoblast and other cell types,[34,91] and maternal folate deficiency in mice inhibits placental mTORC1 and mTORC2 signaling and placental amino acid transport contributing to FGR.[91] Furthermore, both mTORC1 and mTORC2 are positive regulators of trophoblast folate uptake by modulating the cell surface expression of folate receptor-α (FR-α) and the reduced folate carrier.[34,92] Placental folate transport capacity is decreased in human FGR,[93] which may contribute to the restricted fetal growth and intrauterine programming of childhood and adult disease.

SMALL EXTRACELLULAR VESICLES AND microRNA

Extracellular vesicles are membrane-bound particles containing bioactive proteins, lipids, DNA, mRNA, and microRNA (miR) that are secreted from most cells and participate in cell-to-cell communication. Small extracellular vesicles (sEVs), commonly referred to as exosomes, are small (<150 nm in diameter) nanovesicles produced from the endosomal pathway and released on fusion of multivesicular bodies with the plasma membrane. Because of a lack of specific subtypes and mixed origins, the International Society of Extracellular Vesicles has recommended the use of size to categorize extracellular vesicles; therefore, this article refers to this heterogenous population as sEVs.[94]

At present, little is known about the relationship between sEVs, placental or originating from other tissues, and fetal growth. However, mice infused with human total and/or placental sEVs from women with preeclampsia developed hypertension,[95] and mice infused with sEVs from women with GDM became glucose intolerant and insulin resistant.[96] Therefore, it is highly plausible that sEVs regulate fetal growth, at least secondarily to changes in maternal physiology (**Fig. 3**). Indirect support of this hypothesis is found in the differential expression of sEV miR isolated from maternal

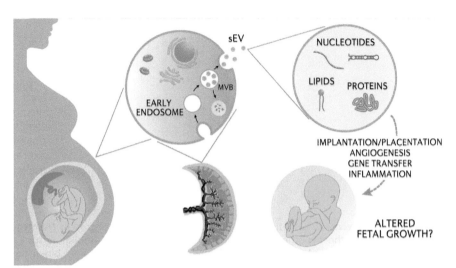

Fig. 3. The influence of small extracellular vesicles on placental function. sEVs are membrane-bound particles containing bioactive proteins, lipids, DNA, mRNA, and miR that are secreted from most cells and participate in cell-to-cell communication. The functions of maternal and placental sEVs remain to be fully established but they are thought to be involved in immune response, angiogenesis, placentation, and the transfer of nucleic acids and proteins important in normal and complicated pregnancies that may influence fetal growth. MVB, multivesicular bodies. (*Courtesy of* KIMEN Design4Research, with permission.)

serum in the second trimester being correlated with birth weight.[97] Further, the fraction of total circulating sEVs that are of placental origin is reduced in FGR, likely because the levels of circulating placental sEVs was correlated with placental weight, suggesting that decreased release of placental sEV may be a result of reduced placental size.[98] The functions of placental sEVs remain to be fully established but they are thought to be involved in immune response, angiogenesis, and the transfer of nucleic acids and proteins important in normal and complicated pregnancies.[99] Placental sEVs containing miR-520c-3p have been reported to inhibit CD44/HA-mediated extravillous trophoblast invasion, suggesting a link between placental sEVs and placentation.[100] sEVs isolated from second trimester cytotrophoblasts contain a significant amount of TNF-α and increase decidual stromal cell transcription and secretion of NF-κB targets, including IL-8.[101] In addition, placental sEVs from women with GDM promote endothelial cytokine release compared with placenta-derived sEVs from normal pregnancies,[102] in agreement with previous studies showing that placental sEVs mediate monocyte recruitment and induce IL-1β production.[103] A direct link between sEVs of maternal or placental origin and abnormal fetal growth remains to be established.

INTERVENTIONS TARGETING PLACENTAL FUNCTION IN FETAL GROWTH RESTRICTION AND FETAL OVERGROWTH
Restoring Uteroplacental Blood Flow in Fetal Growth Restriction

Numerous studies have tested the hypothesis that systemic administration of vasodilators increases uteroplacental blood flow and promotes fetal growth in FGR (**Fig. 4**). Aspirin is a cyclo-oxygenase inhibitor that suppresses the production of thromboxane,

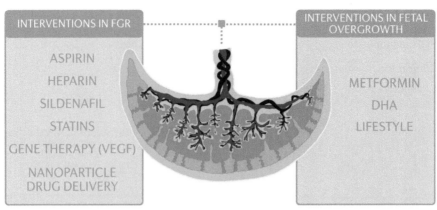

Fig. 4. Clinical interventions targeting placental function to restore fetal growth. Numerous studies have tested the hypothesis that systemic administration of vasodilators such as aspirin, low-molecular-weight heparin, and sildenafil increases uteroplacental blood flow and promotes fetal growth in FGR; however, the results have not been encouraging. Clinical trials to improve fetal growth in FGR pregnancies using statins have been initiated. In addition, gene therapy and nanoparticle drug delivery designed to alter the expression of genes in the uteroplacental circulation and the placenta, including vascular endothelial growth factor (VEGF), is an area of active research. Limited clinical approaches to prevent fetal overgrowth currently exist; however, treatment of GDM and/or maternal obesity with metformin, docosahexaenoic acid (DHA) supplementation, or lifestyle interventions may mitigate fetal overgrowth in high-risk pregnancies. (*Courtesy of* KIMEN Design4Research, with permission.)

which promotes platelet aggregation and functions as a vasoconstrictor. Thus, aspirin has the potential to increase uteroplacental blood flow. Although the evidence on the efficacy of initiating aspirin therapy in early gestation to prevent FGR is conflicting, several meta-analyses suggest that low-dose aspirin (75–100 mg) has a modest effect on reducing the risk for developing preeclampsia and FGR.[104–106] Challenges remain in determining the appropriate timing to initiate treatment (before or after 16 weeks of gestation), defining the optimal dose, and delineating the benefits of aspirin in women with chronic hypertension versus those who develop preeclampsia during late gestation. Further, most of the studies included in the meta-analyses were designed with preeclampsia prevention as a primary end point, with effects on fetal growth as a secondary outcome. In an effort to address these concerns, the Chronic Hypertension and Acetyl Salicylic Acid in Pregnancy (CHASP) trial will compare the efficacy of aspirin (150 mg/d) introduced before 15 weeks of gestation in the prevention of maternal and fetal morbidity and mortality, including FGR, in women with chronic hypertension.[107]

Low-molecular-weight heparin is commonly used in pregnancy as a thromboprophylaxis and for the treatment of venous thromboembolism. Heparin therapy during pregnancy is associated with increased circulating levels of placental growth factor and decreased risk of recurrence of placental-mediated complications in women without thrombophilia.[108] Randomized controlled trials initially showed a potential reduction of the incidence of preeclampsia and FGR; however, recent meta-analyses suggest no benefit.[109,110] Despite early promise in small trials, a recent large trial of the phosphodiesterase type 5 inhibitor sildenafil, Sildenafil TheRapy In Dismal Prognosis Early-onset Fetal Growth Restriction (STIDER), was terminated before completion after several fetal deaths were reported,[111] possibly caused by fetal hypotension as a result of transplacental transfer of sildenafil into fetal circulation.[112] In contrast, a phase II trial (TADAFER) of tadalafil, a phosphodiesterase 5 inhibitor that does not cross the placenta, decreased fetal and infant deaths associated with FGR, although fetal growth velocity and birthweight were unchanged.[113]

Clinical Interventions Targeting Placental Function in Fetal Overgrowth

Significant challenges exist in designing interventions targeting placental function in pregnancies complicated by maternal obesity. As described in this article, placental dysfunction as a result of increased nutrient availability and transport in response to increased insulin level, low adiponectin level, and enhanced mTOR placental signaling may contribute to fetal overgrowth. However, concerns over safety with the use of pharmaceuticals to reduce circulating maternal nutrients have limited the clinical approaches to prevent fetal overgrowth (see **Fig. 4**). Using metformin for glucose control in GDM pregnancies decreased the risk of fetal overgrowth compared with women receiving insulin or glyburide[114] but was recently shown to increase the proportion of small-for-gestation-age infants in women with type 2 diabetes and obesity.[115] Although the cause of reduced infant birthweights is unknown, it is possible those infants did not experience accelerated growth, highlighting the need for early detection of fetal overgrowth to guide clinical decision making. In contrast, metformin did not prevent fetal overgrowth in obese pregnant women.[116] Because metformin is transported across the placenta into fetal circulation, concerns have been raised that metformin may program the fetus for adverse outcomes, including obesity, later in life.[117] However, a recent report showed that children of obese mothers exposed prenatally to metformin had improved cardiovascular profiles compared with placebo-controlled offspring.[118]

The powerful impact of hormonal regulation on placental function and fetal growth was shown by experimentally increasing adiponectin levels in obese mice compared with those observed in normal-weight pregnant mice. Not only did this treatment improve placental function and prevent fetal overgrowth[41] but the long-term programming effects on metabolism, weight gain, glucose intolerance, and cardiac dysfunction were also corrected.[53,54] In human pregnancy, nutrition and lifestyle interventions and dietary supplements have been explored as treatments to reduce fetal overgrowth in pregnancies complicated by maternal obesity or GDM. The UK Pregnancies Better Eating and Activity Trial (UPBEAT) recently reported that a comprehensive intervention targeting improvements in nutrition and physical activity did not reduce the incidence of LGA infants in pregnant women with obesity,[119] although placental storage of fatty acids in droplets was reported to be modestly decreased in women who received the lifestyle intervention.[120] In addition, supplementation with docosahexaenoic acid (DHA) in pregnancy decreases placental inflammation and amino acid transporter expression in obese pregnancies, which may mitigate fetal overgrowth.[121] However, trials assessing the effect of DHA on clinical outcomes related to fetal growth are lacking.

Future Interventional Approaches and Priorities

Targeting the placenta with pharmaceutical interventions and approaches designed to alter placental gene expression is an area of active research. Injection of adenoviral vectors containing vascular endothelial growth factor (VEGF), a potent angiogenic factor, in the uterine artery of sheep was shown to improve uterine blood flow.[122] Gene therapy targeting maternal VEGF is currently being investigated as a therapeutic intervention in early-onset FGR (EVERREST trial).[123] The use of statins, particularly lipophilic statins that readily cross plasma membranes, is contraindicated during pregnancy because of the risk of congenital malformations.[124] Despite recent interest in the use of pravastatin to improve outcomes in preeclampsia and FGR mediated by inhibition of placental sFLT1 secretion,[125] the evidence that pravastatin is beneficial in these 2 pregnancy complications is conflicting.[126,127] Large randomized controlled trials are needed to assess the efficacy of statins in preeclampsia and FGR pregnancies. In addition, innovative approaches using nanoparticles for drug delivery or gene targeting to the placenta represents an emerging area of clinical interest and warrants further investigation.[128]

SUMMARY

Placental regulation of fetal growth involves the integration of multiple hormonal, inflammatory, nutrient, oxygen, and energy-sensing signaling pathways that modulate an array of placental functions, including nutrient transport. As a result, the flux of oxygen and nutrients to the fetus is altered, leading to changes in fetal growth. Placental insulin/IGF-1 and mTOR signaling and transport capacity of certain nutrients are inhibited in FGR and activated in some cases of fetal overgrowth, implicating these placental functions in driving fetal growth. Emerging evidence suggests that circulating total and placenta-derived sEVs and miR may modulate placental function; however, it is currently unknown how these novel signaling systems affect fetal growth. Future research priorities include establishing the role of sEVs in regulating fetal growth and determining the mechanistic role of maternal versus placental sEVs in the development of FGR and fetal overgrowth. Despite a considerable body of evidence linking placental function and fetal growth, clinical interventions specifically designed to restore normal placental function in high-risk pregnancies are lacking. Although novel interventions using placental gene targeting and nanoparticle drug delivery are currently being investigated, the development of future clinically useful therapies to alleviate abnormal fetal growth is likely to depend on a better understanding of the specific placental molecular pathways that regulate fetal growth.

CLINICS CARE POINTS

- FGR and fetal overgrowth increase the risk of perinatal complications and the development of obesity, diabetes, and cardiovascular disease in childhood and later in life.
- Changes in placental function contribute to abnormal fetal growth.
- The understanding of the causes of abnormal fetal growth is limited, and no effective treatments are available.
- Therapeutic strategies designed to restore normal placental function in women with an FGR or LGA fetus have largely been unsuccessful and may potentially harm the fetus.
- Novel interventions using placental gene targeting and nanoparticle drug delivery may be effective therapeutic strategies to restore normal fetal growth in high-risk pregnancies but require rigorous research to determine their clinical usefulness.

CONFLICT OF INTERESTS

The authors declare that there are no competing interests associated with this article.

AUTHOR CONTRIBUTIONS

J.H. Dumolt wrote the article. T.L. Powell and T. Jansson were involved in the planning, organization, and revision of the review.

ACKNOWLEDGMENTS

The authors thank KIMEN Design4Research (kimendesign4research.com) for the graphic design of the figures in this article.

REFERENCES

1. Goldstein RF, Abell SK, Ranasinha S, et al. Association of gestational weight gain with maternal and infant outcomes: a systematic review and meta-analysis. JAMA 2017;317(21):2207–25.
2. Gluckman PD, Hanson MA, Cooper C, et al. Effect of in utero and early-life conditions on adult health and disease. N Engl J Med 2008;359(1):61–73.
3. Reynolds RM, Allan KM, Raja EA, et al. Maternal obesity during pregnancy and premature mortality from cardiovascular event in adult offspring: follow-up of 1 323 275 person years. BMJ 2013;347:f4539.
4. Catalano PM, Ehrenberg HM. The short- and long-term implications of maternal obesity on the mother and her offspring. BJOG 2006;113(10):1126–33.
5. Gluckman PD, Hanson MA, Pinal C. The developmental origins of adult disease. Matern Child Nutr 2005;1(3):130–41.
6. Lao TT, Wong W. The neonatal implications of a high placental ratio in small-for-gestational age infants. Placenta 1999;20(8):723–6.
7. Karsdorp VH, van Vugt JM, van Geijn HP, et al. Clinical significance of absent or reversed end diastolic velocity waveforms in umbilical artery. Lancet 1994; 344(8938):1664–8.
8. Vaughan OR, Rosario FJ, Powell TL, et al. Regulation of placental amino acid transport and fetal growth. Prog Mol Biol Transl Sci 2017;145:217–51.
9. Jansson T, Powell TL. Role of placental nutrient sensing in developmental programming. Clin Obstet Gynecol 2013;56(3):591–601.
10. Turco MY, Moffett A. Development of the human placenta. Development 2019; 146(22):dev163428.
11. Pollheimer J, Vondra S, Baltayeva J, et al. Regulation of placental extravillous trophoblasts by the maternal uterine environment. Front Immunol 2018;9:2597.
12. Leach L, Firth JA. Fine structure of the paracellular junctions of terminal villous capillaries in the perfused human placenta. Cell Tissue Res 1992;268(3): 447–52.
13. Elad D, Levkovitz R, Jaffa AJ, et al. Have we neglected the role of fetal endothelium in transplacental transport? Traffic 2014;15(1):122–6.
14. Burton GJ, Fowden AL. The placenta: a multifaceted, transient organ. Philos Trans R Soc Lond B Biol Sci 2015;370(1663):20140066.
15. James-Allan LB, Arbet J, Teal SB, et al. Insulin stimulates GLUT4 trafficking to the syncytiotrophoblast basal plasma membrane in the human placenta. J Clin Endocrinol Metab 2019;104(9):4225–38.
16. Fang J, Furesz TC, Lurent RS, et al. Spatial polarization of insulin-like growth factor receptors on the human syncytiotrophoblast. Pediatr Res 1997;41(2):258–65.
17. Aye IL, Powell TL, Jansson T. Review: adiponectin–the missing link between maternal adiposity, placental transport and fetal growth? Placenta 2013; 34(Suppl):S40–5.
18. Bowman CJ, Streck RD, Chapin RE. Maternal-placental insulin-like growth factor (IGF) signaling and its importance to normal embryo-fetal development. Birth Defects Res B Dev Reprod Toxicol 2010;89(4):339–49.

19. Roos S, Kanai Y, Prasad PD, et al. Regulation of placental amino acid transporter activity by mammalian target of rapamycin. Am J Physiol Cell Physiol 2009;296(1):C142–50.

20. Martina NA, Kim E, Chitkara U, et al. Gestational age-dependent expression of insulin-like growth factor-binding protein-1 (IGFBP-1) phosphoisoforms in human extraembryonic cavities, maternal serum, and decidua suggests decidua as the primary source of IGFBP-1 in these fluids during early pregnancy. J Clin Endocrinol Metab 1997;82(6):1894–8.

21. Chassen S, Jansson T. Complex, coordinated and highly regulated changes in placental signaling and nutrient transport capacity in IUGR. Biochim Biophys Acta Mol Basis Dis 2020;1866(2):165373.

22. Olausson H, Lof M, Brismar K, et al. Maternal serum concentrations of insulin-like growth factor (IGF)-I and IGF binding protein-1 before and during pregnancy in relation to maternal body weight and composition and infant birth weight. Br J Nutr 2010;104(6):842–8.

23. Gupta MB, Abu Shehab M, Nygard K, et al. IUGR is associated with marked hyperphosphorylation of decidual and maternal plasma IGFBP-1. J Clin Endocrinol Metab 2019;104(2):408–22.

24. Singal SS, Nygard K, Gratton R, et al. Increased insulin-like growth factor binding protein-1 phosphorylation in decidualized stromal mesenchymal cells in human intrauterine growth restriction placentas. J Histochem Cytochem 2018; 66(9):617–30.

25. Calvo MT, Romo A, Gutierrez JJ, et al. Study of genetic expression of intrauterine growth factors IGF-I and EGFR in placental tissue from pregnancies with intrauterine growth retardation. J Pediatr Endocrinol Metab 2004;17(Suppl 3): 445–50.

26. Laviola L, Perrini S, Belsanti G, et al. Intrauterine growth restriction in humans is associated with abnormalities in placental insulin-like growth factor signaling. Endocrinology 2005;146(3):1498–505.

27. Yung HW, Calabrese S, Hynx D, et al. Evidence of placental translation inhibition and endoplasmic reticulum stress in the etiology of human intrauterine growth restriction. Am J Pathol 2008;173(2):451–62.

28. Street ME, Viani I, Ziveri MA, et al. Impairment of insulin receptor signal transduction in placentas of intra-uterine growth-restricted newborns and its relationship with fetal growth. Eur J Endocrinol 2011;164(1):45–52.

29. Jansson N, Rosario FJ, Gaccioli F, et al. Activation of placental mTOR signaling and amino acid transporters in obese women giving birth to large babies. J Clin Endocrinol Metab 2013;98(1):105–13.

30. Shang M, Wen Z. Increased placental IGF-1/mTOR activity in macrosomia born to women with gestational diabetes. Diabetes Res Clin Pract 2018;146:211–9.

31. Jansson N, Nilsfelt A, Gellerstedt M, et al. Maternal hormones linking maternal body mass index and dietary intake to birth weight. Am J Clin Nutr 2008; 87(6):1743–9.

32. Saxton RA, Sabatini DM. mTOR signaling in growth, metabolism, and disease. Cell 2017;168(6):960–76.

33. Rosario FJ, Kanai Y, Powell TL, et al. Mammalian target of rapamycin signalling modulates amino acid uptake by regulating transporter cell surface abundance in primary human trophoblast cells. J Physiol 2013;591(3):609–25.

34. Rosario FJ, Powell TL, Jansson T. mTOR folate sensing links folate availability to trophoblast cell function. J Physiol 2017;595(13):4189–206.

35. Rosario FJ, Gupta MB, Myatt L, et al. Mechanistic target of rapamycin complex 1 promotes the expression of genes encoding electron transport chain proteins and stimulates oxidative phosphorylation in primary human trophoblast cells by regulating mitochondrial biogenesis. Sci Rep 2019;9(1):246.

36. Roos S, Jansson N, Palmberg I, et al. Mammalian target of rapamycin in the human placenta regulates leucine transport and is down-regulated in restricted fetal growth. J Physiol 2007;582(Pt 1):449–59.

37. Chen YY, Rosario FJ, Shehab MA, et al. Increased ubiquitination and reduced plasma membrane trafficking of placental amino acid transporter SNAT-2 in human IUGR. Clin Sci (Lond) 2015;129(12):1131–41.

38. Rosario FJ, Jansson N, Kanai Y, et al. Maternal protein restriction in the rat inhibits placental insulin, mTOR, and STAT3 signaling and down-regulates placental amino acid transporters. Endocrinology 2011;152(3):1119–29.

39. Kavitha JV, Rosario FJ, Nijland MJ, et al. Down-regulation of placental mTOR, insulin/IGF-I signaling, and nutrient transporters in response to maternal nutrient restriction in the baboon. FASEB J 2014;28(3):1294–305.

40. Sati L, Soygur B, Celik-Ozenci C. Expression of mammalian target of rapamycin and downstream targets in normal and gestational diabetic human term placenta. Reprod Sci 2016;23(3):324–32.

41. Aye IL, Rosario FJ, Powell TL, et al. Adiponectin supplementation in pregnant mice prevents the adverse effects of maternal obesity on placental function and fetal growth. Proc Natl Acad Sci U S A 2015;112(41):12858–63.

42. Rosario FJ, Powell TL, Jansson T. Activation of placental insulin and mTOR signaling in a mouse model of maternal obesity associated with fetal overgrowth. Am J Physiol Regul Integr Comp Physiol 2016;310(1):R87–93.

43. Gupta MB, Jansson T. Novel roles of mechanistic target of rapamycin signaling in regulating fetal growth. Biol Reprod 2019;100(4):872–84.

44. Kola B, Grossman AB, Korbonits M. The role of AMP-activated protein kinase in obesity. Front Horm Res 2008;36:198–211.

45. Wang J, Shang LX, Dong X, et al. Relationship of adiponectin and resistin levels in umbilical serum, maternal serum and placenta with neonatal birth weight. Aust N Z J Obstet Gynaecol 2010;50(5):432–8.

46. Haghiac M, Basu S, Presley L, et al. Patterns of adiponectin expression in term pregnancy: impact of obesity. J Clin Endocrinol Metab 2014;99(9):3427–34.

47. Hendler I, Blackwell SC, Mehta SH, et al. The levels of leptin, adiponectin, and resistin in normal weight, overweight, and obese pregnant women with and without preeclampsia. Am J Obstet Gynecol 2005;193(3 Pt 2):979–83.

48. Vernini JM, Moreli JB, Costa RA, et al. Maternal adipokines and insulin as biomarkers of pregnancies complicated by overweight and obesity. Diabetol Metab Syndr 2016;8(1):68.

49. Yamauchi T, Kamon J, Ito Y, et al. Cloning of adiponectin receptors that mediate antidiabetic metabolic effects. Nature 2003;423(6941):762–9.

50. Yoon MJ, Lee GY, Chung JJ, et al. Adiponectin increases fatty acid oxidation in skeletal muscle cells by sequential activation of AMP-activated protein kinase, p38 mitogen-activated protein kinase, and peroxisome proliferator-activated receptor alpha. Diabetes 2006;55(9):2562–70.

51. Jones HN, Jansson T, Powell TL. Full-length adiponectin attenuates insulin signaling and inhibits insulin-stimulated amino Acid transport in human primary trophoblast cells. Diabetes 2010;59(5):1161–70.

52. Aye IL, Gao X, Weintraub ST, et al. Adiponectin inhibits insulin function in primary trophoblasts by PPARalpha-mediated ceramide synthesis. Mol Endocrinol 2014;28(4):512–24.

53. Vaughan OR, Rosario FJ, Powell TL, et al. Normalisation of circulating adiponectin levels in obese pregnant mice prevents cardiac dysfunction in adult offspring. Int J Obes (Lond) 2020;44(2):488–99.

54. Paulsen ME, Rosario FJ, Wesolowski SR, et al. Normalizing adiponectin levels in obese pregnant mice prevents adverse metabolic outcomes in offspring. FASEB J 2019;33(2):2899–909.

55. Pantham P, Aye IL, Powell TL. Inflammation in maternal obesity and gestational diabetes mellitus. Placenta 2015;36(7):709–15.

56. St-Germain LE, Castellana B, Baltayeva J, et al. Maternal obesity and the uterine immune cell landscape: the shaping role of inflammation. Int J Mol Sci 2020; 21(11):3776.

57. Nguyen-Ngo C, Jayabalan N, Salomon C, et al. Molecular pathways disrupted by gestational diabetes mellitus. J Mol Endocrinol 2019;63(3):R51–72.

58. Tenorio MB, Ferreira RC, Moura FA, et al. Cross-talk between oxidative stress and inflammation in preeclampsia. Oxid Med Cell Longev 2019;2019:8238727.

59. Hauguel-de Mouzon S, Guerre-Millo M. The placenta cytokine network and inflammatory signals. Placenta 2006;27(8):794–8.

60. Aye IL, Lager S, Ramirez VI, et al. Increasing maternal body mass index is associated with systemic inflammation in the mother and the activation of distinct placental inflammatory pathways. Biol Reprod 2014;90(6):129.

61. Kelly AC, Powell TL, Jansson T. Placental function in maternal obesity. Clin Sci (Lond) 2020;134(8):961–84.

62. Jones HN, Jansson T, Powell TL. IL-6 stimulates system A amino acid transporter activity in trophoblast cells through STAT3 and increased expression of SNAT2. Am J Physiol Cell Physiol 2009;297(5):C1228–35.

63. Aye IL, Jansson T, Powell TL. TNF-alpha stimulates system A amino acid transport in primary human trophoblast cells mediated by p38 MAPK signaling. Physiol Rep 2015;3(10):e12594.

64. Aye IL, Jansson T, Powell TL. Interleukin-1beta inhibits insulin signaling and prevents insulin-stimulated system A amino acid transport in primary human trophoblasts. Mol Cell Endocrinol 2013;381(1–2):46–55.

65. Jansson T, Wennergren M, Illsley NP. Glucose transporter protein expression in human placenta throughout gestation and in intrauterine growth retardation. J Clin Endocrinol Metab 1993;77(6):1554–62.

66. Acosta O, Ramirez VI, Lager S, et al. Increased glucose and placental GLUT-1 in large infants of obese nondiabetic mothers. Am J Obstet Gynecol 2015; 212(2):227.e1-7.

67. Luscher BP, Marini C, Joerger-Messerli MS, et al. Placental glucose transporter (GLUT)-1 is down-regulated in preeclampsia. Placenta 2017;55:94–9.

68. Sharma D, Shastri S, Sharma P. Intrauterine growth restriction: antenatal and postnatal aspects. Clin Med Insights Pediatr 2016;10:67–83.

69. Rosario FJ, Dimasuay KG, Kanai Y, et al. Regulation of amino acid transporter trafficking by mTORC1 in primary human trophoblast cells is mediated by the ubiquitin ligase Nedd4-2. Clin Sci (Lond) 2016;130(7):499–512.

70. James-Allan LB, Teal S, Powell TL, et al. Changes in placental nutrient transporter protein expression and activity across gestation in normal and obese women. Reprod Sci 2020;27(9):1758–69.

71. Jansson T, Castillo-Castrejon M, Gupta MB, et al. Down-regulation of placental Cdc42 and Rac1 links mTORC2 inhibition to decreased trophoblast amino acid transport in human intrauterine growth restriction. Clin Sci (Lond) 2020;134(1): 53–70.

72. Norberg S, Powell TL, Jansson T. Intrauterine growth restriction is associated with a reduced activity of placental taurine transporters. Pediatr Res 1998; 44(2):233–8.

73. Jansson T, Scholtbach V, Powell TL. Placental transport of leucine and lysine is reduced in intrauterine growth restriction. Pediatr Res 1998;44(4):532–7.

74. Mahendran D, Donnai P, Glazier JD, et al. Amino acid (system A) transporter activity in microvillous membrane vesicles from the placentas of appropriate and small for gestational age babies. Pediatr Res 1993;34(5):661–5.

75. Glazier JD, Cetin I, Perugino G, et al. Association between the activity of the system A amino acid transporter in the microvillous plasma membrane of the human placenta and severity of fetal compromise in intrauterine growth restriction. Pediatr Res 1997;42(4):514–9.

76. Marconi AM, Paolini CL, Stramare L, et al. Steady state maternal-fetal leucine enrichments in normal and intrauterine growth-restricted pregnancies. Pediatr Res 1999;46(1):114–9.

77. Paolini CL, Marconi AM, Ronzoni S, et al. Placental transport of leucine, phenylalanine, glycine, and proline in intrauterine growth-restricted pregnancies. J Clin Endocrinol Metab 2001;86(11):5427–32.

78. Jansson N, Pettersson J, Haafiz A, et al. Down-regulation of placental transport of amino acids precedes the development of intrauterine growth restriction in rats fed a low protein diet. J Physiol 2006;576(Pt 3):935–46.

79. Pantham P, Rosario FJ, Nijland M, et al. Reduced placental amino acid transport in response to maternal nutrient restriction in the baboon. Am J Physiol Regul Integr Comp Physiol 2015;309(7):R740–6.

80. Pantham P, Rosario FJ, Weintraub ST, et al. Down-regulation of placental transport of amino acids precedes the development of intrauterine growth restriction in maternal nutrient restricted baboons. Biol Reprod 2016;95(5):98.

81. Lewis RM, Childs CE, Calder PC. New perspectives on placental fatty acid transfer. Prostaglandins Leukot Essent Fatty Acids 2018;138:24–9.

82. Lewis RM, Wadsack C, Desoye G. Placental fatty acid transfer. Curr Opin Clin Nutr Metab Care 2018;21(2):78–82.

83. Segura MT, Demmelmair H, Krauss-Etschmann S, et al. Maternal BMI and gestational diabetes alter placental lipid transporters and fatty acid composition. Placenta 2017;57:144–51.

84. Lager S, Ramirez VI, Gaccioli F, et al. Protein expression of fatty acid transporter 2 is polarized to the trophoblast basal plasma membrane and increased in placentas from overweight/obese women. Placenta 2016;40:60–6.

85. Magnusson AL, Waterman IJ, Wennergren M, et al. Triglyceride hydrolase activities and expression of fatty acid binding proteins in the human placenta in pregnancies complicated by intrauterine growth restriction and diabetes. J Clin Endocrinol Metab 2004;89(9):4607–14.

86. Gauster M, Hiden U, Blaschitz A, et al. Dysregulation of placental endothelial lipase and lipoprotein lipase in intrauterine growth-restricted pregnancies. J Clin Endocrinol Metab 2007;92(6):2256–63.

87. Chassen SS, Ferchaud-Roucher V, Gupta MB, et al. Alterations in placental long chain polyunsaturated fatty acid metabolism in human intrauterine growth restriction. Clin Sci (Lond) 2018;132(5):595–607.

88. Mishima T, Miner JH, Morizane M, et al. The expression and function of fatty acid transport protein-2 and -4 in the murine placenta. PLoS One 2011;6(10):e25865.

89. Chassen SS, Ferchaud-Roucher V, Palmer C, et al. Placental fatty acid transport across late gestation in a baboon model of intrauterine growth restriction. J Physiol 2020;598(12):2469–89.

90. Welge JA, Warshak CR, Woollett LA. Maternal plasma cholesterol concentration and preterm birth: a meta-analysis and systematic review of literature. J Matern Fetal Neonatal Med 2020;33(13):2291–9.

91. Rosario FJ, Nathanielsz PW, Powell TL, et al. Maternal folate deficiency causes inhibition of mTOR signaling, down-regulation of placental amino acid transporters and fetal growth restriction in mice. Sci Rep 2017;7(1):3982.

92. Rosario FJ, Powell TL, Jansson T. Mechanistic target of rapamycin (mTOR) regulates trophoblast folate uptake by modulating the cell surface expression of FR-alpha and the RFC. Sci Rep 2016;6:31705.

93. Chen YY, Gupta MB, Grattton R, et al. Down-regulation of placental folate transporters in intrauterine growth restriction. J Nutr Biochem 2018;59:136–41.

94. Thery C, Witwer KW, Aikawa E, et al. Minimal information for studies of extracellular vesicles 2018 (MISEV2018): a position statement of the International Society for Extracellular Vesicles and update of the MISEV2014 guidelines. J Extracell Vesicles 2018;7(1):1535750.

95. Han C, Wang C, Chen Y, et al. Placenta-derived extracellular vesicles induce preeclampsia in mouse models. Haematologica 2020;105(6):1686–94.

96. James-Allan LB, Rosario FJ, Barner K, et al. Regulation of glucose homeostasis by small extracellular vesicles in normal pregnancy and in gestational diabetes. FASEB J 2020;34(4):5724–39.

97. Rodosthenous RS, Burris HH, Sanders AP, et al. Second trimester extracellular microRNAs in maternal blood and fetal growth: an exploratory study. Epigenetics 2017;12(9):804–10.

98. Miranda J, Paules C, Nair S, et al. Placental exosomes profile in maternal and fetal circulation in intrauterine growth restriction - Liquid biopsies to monitoring fetal growth. Placenta 2018;64:34–43.

99. Jin J, Menon R. Placental exosomes: a proxy to understand pregnancy complications. Am J Reprod Immunol 2018;79(5):e12788.

100. Takahashi H, Ohkuchi A, Kuwata T, et al. Endogenous and exogenous miR-520c-3p modulates CD44-mediated extravillous trophoblast invasion. Placenta 2017;50:25–31.

101. Taylor SK, Houshdaran S, Robinson JF, et al. Cytotrophoblast extracellular vesicles enhance decidual cell secretion of immune modulators via TNF-alpha. Development 2020;147(17):dev187013.

102. Salomon C, Scholz-Romero K, Sarker S, et al. Gestational diabetes mellitus is associated with changes in the concentration and bioactivity of placenta-derived exosomes in maternal circulation across gestation. Diabetes 2016;65(3):598–609.

103. Atay S, Gercel-Taylor C, Suttles J, et al. Trophoblast-derived exosomes mediate monocyte recruitment and differentiation. Am J Reprod Immunol 2011;65(1):65–77.

104. Roberge S, Bujold E, Nicolaides KH. Aspirin for the prevention of preterm and term preeclampsia: systematic review and metaanalysis. Am J Obstet Gynecol 2018;218(3):287–93.e1.

105. Roberge S, Nicolaides K, Demers S, et al. The role of aspirin dose on the prevention of preeclampsia and fetal growth restriction: systematic review and meta-analysis. Am J Obstet Gynecol 2017;216(2):110–20.e6.

106. Meher S, Duley L, Hunter K, et al. Antiplatelet therapy before or after 16 weeks' gestation for preventing preeclampsia: an individual participant data meta-analysis. Am J Obstet Gynecol 2017;216(2):121–8.e2.

107. Lecarpentier E, Haddad B. Aspirin for the prevention of placenta-mediated complications in pregnant women with chronic hypertension. J Gynecol Obstet Hum Reprod 2020;49:101845.

108. Nawathe A, David AL. Prophylaxis and treatment of foetal growth restriction. Best Pract Res Clin Obstet Gynaecol 2018;49:66–78.

109. Rodger MA, Gris JC, de Vries JIP, et al. Low-molecular-weight heparin and recurrent placenta-mediated pregnancy complications: a meta-analysis of individual patient data from randomised controlled trials. Lancet 2016;388(10060): 2629–41.

110. Mastrolia SA, Novack L, Thachil J, et al. LMWH in the prevention of preeclampsia and fetal growth restriction in women without thrombophilia. A systematic review and meta-analysis. Thromb Haemost 2016;116(5):868–78.

111. Hawkes N. Trial of Viagra for fetal growth restriction is halted after baby deaths. BMJ 2018;362:k3247.

112. Hitzerd E, Broekhuizen M, Mirabito Colafella KM, et al. Placental effects and transfer of sildenafil in healthy and preeclamptic conditions. EBioMedicine 2019;45:447–55.

113. Maki S, Tanaka H, Tsuji M, et al. Safety evaluation of tadalafil treatment for fetuses with early-onset growth restriction (TADAFER): results from the phase II trial. J Clin Med 2019;8(6):856.

114. Tarry-Adkins JL, Aiken CE, Ozanne SE. Comparative impact of pharmacological treatments for gestational diabetes on neonatal anthropometry independent of maternal glycaemic control: a systematic review and meta-analysis. PLoS Med 2020;17(5):e1003126.

115. Feig DS, Donovan LE, Zinman B, et al. Metformin in women with type 2 diabetes in pregnancy (MiTy): a multicentre, international, randomised, placebo-controlled trial. Lancet Diabetes Endocrinol 2020;8(10):834–44.

116. Nascimento IBD, Sales WB, Dienstmann G, et al. Metformin for prevention of cesarean delivery and large-for-gestational-age newborns in non-diabetic obese pregnant women: a randomized clinical trial. Arch Endocrinol Metab 2020; 64(3):290–7.

117. Tarry-Adkins JL, Aiken CE, Ozanne SE. Neonatal, infant, and childhood growth following metformin versus insulin treatment for gestational diabetes: a systematic review and meta-analysis. PLoS Med 2019;16(8):e1002848.

118. Panagiotopoulou O, Syngelaki A, Georgiopoulos G, et al. Metformin use in obese mothers is associated with improved cardiovascular profile in the offspring. Am J Obstet Gynecol 2020;223(2):246.e1–10.

119. Poston L, Bell R, Croker H, et al. Effect of a behavioural intervention in obese pregnant women (the UPBEAT study): a multicentre, randomised controlled trial. Lancet Diabetes Endocrinol 2015;3(10):767–77.

120. Gazquez A, Uhl O, Ruiz-Palacios M, et al. Placental lipid droplet composition: effect of a lifestyle intervention (UPBEAT) in obese pregnant women. Biochim Biophys Acta Mol Cell Biol Lipids 2018;1863(9):998–1005.

121. Lager S, Ramirez VI, Acosta O, et al. Docosahexaenoic acid supplementation in pregnancy modulates placental cellular signaling and nutrient transport capacity in obese women. J Clin Endocrinol Metab 2017;102(12):4557–67.

122. Carr DJ, Wallace JM, Aitken RP, et al. Uteroplacental adenovirus vascular endothelial growth factor gene therapy increases fetal growth velocity in growth-restricted sheep pregnancies. Hum Gene Ther 2014;25(4):375–84.

123. Spencer R, Ambler G, Brodszki J, et al. EVERREST prospective study: a 6-year prospective study to define the clinical and biological characteristics of pregnancies affected by severe early onset fetal growth restriction. BMC Pregnancy Childbirth 2017;17(1):43.

124. Edison RJ, Muenke M. Mechanistic and epidemiologic considerations in the evaluation of adverse birth outcomes following gestational exposure to statins. Am J Med Genet A 2004;131(3):287–98.

125. Brownfoot FC, Tong S, Hannan NJ, et al. Effects of pravastatin on human placenta, endothelium, and women with severe preeclampsia. Hypertension 2015;66(3):687–97 [discussion: 445].

126. Ahmed A, Williams DJ, Cheed V, et al. Pravastatin for early-onset pre-eclampsia: a randomised, blinded, placebo-controlled trial. BJOG 2020;127(4):478–88.

127. Lefkou E, Mamopoulos A, Dagklis T, et al. Pravastatin improves pregnancy outcomes in obstetric antiphospholipid syndrome refractory to antithrombotic therapy. J Clin Invest 2016;126(8):2933–40.

128. Irvin-Choy NS, Nelson KM, Gleghorn JP, et al. Design of nanomaterials for applications in maternal/fetal medicine. J Mater Chem B 2020;8(31):6548–61.

Abnormal Fetal Growth

Small for Gestational Age, Fetal Growth Restriction, Large for Gestational Age: Definitions and Epidemiology

Stefanie E. Damhuis, MD[a,b,]*, Wessel Ganzevoort, MD, PhD[b],
Sanne J. Gordijn, MD, PhD[a]

KEYWORDS

- Fetal growth restriction • Fetal overgrowth • Intrauterine growth restriction
- Large for gestational age • Macrosomia • Placental insufficiency
- Small for gestational age

KEY POINTS

- Fetal growth is a dynamic process, whereas fetal size is a static measurement of past growth.
- Although underlying pathology is more common at the extreme ends of the spectrum of fetal size for gestational age, small or large fetal size does not necessarily indicate pathology and a seemingly appropriate size is not a guarantee for physiology.
- The challenge for the coming decade is to evaluate and implement biometrical and functional markers that identify the compromised or overgrown fetus in the complete spectrum of fetal size.

BACKGROUND

Appropriate placental supply of nutrients and oxygen is essential for fetal growth and development, neonatal health, and lifelong well-being. Conversely, abnormal placental supplies resulting in abnormal fetal growth, including fetal growth restriction (FGR) and fetal overgrowth, is associated with mortality and significant risks to health. In medical literature the terms small for gestational age (SGA) and large for gestational age (LGA) are commonly used to describe abnormal growth. Both SGA and LGA are merely defined by the statistical deviation of fetal size in relation to a reference

[a] Department of Obstetrics and Gynaecology, University Medical Center of Groningen, CB20, Hanzeplein 1, 9700RB Groningen, the Netherlands; [b] Department of Obstetrics and Gynaecology, University Medical Centers Amsterdam, University of Amsterdam, H4, PO Box 22660, Amsterdam 1105 AZ, the Netherlands
* Corresponding author. Department of Obstetrics and Gynecology, Amsterdam University Medical Centers, H4, PO Box 22660, Amsterdam 1105 AZ, the Netherlands.
E-mail addresses: s.e.damhuis@amsterdamumc.nl; s.e.damhuis@umcg.nl

Obstet Gynecol Clin N Am 48 (2021) 267–279
https://doi.org/10.1016/j.ogc.2021.02.002   obgyn.theclinics.com

population. As such, SGA and LGA describe the variation of size rather than an abnormal condition. Moreover, fetal size is frequently used as a misnomer for fetal growth. Size at a certain point in time (static) is the result of the (dynamic) process of past growth. For prenatal care, risk stratification is essential. In this respect it is important to acknowledge that the size of fetuses can be deviant yet constitutionally small or large and thus healthy, whereas fetuses with seemingly normal size can be growth restricted or overgrown. In this article we describe the differences between abnormal and normal fetal size and growth in terms of history, definition, and epidemiology. The 'placental function and the development of fetal overgrowth and fetal growth restriction' is reviewed in the article of Dumolt et al. in this issue.

Fetal growth depends on maternal factors (including maternal health status, nutritional status, smoking, drug use), fetal factors (genetic make-up), and placental function.[1] The common pathophysiologic mechanism of FGR in an otherwise healthy fetus is placental insufficiency in which, as a consequence of impaired placental function, the fetus fails to reach its intrinsic growth potential.[2,3] Placental-related FGR arises most commonly by poor remodeling of the uterine spiral arteries during early pregnancy resulting in maternal vascular malperfusion, but many other types of causal placental lesions exist.[4] In maternal vascular malperfusion the oxygen and nutrient supply is suboptimal because of high resistance flow in the fetoplacental circulation, reduced villus surface (hypoplasia), secondary damage to shear stress, and placental infarcts.[2] As a result, the placenta is unable to provide the fetal demands for appropriate growth and development throughout pregnancy, resulting in a compromised fetus. During delivery, uterine contractions combined with the impaired placental function predisposes the compromised fetus to hypoxic insults and birth asphyxia because the hypoxic stress of labor is less well tolerated. FGR is a major contributor to perinatal morbidity and mortality and carries an increased risk of long-term neurologic and neurodevelopmental complications.[5–7] Moreover, infants born with FGR are at increased risk to develop cardiovascular disease in adult life.[8,9] These long-term implications of FGR are reviewed in the article 'Short and Long Term Implications of SGA,' from Fung et al, in this issue.

On the other side of the size spectrum, the fetus can also experience growth acceleration resulting in excessive size. The Pederson hypothesis states that fetal overgrowth or macrosomia is a consequence of maternal hyperglycemia (because of obesity or diabetes), which stimulates fetal insulin production.[10] However, macrosomia may occur in pregnancies complicated by maternal diabetes despite rigorous glycemic control. It is clear that a relationship exists between maternal metabolic conditions and macrosomia, but the macronutrient metabolism cannot completely explain the phenomenon because lifestyle modification does not always reduce the incidence of macrosomia.[11] Besides glucose metabolism, several maternal and placental factors can affect the supply and uptake of nutrients to the fetus and contribute to fetal overgrowth, including physical activity, race/ethnicity, uteroplacental blood flow, and placental transfer characteristics.[12–14] Some genetic conditions are associated with overgrowth and should also be considered.[15] Fetal overgrowth is associated with a three-fold higher risk for stillbirth independent of maternal diabetes status and represents a risk factor for maternal and fetal trauma during birth and neonatal morbidity and mortality.[16–18] Overgrown newborns from mothers with and without diabetes are at risk for long-term metabolic complications, such as obesity and insulin resistance.[19,20] It is currently unknown what the effect is on neurodevelopmental outcomes because data are limited and contradictory.[21,22]

HISTORY

The description of abnormal fetal growth has changed throughout history. Initially, before ultrasound was available as a diagnostic modality, the term "premature" was commonly used by pediatricians to describe children who were born with a birthweight less than 2500 g, regardless of the estimated period of gestation. In 1961 the process of intrauterine growth retardation was first described, recognizing that the growth of fetuses could be hampered in utero and that occasionally infants were born with a birth weight far less than the expected birth weight for their gestational age.[23] Because the diagnosis was made postpartum, interventions applied to live born infants in the form of special care and treatment by the pediatrician.

In 1958 the first ultrasound images of the fetus were published.[24] Imaging of the fetus in utero allowed the antenatal detection of certain conditions. In 1971 the first cephalometry graph from 13 to 40 weeks was developed and used to identify the growth-restricted fetus by showing a decline of biparietal diameter growth in the third trimester. Serial cephalometry became a standard method of the assessment of fetal growth in developing countries for many years.[25]

Seven years later the value of routine scanning of the obstetric population for accurate dating was demonstrated. It became key to accurately assess gestational age for the later assessment of fetal growth because fetal weight is inextricably linked to gestational age.[26] At the same time, real-time scanners were developed and became widely available for clinicians. Within a space of one or two decades this terra incognita became charted land as more and more fetal structures were visualized and measured and a great number of reference charts of different planes and organs were developed. In the 1980s the standard fetal biometric measurements for assessing growth included the biparietal diameter, head circumference, abdominal circumference, and femur length, which were incorporated into equations for fetal weight and growth predictions according to the models of Hadlock and colleagues,[27] still commonly used today.

Simultaneously the use of Doppler ultrasound to measure fetal flow velocities was rapidly developed and was increasingly used to evaluate fetal well-being. These technological developments led to real-time imaging and color Doppler studies to be incorporated in obstetric care to assess fetal growth and well-being, install appropriate management, and assess the timing of delivery of the compromised fetus. However, it should be noted that the body of randomized evidence to support the widespread use of these parameters is limited. For example, the Cochrane review addressing the use of any Doppler measurement for any clinical situation only reports on little more than 10,000 women.[28]

Macrosomia has also been recognized in literature for more than 100 years and the adverse outcomes related to cephalopelvic disproportion have been well described. However, unlike the rich history of investigations of cephalopelvic disproportion, little attention was paid to the metabolic aspect of large infants. Historically, only short-term and long-term health outcomes were known of infants born with a large birth weight. For instance, children born in the 1920s who were classified as large at birth seemed to have reduced morbidity and mortality in their seventh decade compared with infants with a lower birth weight.[29,30]

The focus on detecting antenatal LGA became of interest during the last four decades, during which time increased metabolic and respiratory risks of being born LGA became apparent. This transformation from being thought to have advantages to conferring risk for adverse outcomes is likely attributable to a change in population welfare, availability and composition of nutrition, and increase in diabetic disorders in pregnancy over the intervening decades. Societal events in the past, including world wars and the great depression, were characterized by limited available nutrition to the wider population.[31,32] Fetuses were thus not likely exposed to over-nourishment in utero, as shown by lower maternal weight gain and obesity rates in pregnancy during these periods compared with current rates.[33,34] Neonates classified as being LGA back then, were more likely to have been long and lean, whereas in recent decades the excess of nutrition in utero leads to long and chubby neonates.

TERMINOLOGY AND DEFINITIONS

Historically there was considerable inconsistency in terms that were used to classify fetuses who do not reach their intrinsic growth potential. Many terms have been described in literature, of which intrauterine growth restriction/retardation was most commonly used for a long period of time. However, because "intrauterine" refers to a location and not to the fetus who is actually affected by the condition, and the fact that "retardation" suggests that a catch-up is possible, FGR was considered to be a more accurate term.[35] From 2016 onward this term has been widely accepted and is increasingly used in research and clinical practice. Not only has the standardization of the terminology been a hurdle, but the establishment of a widely accepted, standard definition for FGR has also been challenging.

Fetal Growth Restriction and Small for Gestational Age

In the absence of a gold standard there was, and to a lesser extent still is, large heterogeneity in the definition of FGR. FGR has been used interchangeably with SGA for decades, although small is not necessarily too small. The attractiveness of the use of SGA lies in its easy application because it is purely a statistical deviation of fetal size, often the 10th percentile, related to a reference chart to define abnormality.[36] Although there is significant overlap between SGA and FGR, the two terms principally refer to a different condition (**Figs. 1** and **2**). Approximately 40% of babies with a fetal size less than the 10th percentile are constitutionally small and healthy, whereas FGR is a pathologic condition where the fetus is deprived of oxygen (hypoxia) and nutrition (starvation), but the baby is not necessarily small.[37] An appropriate for gestational age (AGA) fetus can be growth restricted, if its intrinsic growth potential was higher. Using SGA as a definition for FGR thus leads to overestimation of FGR among SGA and underestimation or failure to diagnose FGR among AGA. In clinical studies SGA is often used as a proxy for FGR in the absence of other available indicators. The proxy concept makes use of the fact that the smaller the fetal size the higher the chance that growth restriction occurred, but it is important to realize that the population is diluted by healthy SGA fetuses and ignores FGR fetuses who are AGA (see **Figs. 1** and **2**).

A 2016 consensus definition was established by experts in the field for the antenatal diagnosis of FGR through a Delphi procedure.[38] The items that were evaluated for inclusion in the definition included parameters of placental function (eg, Doppler velocimetry measurements, decline in size percentile, and serum biomarkers) in addition to fetal biometric measurements/size. This resulted in the inclusion of abnormal Doppler flow profiles and growth trajectory (50-point decline in estimated fetal weight percentile) in the definition in addition to the biometrical measures that were used historically. This definition therefore allows FGR to be diagnosed in SGA and AGA fetuses. Also, the definition distinguishes between very small (less than the third percentile) and small (between the 3rd and 10th percentile). A fetal size less than the third percentile is an isolated criterion to define FGR at any gestational age because these fetuses are at highest risk for stillbirth and neonatal problems, such as hypothermia and

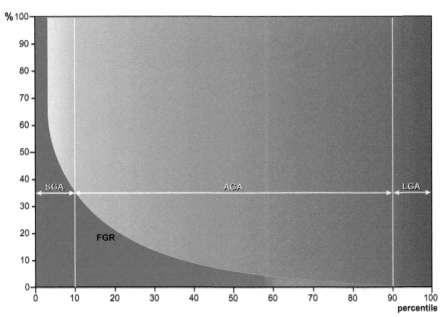

Fig. 1. Schematic depiction of the overlap and difference between FGR and SGA. SGA includes all fetuses with a weight less than the 10th percentile, which is represented in the combined *orange* and *gray* area to the left of the *vertical white line*. FGR represents the *orange* area. The *orange* area fades toward higher growth percentiles because being a little bit growth restricted might not be of clinical relevance and the consensus definition does not apply. AGA, appropriate for gestational age; FGR, fetal growth restriction; LGA, large for gestational age; SGA, small for gestational age. (*Adapted from* Ganzevoort W, Thilaganathan B, Baschat A, Gordijn SJ, Gardosi J. Fetal growth and risk assessment: is there an impasse?; with permission.)

hypoglycemia, regardless of the reason for the severe smallness. It also takes into account that small fetuses with a size between the 3rd and 10th percentile can be healthy in the absence of other indicators pointing toward placental insufficiency as shown in **Table 1**. Using this definition in clinical practice is designed to prevent unnecessary and potentially harmful interventions in the healthy-but-small fetuses and allows the clinician to pick up the compromised AGA fetus and install adequate management. Several studies (among others the DRIGITAT trial [Dutch], Truffle2 trial [European], and RATIO37 trial [Spain]) are ongoing that evaluate the efficacy of adding parameters of placental function to the management algorithm. Results from these trials may validate the theoretic benefit of using a uniform diagnostic definition apart from the obvious advantage of speaking the same language.

Furthermore, the Delphi study definition distinguishes between early and late-onset FGR. The consensus-based agreement is that early onset FGR is diagnosed at or less than 32 weeks and differs from late-onset FGR because of its association with maternal hypertensive disorders, patterns of deterioration, and severity of placental dysfunction.[39] The clinically obvious fetal and maternal manifestations make the identification of fetuses with early onset FGR simple, but this diagnosis poses a serious dilemma to the obstetrician. To solve the problem of the deprived environment the fetus needs to be delivered. However, delivery exposes the neonate to morbidity associated with prematurity, such as respiratory distress syndrome, necrotizing enterocolitis, and neonatal death. Yet, to gain maturity, the fetus should remain in

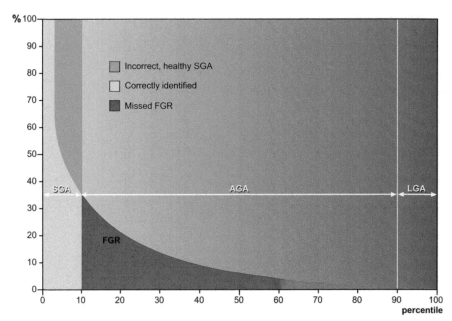

Fig. 2. Schematic overview of the limitations when SGA is used as a definition for FGR. The *dark* and *light green* area represent SGA fetuses. The area highlighted in *light green* represents the SGA fetuses who are correctly identified as being growth restricted. The *dark green* area includes constitutionally small yet healthy fetuses who are thus incorrectly identified as being growth restricted. The area highlighted in *red* represents growth restricted fetuses with a seemingly appropriate size and who will be missed if the definition of SGA is applied. AGA, appropriate for gestational age; FGR, fetal growth restriction; LGA, large for gestational age; SGA, small for gestational age. (*Adapted from* Ganzevoort W, Thilaganathan B, Baschat A, Gordijn SJ, Gardosi J. Fetal growth and risk assessment: is there an impasse?; with permission.)

the deprived environment, risking stillbirth and serious additional morbidity secondary to critical fetal hypoxia because of postponing delivery. "Treat first what kills first," the common medical doctrine, is thus difficult to apply.

Table 1
Consensus-based definitions for early and late FGR in the absence of congenital anomalies

Early FGR: GA <32 wk	Late FGR: GA ≥32 wk
AC/EFW <3rd centile or UA-AEDF	AC/EFW <3rd centile
Or	Or at least 2 out of 3 of the following
1. AC/EFW <10th centile combined with	1. AC/EFW <10th centile
2. UtA-PI >95th centile and/or	2. AC/EFW crossing centiles >2 quartiles on growth centiles
3. UA-PI >95th centile	3. CPR <5th centile or UA-PI >95th centile

Growth centiles are noncustomized centiles.
Abbreviations: AC, fetal abdominal circumference; AEDF, absent end-diastolic flow; CPR, cerebroplacental ratio; EFW, estimated fetal weight; GA, gestational age; PI, pulsatility index; UA, umbilical artery; UtA, uterine artery.
From Gordijn S, Beune I, Thilaganathan B, et al. Consensus definition of fetal growth restriction: a Delphi procedure. Ultrasound in Obstetrics & Gynecology 2016;48(3):333-39; with permission.

Contrary to early onset FGR, the detection and diagnosis of late-onset FGR is neither simple nor obvious, and late-onset FGR is frequently missed. Fetal sizes can be within normal ranges and the measurable cardiovascular changes are less obvious.[40,41] Fetal reserves to withstand impaired placental function are more limited in advanced gestation and acute hypoxemia (and fetal death) may occur before fetal growth has dropped below the 10th percentile for the population on reference charts.[42] Unlike early onset FGR, management of late-onset FGR is less complex because the fetal organs are more mature and the incidence of serious neonatal morbidity from prematurity is low. Thus, delivery is a more attractive option with less downside than earlier in gestation. Routine ultrasonography in the third trimester, however, is not recommended in low-risk pregnancies because it has not been shown to reduce the incidence of severe adverse perinatal outcomes compared with usual care.[43] The detection and management of FGR is described in the article 'Fetal Growth Curves: Is There a Universal Reference?,' from Grantz et al. in this issue.

FGR in singletons differs from FGR in twins and the diagnosis of FGR in stillborn babies raises specific challenges. Consensus definitions have also been established for selective FGR in monochorionic and dichorionic twin pregnancies, diagnosis of FGR in stillbirths, and also for growth restriction in the newborn.[44–46] To further facilitate standardization in growth restriction studies and enable future studies to compare and pool data between study populations, outcomes and baseline characteristics for clinical trials (known as core outcome sets and minimum reporting sets) were developed for FGR and for feeding intervention studies in growth-restricted newborns.[47–49]

Macrosomia and Fetal Overgrowth

In contrast to FGR, no consensus definition for macrosomia exists, nor have there been efforts to standardize study outcomes. In high-income countries, the most commonly used threshold is an estimated fetal weight or birth weight greater than 4500 g, but a cutoff greater than 4000 g is also frequently used.[50–52] These thresholds are not useful for identifying the preterm overgrown fetus because they are not based on population statistics and unrelated to gestational age. The statistical approach considers any fetus or infant weighing greater than the 90th percentile for gestational age as being LGA. However, it has been suggested to restrict the definition to a weight higher than the 97th percentile, because this more accurately identifies newborns who are at the greatest risk for perinatal mortality and morbidity.[53,54] As with FGR, there will be a group of LGA fetuses who are healthy and may not experience adverse effects of their nutritional status and AGA fetuses who actually have a disproportional incline in growth centiles and may be overgrown but remain undetected because their fetal size and/or birth weight remains lower than the threshold. These overgrown fetuses are at risk for metabolic and respiratory problems just after birth and should be monitored.

As in FGR, macrosomia also confers an increased risk for perinatal asphyxia, although the underlying placental and mechanical mechanisms are completely different. In FGR the oxygen supply is insufficient, whereas in macrosomia it is postulated that hyperglycemia and hyperinsulinemia leads to increased intrauterine oxygen demands, especially in infants of mothers with diabetes.[55] Another contributing factor includes the mechanistic complication of cephalopelvic disproportion (leading to prolonged labor and shoulder dystocia), which increases the percentage of women undergoing operative delivery. To assess the risk for operative delivery and assist in the decision making, a grading system has been developed based on absolute weights independent of gestational age. This system suggests that grade 1

(>4000 g) is useful for the identification of increased risks of labor and newborn complications, grade 2 (>4500 g) is predictive of neonatal morbidity, and grade 3 (>5000 g) is an indicator for mortality risk.[53] Timely delivery based on these absolute weights is an intuitive but unproven approach to prevent adverse outcomes from cephalopelvic disproportion. However, relying on an absolute weight cutoff alone will not adequately identify all overgrown fetuses who are at risk for metabolic adverse outcomes. Research is urgently needed to optimize prenatal identification and clinical management of excess fetal growth.

REFERENCE CHARTS

Parameters reflecting placental function (eg, Doppler indices and serum biomarkers currently under investigation) are gaining more importance in the detection of abnormal growth. Nonetheless, the assessment of estimated fetal weight and birth weight for gestational age, and the expression in percentiles to compare current size with a reference or standard population, will remain a significant element of assessing growth. The use of these percentiles requires an appropriate reference. However, as in all aspects of FGR, there is inconsistency with regard to the reference charts used to determine abnormal fetal weight and birth weight. Different reference charts for fetal growth are extensively described in the article 'Evaluation and management of suspected FGR,' from Bruin et al. in this issue.

EPIDEMIOLOGY

The overall incidence of FGR depends on the definition used, and the population being examined. It is estimated that between 3% and 9% of pregnancies in the developed world, and up to 25% of pregnancies in low- and middle-income countries are affected by FGR. In contrast, the incidence of SGA by definition is around 10% and only partly overlaps with FGR.[56,57] The estimated prevalence of FGR throughout the percentile ranges is shown in **Fig. 1** and emphasizes that the lower the weight the higher the chance that FGR occurred. Also, a significant part, if not 50% of all FGR, occurs in AGA. Factors that influence FGR rates in communities include maternal nutritional status, smoking rates, alcohol and drug use, socioeconomic status, maternal activity, maternal disease, air pollution, and genetic make-up.[57] The incidence of FGR is significantly higher in low- and middle-income countries, and this is mainly attributed to a large number of FGR infants born in the Asian continent, which accounts for approximately 75% of all FGR in the world, followed by Africa and South America.[58] Firm statements regarding incidence and timing of FGR are hampered worldwide because of diagnostic inaccuracy. This is exacerbated by the fact that in developing countries, pregnant women do not receive a standard ultrasound for accurate pregnancy dating. When the gestational age is not known with reasonable certainty, a birth weight cannot be used to determine whether there has been growth restriction. This is a problem even when SGA is used as a proxy for FGR, because this may well be caused by preterm birth. The incidence of FGR in sub-Saharan countries may be higher because contributors to FGR, such as maternal malnourishment, and conditions, such as placental malaria and syphilis, are common.[59]

An epidemiologic distinction between early and late-onset FGR is commonly made. The prevalence of early onset FGR is far less (0.5%–1%) compared with late-onset FGR (5%–10%), but the clinical impact is high because there is a high mortality and morbidity rate.[41] Late-onset FGR is associated with lower mortality and morbidity rates, but causes a large absolute number of adverse outcomes because of its higher incidence.[41,60] Moreover, approximately one-third of medically indicated late preterm births may be complicated with FGR.[61]

At the other end of the spectrum, the incidence of women giving birth to large infants has increased in the last four decades.[62–66] The current proportion of macrosomia ($\geq$4000 g) worldwide is approximately 9% and 0.1% for birth weight greater than the 5000 g with a wide variation among countries. Variation is influenced by contributing factors, such as genetics, gestational diabetes, and obesity rates.[67] The highest prevalence is found in Nordic countries where around 20% of the newborns have a birth weight at or greater than the 4000 g.[66] In developing countries the prevalence of macrosomia ($\geq$4000 g) is typically 1% to 5% ranging from 0.5% to 14.9%.[68] Similar to SGA the incidence of LGA by definition is 10%. In the absence of a clear distinction between macrosomia, LGA, and overgrown fetuses and also in the absence of an accurate diagnostic tool to differentiate the overgrown fetuses from healthy LGA, little is known about the incidence throughout the percentile spectrum, but it is plausible that the inverted curve of FGR applies (see **Fig. 1**).

DISCUSSION

Because approximately 9% of pregnancies are affected by FGR and another 9% by fetal overgrowth, the clinical and societal impact of abnormal fetal growth is significant. To make matters worse, accurate detection of FGR and fetal overgrowth is challenging technically (ultrasound is imperfect)[69] as in the way we define the compromised and overgrown fetus.

At present there is no effective treatment to reverse the course of FGR and macrosomia except delivery. FGR is probably the condition among the obstetric entities with the greatest variation in clinical practice, in terms of monitoring, management strategies, and gestational age at delivery. Prenatal recognition of FGR remains a major challenge in daily obstetric practice. Current focus of measurements lies on the nutritional component of fetal deprivation because this is inferred from size measurements. By using the expression FGR it is implied that the nutritional component of the deprivation is the biggest threat. However, the most important outcomes, including the devastating outcome of perinatal mortality, are caused by a deprived oxygen status of the fetus rather than starvation and, unfortunately, fetal serum oxygen levels currently cannot be measured. New techniques for in vivo assessment of fetal oxygenation, such as the magnetic resonance blood oxygen level dependent effect, are currently being investigated as part of the National Institutes of Health–sponsored Human Placenta Project.[70]

Similarly, methods to distinguish healthy large fetuses from overgrown fetuses or to identify overgrown fetuses with appropriate weight are lacking, especially in the absence of maternal diabetes. Beyond the obvious obstetric concerns of obstructed labor, detecting the latter group with normal size is necessary so interventions can be developed to mitigate the associated long-term health risks for the overgrown newborn. Future efforts should focus on the development of a more accurate diagnostic approach that considers fetal body proportion, composition, and metabolic characteristics.

SUMMARY

Abnormal fetal growth has been subjected to different terms and definitions, resulting in varying epidemiology throughout history. Gold standards to detect growth-restricted fetuses and overgrown fetuses are lacking. However, knowledge and understanding about both pathologic conditions has improved significantly in the past years. Better identification of the fetuses at risk, independent of size, is essential to prevent potential harmful interventions in healthy but small fetuses and allow clinicians to appropriately intervene for fetuses with seemingly normal size but who are growth restricted or overgrown.

CLINICS CARE POINTS

- Assessment of fetal growth and defining abnormality is complex. Being of small or large fetal size does not necessarily reflect pathology but puts the fetus at a higher risk and an appropriate size is not a guarantee of normal outcomes.

- Implementation of the established consensus definitions in clinical practice and research facilitates the improvement of accurate identification of compromised fetuses.

DISCLOSURE

The authors S.J. Gordijn and W. Ganzevoort report the in-kind contribution of study materials from Roche Diagnostics for investigator-initiated studies. Author S.E. Damhuis has nothing to disclose.

REFERENCES

1. Maulik D. Fetal growth restriction: the etiology. Clin Obstet Gynecol 2006;49(2):228–35.
2. Mifsud W, Sebire NJ. Placental pathology in early-onset and late-onset fetal growth restriction. Fetal Diagn Ther 2014;36(2):117–28.
3. Kingdom J, Huppertz B, Seaward G, et al. Development of the placental villous tree and its consequences for fetal growth. Eur J Obstet Gynecol Reprod Biol 2000;92(1):35–43.
4. Burton GJ, Jauniaux E. Pathophysiology of placental-derived fetal growth restriction. Am J Obstet Gynecol 2018;218(2):S745–61.
5. Burton GJ, Fowden AL, Thornburg KL. Placental origins of chronic disease. Physiol Rev 2016;96(4):1509–65.
6. Flenady V, Koopmans L, Middleton P, et al. Major risk factors for stillbirth in high-income countries: a systematic review and meta-analysis. Lancet 2011; 377(9774):1331–40.
7. Walker D, Marlow N. Neurocognitive outcome following fetal growth restriction. Arch Dis Child Fetal Neonatal Ed 2008;93(4):F322–5.
8. Barker DJ, Osmond C, Golding J, et al. Growth in utero, blood pressure in childhood and adult life, and mortality from cardiovascular disease. Br Med J 1989; 298(6673):564–7.
9. Leon DA, Lithell HO, Vågerö D, et al. Reduced fetal growth rate and increased risk of death from ischaemic heart disease: cohort study of 15 000 Swedish men and women born 1915-29. BMJ 1998;317(7153):241–5.
10. Pedersen J. The pregnant diabetic and her newborn: problems and management, by Farquhar J. The Williams and Wilkins Company Baltimore; 1968.
11. Nahavandi S, Price S, Sumithran P, et al. Exploration of the shared pathophysiological mechanisms of gestational diabetes and large for gestational age offspring. World J Diabetes 2019;10(6):333.
12. Jansson T, Cetin I, Powell T, et al. Placental transport and metabolism in fetal overgrowth: a workshop report. Placenta 2006;27:109–13.

13. McGrath RT, Glastras SJ, Hocking SL, et al. Large-for-gestational-age neonates in type 1 diabetes and pregnancy: contribution of factors beyond hyperglycemia. Diabetes Care 2018;41(8):1821–8.
14. Wang X, Guan Q, Zhao J, et al. Association of maternal serum lipids at late gestation with the risk of neonatal macrosomia in women without diabetes mellitus. Lipids Health Dis 2018;17(1):78.
15. Brioude F, Toutain A, Giabicani E, et al. Overgrowth syndromes: clinical and molecular aspects and tumour risk. Nat Rev Endocrinol 2019;15(5):299–311.
16. Ju H, Chadha Y, Donovan T, et al. Fetal macrosomia and pregnancy outcomes. Aust N Z J Obstet Gynaecol 2009;49(5):504–9.
17. Esakoff TF, Cheng YW, Sparks TN, et al. The association between birthweight 4000 g or greater and perinatal outcomes in patients with and without gestational diabetes mellitus. Am J Obstet Gynecol 2009;200(6):672.e1–4.
18. Carter EB, Stockburger J, Tuuli MG, et al. Large-for-gestational age and stillbirth: is there a role for antenatal testing? Ultrasound Obstet Gynecol 2019;54(3): 334–7.
19. Evagelidou EN, Kiortsis DN, Bairaktari ET, et al. Lipid profile, glucose homeostasis, blood pressure, and obesity-anthropometric markers in macrosomic offspring of nondiabetic mothers. Diabetes Care 2006;29(6):1197–201.
20. Seidman DS, Laor A, Gale R, et al. A longitudinal study of birth weight and being overweight in late adolescence. Am J Dis Child 1991;145(7):779–81.
21. Paulson JF, Mehta SH, Sokol RJ, et al. Large for gestational age and long-term cognitive function. Am J Obstet Gynecol 2014;210(4):343.e1–4.
22. Adane AA, Mishra GD, Tooth LR. Diabetes in pregnancy and childhood cognitive development: a systematic review. Pediatrics 2016;137(5):e20154234.
23. Warkany J, Monroe BB, Sutherland BS. Intrauterine growth retardation. Am J Dis Child 1961;102(2):249–79.
24. Donald I, Macvicar J, Brown T. Investigation of abdominal masses by pulsed ultrasound. Lancet 1958;271(7032):1188–95.
25. Campbell S, Dewhurst C. Diagnosis of the small-for-dates fetus by serial ultrasonic cephalometry. Lancet 1971;298(7732):1002–6.
26. Grennert L, Persson P-H, Gennser G, et al. Benefits of ultrasonic screening of a pregnant population. Acta Obstet Gynecol Scand 1978;57(sup78):5–14.
27. Hadlock FP, Harrist RB, Sharman RS, et al. Estimation of fetal weight with the use of head, body, and femur measurements: a prospective study. Am J Obstet Gynecol 1985;151(3):333–7.
28. Alfirevic Z, Stampalija T, Dowswell T. Fetal and umbilical Doppler ultrasound in high-risk pregnancies. Cochrane Database Syst Rev 2017;6. https://doi.org/10. 1002/14651858.CD007529.
29. Hales CN, Barker DJ, Clark PM, et al. Fetal and infant growth and impaired glucose tolerance at age 64. Br Med J 1991;303(6809):1019–22.
30. Barker DJ, Hales CN, Fall C, et al. Type 2 (non-insulin-dependent) diabetes mellitus, hypertension and hyperlipidaemia (syndrome X): relation to reduced fetal growth. Diabetologia 1993;36(1):62–7.
31. Granados JAT, Roux AVD. Life and death during the great depression. Proc Natl Acad Sci U S A 2009;106(41):17290–5.
32. Roseboom T, de Rooij S, Painter R. The Dutch famine and its long-term consequences for adult health. Early Hum Dev 2006;82(8):485–91.
33. Gunderson EP, Abrams B. Epidemiology of gestational weight gain and body weight changes after pregnancy. Epidemiol Rev 1999;21(2):261–75.

34. Gunderson EP. Childbearing and obesity in women: weight before, during, and after pregnancy. Obstet Gynecol Clin North Am 2009;36(2):317–32.
35. Gordijn SJ, Beune IM, Ganzevoort W. Building consensus and standards in fetal growth restriction studies. Best Pract Res Clin Obstet Gynaecol 2018;49:117–26.
36. Lausman A, Kingdom J, Gagnon R, et al. Intrauterine growth restriction: screening, diagnosis, and management. J Obstet Gynaecol Can 2013;35(8): 741–8.
37. Khalil AA, Morales-Rosello J, Morlando M, et al. Is fetal cerebroplacental ratio an independent predictor of intrapartum fetal compromise and neonatal unit admission? Am J Obstet Gynecol 2015;213(1):54.e1–10.
38. Gordijn S, Beune I, Thilaganathan B, et al. Consensus definition of fetal growth restriction: a Delphi procedure. Ultrasound Obstet Gynecol 2016;48(3):333–9.
39. Lees C, Marlow N, Arabin B, et al. Perinatal morbidity and mortality in early-onset fetal growth restriction: cohort outcomes of the trial of randomized umbilical and fetal flow in Europe (TRUFFLE). Ultrasound Obstet Gynecol 2013;42(4):400–8.
40. Oros D, Figueras F, Cruz-Martinez R, et al. Longitudinal changes in uterine, umbilical and fetal cerebral Doppler indices in late-onset small-for-gestational age fetuses. Ultrasound Obstet Gynecol 2011;37(2):191–5.
41. Crovetto F, Triunfo S, Crispi F, et al. First-trimester screening with specific algorithms for early- and late-onset fetal growth restriction. Ultrasound Obstet Gynecol 2016;48(3):340–8.
42. Figueras F, Caradeux J, Crispi F, et al. Diagnosis and surveillance of late-onset fetal growth restriction. Am J Obstet Gynecol 2018;218(2):S790–802.
43. Henrichs J, Verfaille V, Jellema P, et al. Effectiveness of routine third trimester ultrasonography to reduce adverse perinatal outcomes in low risk pregnancy (the IRIS study): nationwide, pragmatic, multicentre, stepped wedge cluster randomised trial. BMJ 2019;367:l5517.
44. Beune IM, Bloomfield FH, Ganzevoort W, et al. Consensus based definition of growth restriction in the newborn. J Pediatr 2018;196:71–6.e1.
45. Khalil A, Beune I, Hecher K, et al. Consensus definition and essential reporting parameters of selective fetal growth restriction in twin pregnancy: a Delphi procedure. Ultrasound Obstet Gynecol 2019;53(1):47–54.
46. Beune IM, Damhuis SE, Ganzevoort W, et al. Consensus definition of fetal growth restriction in intrauterine fetal death: a Delphi procedure. Arch Pathol Lab Med 2020;145(4):428–36.
47. Healy P, Gordijn SJ, Ganzevoort W, et al. A core outcome set for the prevention and treatment of fetal GROwth restriction: deVeloping Endpoints: the COS-GROVE study. Am J Obstet Gynecol 2019;221(4):339.e1–10.
48. Damhuis SE, Bloomfield FH, Khalil A, et al. A core outcome set and minimum reporting set for intervention studies in growth restriction in the NEwbOrN: the COS-NEON study. Pediatr Res 2020;1–8.
49. Khalil A, Gordijn SJ, Beune IM, et al. Essential variables for reporting research studies on fetal growth restriction: a Delphi consensus. Ultrasound Obstet Gynecol 2019;53(5):609–14.
50. Modanlou HD, Dorchester WL, Thorosian A, et al. Macrosomia: maternal, fetal, and neonatal implications. Obstet Gynecol 1980;55(4):420–4.
51. Boyd ME, Usher RH, McLean FH. Fetal macrosomia: prediction, risks, proposed management. Obstet Gynecol 1983;61(6):715–22.
52. Langer O, Berkus MD, Huff RW, et al. Shoulder dystocia: should the fetus weighing≥ 4000 grams be delivered by cesarean section? Am J Obstet Gynecol 1991;165(4):831–7.

53. Boulet SL, Alexander GR, Salihu HM, et al. Macrosomic births in the United States: determinants, outcomes, and proposed grades of risk. Am J Obstet Gynecol 2003;188(5):1372–8.
54. Xu H, Simonet F, Luo ZC. Optimal birth weight percentile cut-offs in defining small- or large-for-gestational-age. Acta Paediatr 2010;99(4):550–5.
55. Mimouni F, Miodovnik M, Siddiqi TA, et al. Perinatal asphyxia in infants of insulin-dependent diabetic mothers. J Pediatr 1988;113(2):345–53.
56. Suhag A, Berghella V. Intrauterine growth restriction (IUGR): etiology and diagnosis. Curr Obstet Gynecol Rep 2013;2(2):102–11.
57. Romo A, Carceller R, Tobajas J. Intrauterine growth retardation (IUGR): epidemiology and etiology. Pediatr Endocrinol Rev 2009;6(Suppl 3):332–6.
58. De Onis M, Blössner M, Villar J. Levels and patterns of intrauterine growth retardation in developing countries. Eur J Clin Nutr 1998;52:S5.
59. Schantz-Dunn J, Nour NM. Malaria and pregnancy: a global health perspective. Rev Obstet Gynecol 2009;2(3):186.
60. Figueras F, Gardosi J. Intrauterine growth restriction: new concepts in antenatal surveillance, diagnosis, and management. Am J Obstet Gynecol 2011;204(4):288–300.
61. Carreno CA, Costantine MM, Holland MG, et al. Approximately one-third of medically indicated late preterm births are complicated by fetal growth restriction. Am J Obstet Gynecol 2011;204(3):263.e1–4.
62. Ananth CV, Wen SW. Trends in fetal growth among singleton gestations in the United States and Canada, 1985 through 1998. Semin Perinatol 2002;26(4):260–7. Elsevier.
63. Bergmann RL, Richter R, Bergmann KE, et al. Secular trends in neonatal macrosomia in Berlin: influences of potential determinants. Paediatr Perinat Epidemiol 2003;17(3):244–9.
64. Bonellie SR, Raab GM. Why are babies getting heavier? Comparison of Scottish births from 1980 to 1992. BMJ 1997;315(7117):1205.
65. Kramer MS, Morin I, Yang H, et al. Why are babies getting bigger? Temporal trends in fetal growth and its determinants. J Pediatr 2002;141(4):538–42.
66. Ørskou J, Kesmodel U, Henriksen TB, et al. An increasing proportion of infants weigh more than 4000 grams at birth. Acta Obstet Gynecol Scand 2001;80(10):931–6.
67. Chauhan SP, Grobman WA, Gherman RA, et al. Suspicion and treatment of the macrosomic fetus: a review. Am J Obstet Gynecol 2005;193(2):332–46.
68. Koyanagi A, Zhang J, Dagvadorj A, et al. Macrosomia in 23 developing countries: an analysis of a multicountry, facility-based, cross-sectional survey. Lancet 2013;381(9865):476–83.
69. Milner J, Arezina J. The accuracy of ultrasound estimation of fetal weight in comparison to birth weight: a systematic review. Ultrasound 2018;26(1):32–41.
70. Turk EA, Stout JN, Ha C, et al. Placental MRI: developing accurate quantitative measures of oxygenation. Top Magn Reson Imaging 2019;28(5):285–97.

Fetal Growth Curves
Is There a Universal Reference?

Katherine L. Grantz, MD, MS

KEYWORDS

- Fetal size • Estimated fetal weight • Fetal growth • Growth variation
- Ultrasound reference

KEY POINTS

- There are 3 modern, prospective fetal growth standards that are similar in scope but demonstrate variation in fetal growth.
- Different fetal growth references identify different proportions of fetuses as small-for-gestational-age or large-for-gestational-age.
- A universal reference would make comparison of fetal growth simpler for clinical use and for comparison across populations but may misclassify small-for-gestational-age or large-for-gestational-age fetuses.

INTRODUCTION

To answer the question, Does 1 fetal growth reference fit all populations? it is first necessary to know the purpose of the reference. Fetal size is important because fetal growth restriction and small-for-gestational-age (SGA) as well as macrosomia and large-for-gestational-age (LGA) fetal sizes are associated with increased risks of perinatal morbidity and mortality.[1,2] A range of 10th to 90th percentiles traditionally has been considered appropriate-for-gestational-age, with SGA or LGA often defined as less than 10th or greater than 90th percentiles, respectively.[3] Pathologic fetal growth however, follows more of a gradient, and different percentile cutoffs result in different portions of fetuses who are constitutionally small and not growth restricted, and vice versa for larger fetuses. For instance, a study of UK term singleton births found increased risks of stillbirth and infant death with birthweight up to the 25th percentile and greater than the 85th percentile, suggesting that the commonly used 10th percentile and 90th percentile cutpoints miss fetuses at risk for death.[4] Another study in the

Financial support: This research was supported by the Intramural Research Program of the *Eunice Kennedy Shriver* National Institute of Child Health and Human Development, National Institutes of Health (Contract Numbers: HHSN275200800013C; HHSN275200800002I; HHSN27500006; HHSN275200800003IC; HHSN275200800014C; HHSN275200800012C; HHSN275200800028C; and HHSN275201000009C).

Division of Intramural Population Health Research, *Eunice Kennedy Shriver* National Institute of Child Health and Human Development, National Institutes of Health, 6710B Rockledge Drive, MSC 7004, Bethesda, MD 20892, USA

E-mail address: katherine.grantz@nih.gov

Obstet Gynecol Clin N Am 48 (2021) 281–296
https://doi.org/10.1016/j.ogc.2021.02.003
0889-8545/21/Published by Elsevier Inc.

obgyn.theclinics.com

Netherlands found that although risk of perinatal mortality was highest in the less than 2.3rd percentile followed by the 2.3rd percentile to less than 5th percentile, and the 5th percentile to less than 10th percentile, perinatal mortality had a U-shaped relationship, with a nadir at the 80th to 84th percentiles for births between 28 weeks and 43 weeks.[5] These studies (albeit of birthweight) indicate that although risks for perinatal mortality are higher at the extremes, risk is more continual in the middle of the curve. Therefore, the choice in cutpoints for a fetal growth reference likely depends on how it is being used and on trade-offs between sensitivity and specificity. This decision may differ in clinical settings compared with use in a public health context to monitor and compare populations' health and development. Ideally the 25th percentile of a population reference is used to identify the most fetuses at risk for perinatal morbidity and mortality, but for clinical use, the cutpoint depends on the health care system capacity. Using the 25th percentile estimated fetal weight (EFW) instead of 10th percentile SGA would identify more fetuses at risk of growth restriction and associated morbidity and mortality but could have large cost and health care utilization implications due to increased antenatal surveillance and obstetric intervention. Furthermore, there is potential for increased risk of iatrogenic earlier delivery with associated harm.

Another consideration when selecting a fetal growth reference is to understand how the fetal growth reference that is chosen for clinical use performs in a local population. Three diverse, modern cohort studies with longitudinal fetal measurements recently have been undertaken: International Fetal & Newborn Growth Consortium for the 21st Century (INTERGROWTH-21st) Project,[6,7] the *Eunice Kennedy Shriver* National Institute of Child Health and Human Development (NICHD) Fetal Growth Studies[8–10] and the World Health Organization Multicentre Growth Reference Study (WHO Fetal).[11,12] The objective of this review is to compare these new fetal growth references in context with references in current clinical use and discuss considerations when choosing a reference for clinical practice.

BACKGROUND

A growth chart is used as a reference against which to assess growth and calculate the percentile of size for a given gestational age. Intrauterine growth charts are based on EFW using obstetric sonogram measurements, and birthweight growth charts are based on measured birthweight. Common US birthweight charts include those by Alexander and colleagues[13] and a revised reference by Duryea and colleagues,[14] which were based on improved obstetric estimates of gestational age. Ultrasound fetal weight estimates and birthweight are highly correlated (r = 0.80–0.91) but are not equivalent.[15] EFW is known to differ from birthweight by 100 g or more and can be inaccurate especially at the extremes of EFW, less than 2000 g and greater than 4000 g.[15] Birthweight-for-gestational age percentiles are not as clinically useful for prenatal fetal growth assessment because infants who deliver preterm are more likely to be growth restricted and, therefore, birthweight references inaccurately describe the preterm growth of fetuses who go on to deliver at term.[16,17] Therefore, ultrasound-derived references tend to be preferred to birthweight references for clinical antepartum monitoring. An important point is that growth references depend on accurate gestational age assessment. Unknown gestational age or an error in gestational age calculation may lead to misclassification of SGA and LGA fetuses.

DEFINITIONS

There are 4 types of intrauterine growth charts: (1) population-based intrauterine growth references similar in concept to infant and child growth charts, where a population is used to estimate percentiles; (2) customized growth charts, where growth percentiles are adjusted for a set of characteristics known to be associated with birthweight (eg, race/ethnicity, parity, sex, and maternal height and weight); (3) individualized growth charts where a fetal growth trajectory is calculated based on 2 previous growth measurements; and (4) conditional percentile assessment, where the fetal growth percentile is based on a previous measurement. Fetal growth references that are customized for maternal and fetal characteristics are posited to help differentiate constitutional from pathologic growth at the extremes.[18] There is debate, however, about whether SGA and LGA defined by customized growth charts are an improvement over population-based growth charts because customization has not been found to improve prediction of perinatal morbidity and mortality consistently.[17,19,20] Individualized fetal growth references identify the growth potential for an individual fetus consistent with a personalized medicine approach.[21–23] Although conceptually appealing, this approach has not been adopted widely in clinical practice. The conditional fetal growth percentile approach conditions individualized ranges for a subsequent fetal growth measurement on a previous fetal growth measurement, resulting in ranges that were narrower than and shifted from reference range centiles for the entire population.[24,25] The addition of conditional growth centiles to size centiles recently was found to improve the prediction of adverse perinatal outcomes in fetuses less than 10th percentile, which is promising.[26] Some of these approaches, however, require serial ultrasounds, which not always are available, and population-based references remain in wide use.

FETAL GROWTH REFERENCES

There are many ultrasound-based fetal weight references with some of the more common ones used in clinical practice presented in **Table 1**. Studies with smaller sample sizes are limited because the percentiles at the extremes (eg,10th and 90th) have less precision. It is difficult to estimate an appropriate sample size for developing fetal growth references, but several hundred observations have been estimated to be needed.[27] Growth references that use retrospective ultrasound data have the advantage of larger sample sizes but may be limited by selection bias; in other words, the reason why an ultrasound was obtained at a given gestational age may influence the fetal size measurement by an unknown amount. For growth references that use cross-sectional ultrasound data, each woman contributes data from only 1 ultrasound examination. Therefore, cross-sectional references can indicate fetal size but not fetal growth velocity. Some birthweight references are used clinically for monitoring intrauterine fetal growth with inherent limitations, as discussed previously.[28,29] Longitudinal references are necessary to assess fetal growth and the older, larger studies were performed outside the United States in predominantly white women (see **Table 1**). Furthermore, older fetal growth references have been found to have substantial heterogeneity in their methodology with a wide range of quality that may limit their clinical use.[30] Until recently, there was a lack of prospective longitudinal fetal growth studies in diverse populations.

More recently, 3 diverse, modern cohort studies with longitudinal fetal measurements have been undertaken: INTERGROWTH,[6,7] NICHD,[8–10] and WHO Fetal.[11,12] INTERGROWTH was completed in 8 countries (Brazil, China, India, Italy, Kenya, Oman, United Kingdom, and United States), WHO Fetal in 10 countries (Argentina, Brazil, Democratic Republic of the Congo, Denmark, Egypt, France, Germany, India, Norway, and Thailand), and NICHD at 12 US sites (New York [2], New Jersey, Delaware, Rhode Island, Massachusetts, South Carolina, Alabama, Illinois, and California [3]). These studies were similar in that healthy women who were positioned for optimal fetal growth

Table 1
Selected population-based birthweight and estimated fetal weight references

Authors, Location (y)	Inclusion Criteria and Dates[a]; Data Source	Sample Size[b]; Retrospective or Prospective; Cross-sectional or Longitudinal	Considerations for Use
Altman and Chitty, UK (1994)[27]	Pregnancies from European and Afro-Caribbean ethnic groups with accurate pregnancy dating; fetal biometric measurement from a single examination at 12–42 wk at a single hospital	663; prospective; cross-sectional	Although statistically rigorous methods used, single center may not be representative of fetal growth in local populations; cross-sectional references indicate fetal size but do not assess fetal growth.
Brenner et al, North Carolina and Ohio (1976)[28]	Weight of aborted fetuses 8–21 menstrual wk (1972–1975) at single hospital in North Carolina and birthweight for deliveries 21–44 menstrual wk (1962–1969) at single hospital in Ohio	430 aborted fetuses (8–21 menstrual wk) and 30,772 deliveries (21–44 wk); retrospective; cross-sectional	Birthweight references inaccurately describe the preterm growth of fetuses who go on to deliver at term.
Buck Louis et al, US (2015)[8,9]	Low-risk pregnancies from 4 racial/ethnic groups with accurate dating (2009–2013); randomized among 4 ultrasound schedules with fetal biometric measurements taken at 6 examinations from 10 wk to 41 wk; 12 community and perinatal centers	1737; prospective; longitudinal	NICHD; racially/ethnic diverse; rigorous credentialing of sonographers, use of standardized protocol, highly accurate and reliable measurements on quality assurance[60]
Di Battista et al, Italy (2000)[61]	Low-risk pregnancies with accurate dating and at least 5 (and up to 9) examinations (1987–1990); fetal biometric measurements taken between 12th and 40th wk at 2 obstetric units, which are major public health centers	238; unclear; longitudinal	Smaller sample size may decrease precision in the centiles; homogeneous population may not be representative of fetal growth in local populations.

(continued on next page)

Table 1 (continued)			
Authors, Location (y)	**Inclusion Criteria and Dates[a]; Data Source**	**Sample Size[b]; Retrospective or Prospective; Cross-sectional or Longitudinal**	**Considerations for Use**
Gallivan et al, U.K. (1993)[62]	Low-risk pregnancies with accurate dating (1987–1990); fetal biometric measurements taken at examinations approximately 2-wk intervals from 26 wk until delivery at 2 hospitals	67; prospective; longitudinal	Smaller sample size may decrease precision in the centiles; homogeneous population may not be representative of fetal growth in local populations.
Hadlock et al, Texas (1991)[39]	Low-risk pregnancies from white middle-class patients with certain menstrual history; fetal biometric measurement taken at a single examination from 10 wk to 41 wk at a single hospital	392; prospective; cross-sectional	Homogeneous population may not be representative of fetal growth in local populations; cross-sectional references indicate fetal size but do not assess fetal growth.
Jeanty et al, Belgium (1984)[63]	Low-risk pregnancies from white middle-class patients who were university personnel with certain menstrual history; fetal biometric measurements taken at 6–24 examinations at a single hospital	48; prospective; longitudinal	Smaller sample size may decrease precision in the centiles; homogeneous population may not be representative of fetal growth in local populations.
Johnsen et al, Norway (2006)[64]	Low-risk pregnancies with accurate dating; fetal biometric measurements taken at 4–5 examinations at least 3 wk apart from 20 to 42 wk at single antenatal clinic	634; prospective; longitudinal	Homogeneous population may not be representative of fetal growth in local populations.
Kiserud et al, international (2017)[11,12]	Low-risk pregnancies with accurate dating (2009–2014); fetal biometric measurements taken approximately every 4 wk from 14 to 40 wk, 10 countries	1,362; prospective; longitudinal	WHO; diverse; rigorous credentialing of sonographers, use of standardized protocol

(continued on next page)

Table 1
(continued)

Authors, Location (y)	Inclusion Criteria and Dates[a]; Data Source	Sample Size[b]; Retrospective or Prospective; Cross-sectional or Longitudinal	Considerations for Use
Marsal et al, Sweden and Denmark (1996)[65]	Low-risk pregnancies; fetal biometric measurements taken approximately every 3–4 wk at 4 perinatal centers	86; prospective; longitudinal	Smaller sample size may decrease precision in the centiles; homogeneous population may not be representative of fetal growth in local populations.
Mongelli and Gardosi, UK (1995)[66]	Low-risk pregnancies; fetal biometric measurements taken approximately every 2–3 wk starting from 24 wk to 32 wk for a maximum of 4 examinations at a single center	226; prospective; longitudinal	Homogeneous population may not be representative of fetal growth in local populations; EFW was calculated using a modified Hadlock formula.
Nasrat and Bondagii, Saudi Arabia (2005)[67]	Arab women with certain menstrual history and without insulin requiring diabetes (1995–2002); all examinations from a single hospital over the study period	Approximately 1150; retrospective; cross-sectional	Retrospective ultrasound data may be limited by selection bias, or the reason for why an ultrasound was obtained at a given gestational age may influence the fetal size measurement by an unknown amount; cross-sectional references indicate fetal size but do not assess fetal growth.
Salomon et al, France (2006)[68]	Low-risk pregnancies from examinations taken by trained operators during a 1-year period across France	19,647; unknown; cross-sectional	Single country may not be representative of fetal growth in local populations; cross-sectional references indicate fetal size but do not assess fetal growth.

(continued on next page)

Table 1
(continued)

Authors, Location (y)	Inclusion Criteria and Dates[a]; Data Source	Sample Size[b]; Retrospective or Prospective; Cross-sectional or Longitudinal	Considerations for Use
Snijders and Nicolaides, UK (1994)[69]	Women selected with low-risk pregnancies and known menstrual histories (1987–1993); 40 patients included for each 7-d interval from 14 wk to 40 wk; database from single hospital	1040; retrospective; cross-sectional	Retrospective ultrasound data may be limited by selection bias, or the reason for why an ultrasound was obtained at a given gestational age may influence the fetal size measurement by an unknown amount; cross-sectional references indicate fetal size but do not assess fetal growth.
Stirnemann et al, international (2017)[7]	Low-risk pregnancies with accurate dating (2009–2014); fetal biometric measurements taken at examinations approximately every 5 wk from 9 wk to 14 wk until 40 wk, 8 countries	4321; prospective; longitudinal	INTERGROWTH; created new EFW formula using head and abdominal circumference; diverse; rigorous credentialing of sonographers; use of standardized protocol; separate reference for fetal biometrics[6]
Williams et al, California (1982)[29]	Birthweight from matched birth, death, and fetal death certificates from the Center for Health Statistics of the California Department of Health Services (1970–1976)	2,288,806; retrospective; cross-sectional	Birthweight references inaccurately describe the preterm growth of fetuses who go on to deliver at term. Computer screening method applied to correct errors in gestational age.

[a] Dates not provided for some studies.
[b] Sample size is for number included in construction of the fetal growth reference after inclusions and exclusions from the study sample.

and had a known last menstrual period underwent serial ultrasounds across pregnancy for fetal biometric measurement, although specific inclusion and exclusion criteria varied. A minor difference was that statistical analytical approaches varied among the 3 studies.[31] It also is important to note that INTERGROWTH created a new EFW formula based only on head circumference (HC) and abdominal circumference (AC), whereas NICHD and WHO Fetal used the Hadlock 1985 formula based on HC, AC, and femur length (FL).[7,32]

The 3 studies varied in their approach as to whether to create a unified fetal growth curve for their studies. The INTERGROWTH and WHO Fetal studies followed similar procedures as the WHO Multicentre Growth Reference Study (MGRS) Child Growth Standards which derived a single international growth chart for boys and girls ages 0 to 5 years.[33,34] The INTERGROWTH and WHO Fetal studies differed, however, in their aims at assessing whether there were significant differences between populations. INTERGROWTH operated according to the concept that if conditions were equally optimized, human fetuses grow the same. They, therefore, did not test statistical significance as to whether there were any differences between populations but evaluated the similarities between fetal growth among the sites. A standardized site difference at different gestational ages was calculated and fetal growth was considered similar if the standardized site difference was within a somewhat arbitrary range of -0.5 to 0.5 SD. Correspondingly, they pooled their contributors according to likeness of growth, that is, that variation was within a pragmatically set limit (a coefficient of SDs).[35] Thus, INTERGROWTH prescribed to the concept that 1 reference fits all. The WHO Fetal, on the other hand, aimed at assessing whether there were significant differences between populations and found that differences existed.[11] The WHO Fetal reached a different conclusion from both INTERGROWTH and the World Health Organization (WHO) child growth studies, which reported that it is possible to establish and use 1 reference, including multiple populations, but that the use and interpretation have to take into account that populations are significantly different.[36] The NICHD study was designed to assess differences in fetal growth not among countries but among racial/ethnic groups, given the well-described differences in AC and FL in children and adults of differing racial/ethnic groups.[8,37,38]

When comparing the results of INTERGROWTH, NICHD, and WHO Fetal studies directly, the percentiles for fetal biometrics and EFW varied among the studies.[31] Differences in EFW are presented in **Fig. 1** and **Table 2** (no statistical testing was performed). The 50th percentile EFW for INTERGROWTH was smaller beginning at 26 weeks of gestation than the 50th percentile EFW for WHO Fetal and all racial/ethnic groups in NICHD, with differences persisting through 40 weeks. At 32 weeks of gestation, a time when a growth ultrasound may be obtained, the 50th percentile for EFW was 1755 g in INTERGROWTH and 1901 g in WHO Fetal, a difference of 146 g; and 1960 g for non-Hispanic white, 1879 g for Hispanic, 1830 g for Asian or Pacific Islander, and 1837 g for non-Hispanic black women in the NICHD study, a difference from INTERGROWTH ranging from 75 g to 205 g. The implications of these differences are that different proportions of SGA and LGA are identified in a local population, depending on which fetal growth curve is used as a reference.

Similarly, the WHO Fetal found EFW and growth trajectory variation were significantly different the among 10 countries.[11] **Fig. 2** demonstrates that the 90th percentile of EFW varied across the countries, indicating that again, a different proportion of LGA is identified in a local population when using a unified international growth curve. These findings are in line with the NICHD study group demonstration that different proportions of healthy nonwhite fetuses from low-risk pregnancies would be identified as SGA less than the 5th percentile using a non-Hispanic white or unified standard, which is notable because the older Hadlock and colleagues 1991 study included only white women.[9,39]

CONSIDERATIONS

The findings from 3 modern, multicenter fetal growth reference studies, INTERGROWTH, NICHD, and WHO Fetal, demonstrate wide variation in fetal growth among

Standards for Estimated Fetal Weight 24-40 Wk

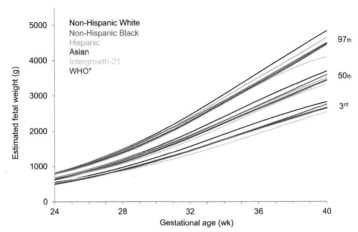

Fig. 1. Variation in EFW among 3 studies. Standards for EFW 24 weeks to 40 weeks. INTER-GROWTH, NICHD, and WHO Fetal, for 24 weeks to 40 weeks of gestation. Estimated 3rd, 50th, and 97th percentiles for fetal weight by study. *Values are the 2.5th and 97.5th for the WHO Fetal. Also, NICHD and WHO Fetal calculated EFW from HC, AC, and FL using the Hadlock 1985 formula,[32] whereas INTERGROWTH created a new formula,[7] based only on HC and AC. (*From* Fetal growth standards: the NICHD fetal growth study approach in context with INTERGROWTH-21st and the World Health Organization Multicentre Growth Reference Study. American Journal of Obstetrics and Gynecology, 2018, with permission.)

different countries and racial and ethnic groups. Variations in fetal growth are similar to variations observed in child growth and that also persist in adult populations.[33,34,40] Body proportion as measured by ratio of sitting height to height and mean stature for adult populations differ across 4 geographic areas, including Australia/New Zealand/Papua New Guinea, Africa, Europe, and Asia.[41] In the United States, black people have shorter sitting height and longer leg length for a similar mean height compared with white people.[42] The racial and ethnic differences in neonatal anthropometry in the NICHD study were not explained by differences in individual socioeconomic factors.[43] These findings indicate that differences among the 3 fetal growth studies may be explained in large part by differences in the international case mix and support the concept that there is natural genetic or inherent variation in fetal growth.

The determinants of fetal growth, however, are not fully understood.[44,45] Normal regional and ethnic variations in body size and proportion likely are due to a combination of genetic and environmental factors.[41] In twin and intergenerational studies, up to 40% of birth size is estimated to be heritable, with fetal genetic factors explaining 31% of variation in birthweight and length and maternal genetic factors explaining 22% and 19%, respectively.[44,46] Africans and East Asians have higher birthweight-lowering genetic variants than Europeans, consistent with the finding that 50th percentile EFW and birthweight were lower in these groups in the NICHD Fetal Growth Studies.[8,47] A genome-wide association study also found a novel genome-wide locus that was associated with reduced fetal weight, manifested by decreased HC but not AC or FL.[48] Genetic factors associated with fetal growth are influenced by environmental factors displaying a developmental plasticity and natural variation in fetal growth.[49,50] It may not be optimal size but optimal adaptation that is important.

Table 2
Fiftieth percentiles for fetal anthropometric measurements by gestational age for the 3 studies[a]

Gestational Age (wk) [b]	Estimated Fetal Weight [c] (g), Fiftieth Percentiles					
	NICHD White	NICHD Hispanic	NICHD Asian	NICHD Black	INTERGROWTH	WHO Fetal
24	674	651	640	647	668	665
25	787	758	745	751	756	778
26	912	876	862	866	856	902
27	1050	1007	990	994	969	1039
28	1202	1151	1132	1134	1097	1189
29	1369	1311	1287	1289	1239	1350
30	1552	1486	1456	1459	1396	1523
31	1749	1676	1637	1642	1568	1707
32	1960	1879	1830	1837	1755	1901
33	2180	2090	2031	2040	1954	2103
34	2408	2307	2238	2247	2162	2312
35	2637	2521	2448	2452	2378	2527
36	2864	2731	2656	2654	2594	2745
37	3086	2935	2862	2854	2806	2966
38	3299	3134	3065	3054	3006	3186
39	3502	3330	3263	3256	3186	3403
40	3693	3525	3455	3466	3338	3617

[a] The NICHD,[8,9] INTERGROWTH,[6,7] and WHO Fetal.[11,12]
[b] Results were reported for the exact day (eg, 16.0 wk).
[c] Note that NICHD and WHO Fetal calculated EFW from HC, AC, and FL using the Hadlock 1985 formula,[32] whereas INTERGROWTH created a new formula,[7] based only on HC and AC.
   Data from Fetal growth standards: the NICHD fetal growth study approach in context with INTERGROWTH-21st and the World Health Organization Multicentre Growth Reference Study. American Journal of Obstetrics and Gynecology, 2018.[31]

Given the natural variation in fetal growth and differences in fetal growth percentiles among references, selecting a universal reference would make comparison of fetal growth simpler for clinical use and for comparison across populations. The disadvantage of a universal reference, however, is that it may describe fetal growth in local populations inaccurately, leading to misclassification of fetuses as SGA and LGA. Fetal growth is influenced by maternal and paternal characteristics, which are known to vary by country and adapt to many external factors, including altitude, nutrition, and other environmental conditions.[18,51,52] For example, the INTERGROWTH and WHO Fetal references were developed in populations living at altitudes less than 1600 m and 1500 m, respectively, and may perform differently for populations living at higher altitude.[7,11] The WHO Fetal also demonstrated that there was more variation in fetal growth in the higher percentiles (eg, 90th) than in the lower percentiles (eg, 2.5th, 5th, and 10th), indicating that the upper percentiles may need more adjustment (ie, customization) at the population level.[11] Country as a proxy for local ethnic mix has been found the most important factor in predicting adverse outcomes in infants compared with customizing for additional individual characteristics.[53] Therefore, it is critical to test how a fetal growth reference performs in relation to clinically meaningful outcomes, including neonatal morbidity and mortality, in the local population to which it is being applied.

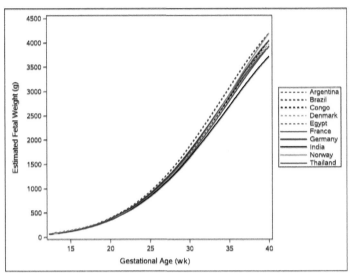

Fig. 2. Variation in EFW among countries in the WHO Fetal. The 90th percentiles for EFW for the 10 participating countries in the WHO Fetal.[11] These findings indicate that a different proportion of LGA are identified in a local population when using a unified international growth curve. (From The World Health Organization Fetal Growth Charts: A Multinational Longitudinal Study of Ultrasound Biometric Measurements and Estimated Fetal Weight. PLOS Medicine, 2017.)

The process of selecting a national reference for fetal growth may be borrowed from the process of selecting a reference for child growth. The Centers for Disease Control and Prevention (CDC) and American Academy of Pediatrics recommend US health care providers use the population-based WHO standard charts for children from birth until ages 2 years, and the 2000 CDC growth reference charts for children ages 2 years to 20 years.[54] The INTERGROWTH and WHO Fetal growth charts were created with the intention of being used internationally. Only INTERGROWTH included a US site, whereas the NICHD study was performed only in the United States but with similar study procedures as the WHO, so the data eventually could be combined. Currently, the WHO recommends use of their fetal growth reference for clinical use in all countries with the caveat that the charts should be tested and monitored for performance in local populations. The American College of Obstetricians and Gynecologists does not refer to a specific fetal growth reference when defining fetal growth restriction or LGA whereas the Society for Maternal-Fetal Medicine recommends use of population-based fetal growth references (such as Hadlock).[1,2,55] The Hadlock reference included only white women from a single center, which may not represent fetal growth in other race/ethnic groups, and, given that it was a cross-sectional reference, 1-time measurement of fetal growth (ie, EFW percentile at a given gestational age) indicates only size.[39] In order to know how a fetus arrived at an EFW, at least 2 measurements separated in time are needed to estimate a trajectory. Consideration of other factors, such as abnormal Doppler velocimetry, amniotic fluid assessment or maternal complications, and clinical judgment, also are important determinants for clinical monitoring and intervention.[56] The newer prospective fetal growth curves also allow estimation of fetal growth velocity, which has potential to better distinguish pathologic from normal fetal growth.[57-59]

SUMMARY

There are 3 modern, prospective fetal growth standards that are similar in scope but demonstrate variation in fetal growth. Different fetal growth charts classify different proportions of fetuses as below or above a cutoff point (eg, below the 10th percentile or greater than the 90th percentile). It is important to know how a growth reference performs in a local population in relation to important clinical outcomes, including fetal morbidity and mortality when implementing in clinical practice. Whether adjusting these population-based fetal growth references further by customization or individualization with conditional growth improves detection of perinatal morbidity and mortality requires future study.

CLINICS CARE POINTS

- Ultrasound references tend to be preferred to birthweight references for clinical antepartum monitoring because infants who deliver preterm are more likely to be growth restricted, and, therefore, birthweight references inaccurately describe the preterm growth of fetuses who go on to deliver at term.

- Different fetal growth references classify different proportions of fetuses as below or above a cutoff point (eg, below the 10th percentile or greater than the 90th percentile).

- Fetal growth references should be tested and monitored for performance in local populations.

ACKNOWLEDGMENT

The author would like to acknowledge Professor Torvid Kiserud, University of Bergen, and Haukeland University Hospital, Bergen, Norway, for his critical review.

DISCLOSURE

The author has nothing to disclose.

DISCLAIMER

K.L. Grantz is a US federal government employee. The named author alone is responsible for the views expressed in this article, which do not necessarily represent the decisions or the stated policy of the NICHD.

REFERENCES

1. ACOG Practice Bulletin No. 204: fetal growth restriction. Obstet Gynecol 2019; 133(2):e97–109.
2. Committee on Practice, B-O. Macrosomia: ACOG practice bulletin, number 216. Obstet Gynecol 2020;135(1):e18–35.
3. Battaglia FC, Lubchenco LO. A practical classification of newborn infants by weight and gestational age. J Pediatr 1967;71(2):159–63.
4. Iliodromiti S, Mackay DF, Smith GC, et al. Customised and noncustomised birth weight centiles and prediction of stillbirth and infant mortality and morbidity: a cohort study of 979,912 term singleton pregnancies in Scotland. PLoS Med 2017;14(1):e1002228.

5. Vasak B, Koenen SV, Koster MP, et al. Human fetal growth is constrained below optimal for perinatal survival. Ultrasound Obstet Gynecol 2015;45(2):162–7.

6. Papageorghiou AT, Ohuma EO, Altman DG, et al. International standards for fetal growth based on serial ultrasound measurements: the Fetal Growth Longitudinal Study of the INTERGROWTH-21st Project. Lancet 2014;384(9946):869–79.

7. Stirnemann J, Villar J, Salomon LJ, et al. International estimated fetal weight standards of the INTERGROWTH-21st project. Ultrasound Obstet Gynecol 2017; 49(4):478–86.

8. Buck Louis GM, Grewal J, Albert PS, et al. Racial/ethnic standards for fetal growth: the NICHD fetal growth studies. Am J Obstet Gynecol 2015;213(4): 449.e1-41.

9. Buck Louis GM, Grewal J. Clarification of estimating fetal weight between 10-14 weeks gestation, NICHD fetal growth studies. Am J Obstet Gynecol 2017;217(1): 96–101.

10. Grewal J, Grantz KL, Zhang C, et al. Cohort profile: NICHD fetal growth studies-singletons and twins. Int J Epidemiol 2018;47(1):25-25l.

11. Kiserud T, Piaggio G, Carroli G, et al. The World Health Organization fetal growth charts: a multinational longitudinal study of ultrasound biometric measurements and estimated fetal weight. PLoS Med 2017;14(1):e1002220.

12. Kiserud T, Piaggio G, Carroli G, et al. Correction: the World Health Organization fetal growth charts: a multinational longitudinal study of ultrasound biometric measurements and estimated fetal weight. PLoS Med 2017;14(3):e1002284.

13. Alexander GR, Himes JH, Kaufman RB, et al. A United States national reference for fetal growth. Obstet Gynecol 1996;87(2):163–8.

14. Duryea EL, Hawkins JS, Mcintire DD, et al. A revised birth weight reference for the United States. Obstet Gynecol 2014;124(1):16–22.

15. Barel O, Vaknin Z, Tovbin J, et al. Assessment of the accuracy of multiple sonographic fetal weight estimation formulas: a 10-year experience from a single center. J Ultrasound Med 2013;32(5):815–23.

16. Gardosi JO. Prematurity and fetal growth restriction. Early Hum Dev 2005; 81(1):43–9.

17. Zhang J, Sun K. Invited commentary: the incremental value of customization in defining abnormal fetal growth status. Am J Epidemiol 2013;178(8):1309–12.

18. Gardosi J. Customized fetal growth standards: rationale and clinical application. Semin Perinatol 2004;28(1):33–40.

19. Hutcheon JA, Zhang X, Platt RW, et al. The case against customised birthweight standards. Paediatr Perinat Epidemiol 2011;25(1):11–6.

20. Carberry AE, Raynes-Greenow CH, Turner RM, et al. Customized versus population-based birth weight charts for the detection of neonatal growth and perinatal morbidity in a cross-sectional study of term neonates. Am J Epidemiol 2013; 178(8):1301–8.

21. Deter RL, Rossavik IK, Harrist RB. Development of individual growth curve standards for estimated fetal weight: I. Weight estimation procedure. J Clin Ultrasound 1988;16(4):215–25.

22. Deter RL, Rossavik IK, Carpenter RJ. Development of individual growth standards for estimated fetal weight: II. Weight prediction during the third trimester and at birth. J Clin Ultrasound 1989;17(2):83–8.

23. Deter RL, Lee W, Yeo L, et al. Individualized growth assessment: conceptual framework and practical implementation for the evaluation of fetal growth and neonatal growth outcome. Am J Obstet Gynecol 2018;218(2S):S656–78.

24. Owen P, Ogston S. Conditional centiles for the quantification of fetal growth. Ultrasound Obstet Gynecol 1998;11(2):110–7.
25. Royston P. Calculation of unconditional and conditional reference intervals for foetal size and growth from longitudinal measurements. Stat Med 1995;14(13): 1417–36.
26. Karlsen HO, Johnsen SL, Rasmussen S, et al. Prediction of adverse perinatal outcome of small-for-gestational-age pregnancy using size centiles and conditional growth centiles. Ultrasound Obstet Gynecol 2016;48(2):217–23.
27. Altman DG, Chitty LS. Charts of fetal size: 1. Methodology. Br J Obstet Gynaecol 1994;101(1):29–34.
28. Brenner WE, Edelman DA, Hendricks CH. A standard of fetal growth for the United States of America. Am J Obstet Gynecol 1976;126(5):555–64.
29. Williams RL, Creasy RK, Cunningham GC, et al. Fetal growth and perinatal viability in California. Obstet Gynecol 1982;59(5):624–32.
30. Ioannou C, Talbot K, Ohuma E, et al. Systematic review of methodology used in ultrasound studies aimed at creating charts of fetal size. BJOG 2012;119(12): 1425–39.
31. Grantz KL, Hediger ML, Liu D, et al. Fetal growth standards: the NICHD fetal growth study approach in context with INTERGROWTH-21st and the World Health Organization Multicentre Growth Reference Study. Am J Obstet Gynecol 2018;218(2S):641–55.e28.
32. Hadlock FP, Harrist RB, Sharman RS, et al. Estimation of fetal weight with the use of head, body, and femur measurements–a prospective study. Am J Obstet Gynecol 1985;151(3):333–7.
33. WHO child growth standards based on length/height, weight and age. Acta Paediatr Suppl 2006;450:76–85.
34. De Onis M, Garza C, Victora CG, et al. The WHO Multicentre Growth Reference Study: planning, study design, and methodology. Food Nutr Bull 2004;25(1 Suppl):S15–26.
35. Villar J, Papageorghiou AT, Pang R, et al. The likeness of fetal growth and newborn size across non-isolated populations in the INTERGROWTH-21st project: the fetal growth longitudinal study and newborn cross-sectional study. Lancet Diabetes Endocrinol 2014;2(10):781–92.
36. Kiserud T, Benachi A, Hecher K, et al. The World Health Organization fetal growth charts: concept, findings, interpretation, and application. Am J Obstet Gynecol 2018;218(2S):S619–29.
37. Malina RM, Brown KH, Zavaleta AN. Relative lower extremity length in Mexican American and in American black and white youth. Am J Phys Anthropol 1987; 72(1):89–94.
38. Wulan SN, Westerterp KR, Plasqui G. Ethnic differences in body composition and the associated metabolic profile: a comparative study between Asians and Caucasians. Maturitas 2010;65(4):315–9.
39. Hadlock FP, Harrist RB, Martinez-Poyer J. In utero analysis of fetal growth: a sonographic weight standard. Radiology 1991;181(1):129–33.
40. Natale V, Rajagopalan A. Worldwide variation in human growth and the World Health Organization growth standards: a systematic review. BMJ Open 2014; 4(1):e003735.
41. Bogin B, Varela-Silva MI. Leg length, body proportion, and health: a review with a note on beauty. Int J Environ Res Public Health 2010;7(3):1047–75.

42. Heymsfield SB, Peterson CM, Thomas DM, et al. Why are there race/ethnic differences in adult body mass index-adiposity relationships? A quantitative critical review. Obes Rev 2016;17(3):262–75.

43. Lambert C, Gleason JL, Pugh SJ, et al. Maternal socioeconomic factors and racial/ethnic differences in neonatal Anthropometry. Int J Environ Res Public Health 2020;17(19):7323.

44. Lunde A, Melve KK, Gjessing HK, et al. Genetic and environmental influences on birth weight, birth length, head circumference, and gestational age by use of population-based parent-offspring data. Am J Epidemiol 2007;165(7):734–41.

45. Kramer MS. Determinants of low birth weight: methodological assessment and meta-analysis. Bull World Health Organ 1987;65(5):663–737.

46. Clausson B, Lichtenstein P, Cnattingius S. Genetic influence on birthweight and gestational length determined by studies in offspring of twins. BJOG 2000; 107(3):375–81.

47. Tekola-Ayele F, Workalemahu T, Amare AT. High burden of birthweight-lowering genetic variants in Africans and Asians. BMC Med 2018;16(1):70.

48. Tekola-Ayele F, Zhang C, Wu J, et al. Trans-ethnic meta-analysis of genome-wide association studies identifies maternal ITPR1 as a novel locus influencing fetal growth during sensitive periods in pregnancy. PLoS Genet 2020;16(5):e1008747.

49. Hanson MA, Gluckman PD. Early developmental conditioning of later health and disease: physiology or pathophysiology? Physiol Rev 2014;94(4):1027–76.

50. Hanson M, Kiserud T, Visser GH, et al. Optimal fetal growth: a misconception? Am J Obstet Gynecol 2015;213(3):332.e1-4.

51. Gluckman PD, Hanson MA, Buklijas T. A conceptual framework for the developmental origins of health and disease. J Dev Orig Health Dis 2010;1(1):6–18.

52. Frisancho AR. Developmental functional adaptation to high altitude: review. Am J Hum Biol 2013;25(2):151–68.

53. Mikolajczyk RT, Zhang J, Betran AP, et al. A global reference for fetal-weight and birthweight percentiles. Lancet 2011;377(9780):1855–61.

54. WHO Growth Standards Are Recommended for Use with Children Younger Than Aged 2 Years in the United States. 2021. Available at: https://www.cdc.gov/nccdphp/dnpao/growthcharts/who/recommendations/index.htm.

55. Society for Maternal-Fetal Medicine. Electronic Address, PSO, Martins JG, Biggio JR, Abuhamad A. Society for Maternal-Fetal Medicine Consult Series #52: Diagnosis and management of fetal growth restriction: (Replaces Clinical Guideline Number 3, April 2012). Am J Obstet Gynecol 2020;223(4):B2–17.

56. ACOG Practice bulletin no. 134: fetal growth restriction. Obstet Gynecol 2013; 121(5):1122–33.

57. Grantz KL, Kim S, Grobman WA, et al. Fetal growth velocity: the NICHD fetal growth studies. Am J Obstet Gynecol 2018;219(3):285.e1–36.

58. Sovio U, White IR, Dacey A, et al. Screening for fetal growth restriction with universal third trimester ultrasonography in nulliparous women in the Pregnancy Outcome Prediction (POP) study: a prospective cohort study. Lancet 2015; 386(10008):2089–97.

59. Ohuma EO, Villar J, Feng Y, et al, Newborn Growth Consortium for the 21st, C. Fetal growth velocity standards from the fetal growth longitudinal study of the INTERGROWTH-21(st) project. Am J Obstet Gynecol 2021;224(2):208.e1-e18.

60. Hediger ML, Fuchs KM, Grantz KL, et al. Ultrasound quality assurance for singletons in the national institute of child health and human development fetal growth studies. J Ultrasound Med 2016;35(8):1725–33.

61. Di Battista E, Bertino E, Benso L, et al. Longitudinal distance standards of fetal growth. Intrauterine and Infant Longitudinal Growth Study: IILGS. Acta Obstet Gynecol Scand 2000;79(3):165–73.
62. Gallivan S, Robson SC, Chang TC, et al. An investigation of fetal growth using serial ultrasound data. Ultrasound Obstet Gynecol 1993;3(2):109–14.
63. Jeanty P, Cantraine F, Romero R, et al. A longitudinal study of fetal weight growth. J Ultrasound Med 1984;3(7):321–8.
64. Johnsen SL, Rasmussen S, Wilsgaard T, et al. Longitudinal reference ranges for estimated fetal weight. Acta Obstet Gynecol Scand 2006;85(3):286–97.
65. Marsal K, Persson PH, Larsen T, et al. Intrauterine growth curves based on ultrasonically estimated foetal weights. Acta Paediatr 1996;85(7):843–8.
66. Mongelli M, Gardosi J. Longitudinal study of fetal growth in subgroups of a low-risk population. Ultrasound Obstet Gynecol 1995;6(5):340–4.
67. Nasrat H, Bondagji NS. Ultrasound biometry of Arabian fetuses. Int J Gynaecol Obstet 2005;88(2):173–8.
68. Salomon LJ, Duyme M, Crequat J, et al. French fetal biometry: reference equations and comparison with other charts. Ultrasound Obstet Gynecol 2006;28(2):193–8.
69. Snijders RJ, Nicolaides KH. Fetal biometry at 14-40 weeks' gestation. Ultrasound Obstet Gynecol 1994;4(1):34–48.

Fetal Growth and Stillbirth

Jessica M. Page, MD, MSCI[a,*], Nathan R. Blue, MD[b],
Robert M. Silver, MD[c]

KEYWORDS

- Stillbirth • Fetal death • Fetal growth restriction

KEY POINTS

- Fetal growth restriction is a strong risk factor for stillbirth.
- The interval between fetal death and recognition of the fetal death may exaggerate the association between fetal growth restriction and stillbirth.
- Further work is needed to identify those pregnancies at highest risk of placental insufficiency and stillbirth.
- Antenatal surveillance and early delivery may reduce the risk of stillbirth in pregnancies affected by fetal growth restriction.
- Stillbirths with fetal growth restriction should be evaluated with fetal autopsy, placental pathology, genetic testing, antiphospholipid antibody testing, and fetal-maternal hemorrhage testing.

INTRODUCTION

Stillbirth is one of the most devastating obstetric outcomes for both families and clinicians. In the United States, stillbirth is defined as fetal death at 20 weeks' gestation or later and occurs in approximately 1 per 160 deliveries.[1] The stillbirth rate has remained largely stable in the United States and exceeds that of many other high-resource countries.[2,3] At least one-quarter of US stillbirths are potentially preventable with many of these cases, including intrapartum losses, complications of maternal medical conditions, and placental insufficiency.[4] A large proportion of stillbirths is attributed to placental insufficiency and represents an important target for prevention. Placental causes of death were the most common cause of fetal death (28%) in US fetal death certificate reporting.[5] In a well-characterized multicenter US stillbirth study, placental causes of fetal death were also common, occurring in 23.6% of cases.[6] One of the

[a] Maternal-Fetal Medicine, Intermountain Healthcare, University of Utah, 5121 South Cottonwood Street, Suite 100, Murray, UT 84107, USA; [b] Maternal-Fetal Medicine, Intermountain Healthcare, University of Utah, 30 North 1900 East, 2A200, Salt Lake City, UT 84132, USA; [c] Maternal-Fetal Medicine, University of Utah, 30 North 1900 East, 2A200, Salt Lake City, UT 84132, USA
* Corresponding author.
E-mail address: jessica.page@hsc.utah.edu
Twitter: @Nateyblue (N.R.B.)

Obstet Gynecol Clin N Am 48 (2021) 297–310
https://doi.org/10.1016/j.ogc.2021.03.001
0889-8545/21/© 2021 Elsevier Inc. All rights reserved.

most common clinical manifestations of placental insufficiency is diminished fetal growth. Fetal growth restriction (FGR) is one of the best-characterized risk factors for stillbirth. Here the authors discuss FGR as it pertains to stillbirth.

FEATURES OF FETAL GROWTH RESTRICTION UNIQUE TO STILLBIRTH

FGR has been associated with stillbirth in many retrospective studies. Small-for-gestational-age (SGA) infants are more common following stillbirths as compared with livebirths, particularly at preterm gestational ages.[7] Also, the risk of fetal death is increased when FGR occurs as a result of placental insufficiency rather than as an association with maternal small stature or obstetric or medical comorbidities.[8] Poor fetal growth has also had a strong association with stillbirth in case control studies, with Frøen and colleagues[9] reporting an odds ratio (OR) of 7.0 (95% confidence interval [CI]: 3.3–15.1). The increased risk of stillbirth is more pronounced with increasing severity of FGR in population-based studies as well.[10] Prospective studies also demonstrate an increased risk of stillbirth, with Hirst and colleagues[11] reporting a hazard ratio of 4.6 (95% CI: 3.4–6.2). In an analysis of prospectively ascertained perinatal outcomes of SGA versus appropriately grown infants at term, the incidence of stillbirth was 3.5 per 1000 among SGA infants as compared with 0.9 per 1000 in non-SGA infants.[12] This association was also demonstrated when including preterm deliveries, with an adjusted OR of 3.98 (95% CI: 2.92–5.42).[13] In meta-analysis, SGA had a population attributable risk of 23% for stillbirth in high-income countries.[14]

Stillbirth can be associated with FGR and SGA via many pathophysiologic pathways. FGR is usually considered a marker for placental insufficiency. Placental insufficiency can occur when the placenta functions suboptimally because of abnormal development or damage during the pregnancy. FGR is also associated with placental insufficiency as a result of maternal medical or obstetric complications. The most common obstetric complications include chronic hypertension, renal disease, pregestational diabetes, and systemic lupus erythematosus. Exposures to tobacco or other illicit drugs can also result in placental insufficiency because of reduced uterine blood flow. Maternal infections, such as syphilis, cytomegalovirus, and malaria, can also cause placental damage through an inflammatory pathway. Obstetric complications that are associated with placental insufficiency include preeclampsia, abruption, and multiple gestation, particularly when monochorionicity is present. Placental insufficiency, regardless of the clinical scenario, results in reduced blood, oxygen, and nutrient passage to the fetus, which underlies the biologic association with stillbirth.

Determining the Timing of Stillbirth

Concern has been raised regarding the strength of the association of FGR with stillbirth given the difficulty of accurate determination of gestational age in the setting of fetal death. Often the exact gestational age at fetal death is not known and some time has elapsed from the time of death to the time of delivery. This delay in diagnosis can overestimate the gestational age of the fetus and incorrectly identify a fetus as growth restricted given that the birthweight is smaller than expected for the gestational age at delivery. Indeed, SGA is often used as a proxy for FGR in the setting of stillbirth, as there is not always a preceding clinical history of FGR that was well documented. This results in nearly a quarter of stillbirths being associated with poor fetal growth or SGA, which is substantially higher than other associations.[14,15]

Work has been done to address the discrepancy between the gestational age at the time of death compared with the assigned gestational age at the time of delivery. A prospective case-control study of stillbirths and live births at 5 clinical centers in the

United States determined the likely age of fetal death by taking into account several clinical criteria. First, the reliability of the estimated due date was evaluated. If the due date was well established by menstrual or ultrasound dating, it was taken into account. Second, the time interval from the last documented evidence of fetal viability to the time of documented fetal death was considered. Last, information regarding the degree of fetal maceration and the fetal foot length was used to provide additional insight into the likely date of death and interval before delivery.[16] These data points were integrated to determine an estimated date of death, which was considered precise in 47% of cases evaluated where reliable dating criteria and an interval of 1 week or less from the date of death had occurred.[16] This algorithm also had good correlation with fetal foot length with agreement within 2 weeks in 75% of cases.[17]

A series of 533 stillbirths with fetal autopsy investigated the relationship between the time interval from fetal death to delivery as well as from delivery to autopsy. Fetal tissue maceration is associated with longer in utero retention from the time of death to delivery. Man and colleagues[18] demonstrated that there was a higher proportion of fetal tissue maceration in the cohort that was classified as SGA with an artifactual reduction in birthweight of approximately −0.8 standard deviations. They also noted an additional decrease in weight from the time of delivery to the time of autopsy with an average 12% reduction. This was related to the length of time elapsed between delivery and postmortem examination, highlighting the importance of noting the delivery weight and accounting for the elapsed time in utero from fetal death to delivery.

A prospective study of stillbirths in the United States used the above referenced algorithm for determining the gestational age at fetal death, incorporating time of death interval, fetal autopsy findings, and reliability of dating criteria.[19] This study demonstrated that stillbirth was associated with SGA when evaluated with population (OR 3.0), ultrasound (OR 4.7), and individualized (OR 4.6) normative curves. This association persisted when adjusting for known prepregnancy stillbirth risk factors and in both preterm and term deliveries. This study demonstrated that the association of placental insufficiency and thus FGR with stillbirth persists even after accounting for the pitfalls of accurately diagnosing FGR in stillbirths.

STILLBIRTH RISK STRATIFICATION IN THE SETTING OF FETAL GROWTH RESTRICTION

It is important to note that FGR is a clinical indicator of placental insufficiency and is thus a risk factor for stillbirth rather than a cause. The underlying cause in this case would be placental insufficiency. Unfortunately, there are limited clinical tools with which to predict and detect placental insufficiency. Currently, tools for detection of placental insufficiency include ultrasound and biochemical markers.

A detailed discussion of routine ultrasonography for identification of FGR as well as the various growth standards by which to diagnose FGR is presented in Katherine L. Grantz's article, "Fetal Growth Curves: Is There a Universal Reference?"; Katie Stephens and colleagues' article, "Routine Third Trimester Sonogram: Friend or Foe," in this issue, and thus the authors briefly review the issues as they pertain to stillbirth here. Of particular interest is identifying those pregnancies at highest risk of stillbirth that do not have other risk factors and so will not have a standard indication for serial screening measures. This otherwise low-risk population is in need of an effective screening test that would identify those at a heightened risk of stillbirth and would benefit most from obstetric intervention. Fetal growth monitoring by way of fundal height measurement and fetal growth ultrasound is the most commonly used measure of placental function in current obstetric practice. Surveillance with fundal height measurement is used essentially universally in practice, whereas, in contrast, serial ultrasound for fetal growth is generally reserved for pregnancies with medical or obstetric risk factors.[20] Randomized trials and meta-analysis of universal third-trimester ultrasound in otherwise low-risk pregnancies did not demonstrate maternal or fetal benefits to screening.[21,22] This may be due in part to lack of a standard definition of FGR and of a standard intervention. In addition, it is difficult to power a trial to show a reduction in stillbirth, as it is a relatively rare event, occurring in approximately 1 per 200 deliveries in high-resource settings.[23] Of course, identification of a small fetus is only the first step in assessing fetal status, as up to 70% of FGR fetuses are healthy and constitutionally small.[24]

Among fetuses diagnosed with FGR, additional sonographic tools are used to risk stratify them based on the likelihood of fetal death. One approach is evaluation of each biometric parameter, as adverse outcomes are best correlated with the fetal abdominal circumference measurement.[25,26] By this approach, a smaller abdominal circumference measurement would be interpreted as conferring a higher risk for placental insufficiency and thus fetal death. Physiologically, when placental insufficiency is present, reduced oxygen and nutrients are available, and the fetal circulation preferentially shunts blood flow to the fetal brain, heart, and adrenal glands, resulting in reduced fat and liver glycogen storage, leading to a small abdominal circumference despite normal fetal head measurements (biparietal diameter, head circumference).

Additional sonographic methods are used to further risk stratify growth-restricted fetuses to determine those at highest risk of fetal death. The first of these strategies is assessment of amniotic fluid volume. Placental insufficiency reduces blood flow to the fetus with subsequent cephalization of blood flow, as discussed above. Placental insufficiency reduces renal perfusion and thus urination and amniotic fluid volume. Low amniotic fluid volume is termed oligohydramnios and is defined as a single deepest vertical pocket measurement of less than 2 cm. The impact of oligohydramnios on outcomes in FGR pregnancies has not been extensively studied. The PORTO study prospectively studied 1100 FGR pregnancies and investigated characteristics associated with adverse perinatal outcomes.[27] They demonstrated that oligohydramnios was not predictive of adverse outcomes unless the fetus was also less than the third percentile. However, there is strong biologic plausibility that oligohydramnios in combination with FGR poses a higher risk for fetal death via either worsening placental insufficiency or cord compression. Thus, current guidelines recommend delivery between 34 weeks 0 days and 37 weeks 6 days for pregnancies affected with both FGR and oligohydramnios.[28,29]

Doppler velocimetry can also assist in further fetal death risk stratification. Umbilical artery Doppler measurement assesses the impedance of blood flow from the fetus to the placenta throughout the fetal cardiac cycle.[30] In the setting of placental insufficiency, placental impedance to blood flow increases, resulting in reduced return of deoxygenated blood to the placenta.[30] Increasing placental resistance results in an elevation in the pulsatility index, resistance index, and systolic-to-diastolic ratio. All of these measures have been used in various studies, and an abnormal value is defined as those above the 95%ile for gestational age or those with absent or reversed end-diastolic velocity.[29] Assessment of umbilical artery Doppler velocimetry can help to distinguish those fetuses with pathologic placental insufficiency from those who are healthy.[27] In fact, incorporating use of umbilical artery Doppler velocimetry reduces the risk of perinatal death, induction of labor, and cesarean delivery.[31,32] Deterioration in umbilical artery Doppler measurement is associated with an increased risk of stillbirth, with a risk of 6.8% for absent end diastolic flow (AEDF) and 19% for reversed end diastolic flow (REDF).[33] These risks for fetal death exceed the risks of severe infant morbidity or mortality at 33 to 34 weeks for AEDF and 30 to 32 weeks for REDF, resulting in recent recommendations for delivery at these gestational ages for each of these groups.[29,34] Umbilical artery Doppler measurement is more predictive of adverse outcomes in cases of early-onset FGR rather than late-onset FGR.[35] Given this, it is important to use additional modalities to monitor fetal status when FGR develops at later gestational ages.

Ideally, a biochemical marker could be assessed in pregnancy that would identify high-risk gestations for placental insufficiency and thus stillbirth. Research efforts have focused primarily on placental proteins. Of these, pregnancy-associated plasma protein-A (PAPP-A) has been studied as an early biochemical marker of placental insufficiency.[36,37] Meta-analysis of PAPP-A as a predictor of fetal death also showed promise with PAPP-A level less than 0.4 multiples of the median (MoM) having a post-test probability of 1.75% for antepartum stillbirth because of placental abruption or growth restriction versus a value of 0.13% with a normal PAPP-A.[36] Patients with a PAPP-A level less than the fifth percentile have also been shown to have a higher chance of fetal death after 24 weeks' gestation (adjusted OR 2.15). However, the positive predictive value for stillbirth after 24 weeks' gestation was low at 58%.[38] A Cochrane Review examining 3 randomized controlled trials of biochemical markers for placental dysfunction (estrogen and human placental lactogen) demonstrated that there was no evidence that use of these biochemical markers was predictive of stillbirth or other adverse perinatal outcomes.[39] Maternal serum alpha-fetoprotein (AFP) has been identified as a second-trimester marker for placental insufficiency. A systematic review of 11 studies showed an increased risk of fetal death in patients with an elevated AFP level. An AFP level of greater than or equal to 2.5 MoM, corresponding to the 97th percentile, resulted in relative risks ranging from 4.4 to 21.0 for fetal death. Additional information on this topic is reviewed elsewhere.[40] There is ongoing investigation into new, novel biomarkers of placental insufficiency. Recently, Cleaton and colleagues[41] demonstrated that deltalike homolog 1, a growth factor involved in adipose homeostasis, is expressed in decreased amounts in maternal serum in the setting of FGR with abnormal umbilical artery Doppler flow. All things considered, there are no biomarkers currently available with sufficient test performance for predicting risk of stillbirth or placental insufficiency.

INTERVENTIONS TO PREVENT STILLBIRTH IN THE SETTING OF PLACENTAL INSUFFICIENCY

Given the lack of effective risk-stratification tools in low-risk pregnancies, use of stillbirth prevention interventions remains guided by maternal and obstetric risk factors. Interventions that have been studied for stillbirth risk reduction include medical treatment and antenatal surveillance. Use of these tools quickly becomes controversial, as clinicians and patients balance the desire to explore all options to ensure fetal safety with the cost, anxiety, and potential for iatrogenic harm inherent to these measures of (sometimes) unproven efficacy.

First, optimization of maternal medical conditions and modifiable risk factors should be addressed before conception, including encouragement of maternal weight loss, cessation of smoking, alcohol, and illicit substances, and appropriate interpregnancy interval. Pregestational diabetes, hypertension, and systemic lupus erythematosus are among the most crucial to maternal/fetal well-being. Finally, although multiple gestation is not a modifiable risk factor from a patient's perspective, efforts should be made to achieve singleton pregnancies when artificial reproductive technologies are used.

Medication treatment is aimed at improving placental function via either reduction in inflammation or enhanced blood flow. In some instances, data for these approaches have been extrapolated from treatment of antiphospholipid syndrome or preeclampsia prevention. Low-dose aspirin has been shown to reduce stillbirth risk, but benefit may be due to reductions in preeclampsia, spontaneous preterm birth, FGR, and placental insufficiency. A meta-analysis of 40 trials included 33,098 women treated with low-dose aspirin demonstrated a 14% reduction in fetal or neonatal deaths. These data points must be interpreted with caution, as preeclampsia was the primary outcome rather than fetal death.[42] Accordingly, the American College of Obstetrics and Gynecology does not recommend aspirin use for stillbirth prevention unless risk factors for preeclampsia are also present.[43] Recently, the US Preventive Services Task Force (USPSTF) evaluated the available randomized controlled trials of aspirin use for preeclampsia prevention. Their work demonstrated a 20% risk reduction in preterm birth, 18% reduction in SGA/FGR, and a 21% reduction in perinatal mortality.[44,45] The USPSTF states that more data are needed to define the populations that will benefit most from aspirin prophylaxis. Low-molecular-weight heparin (LMWH) has also been studied for the prevention of fetal death. One randomized clinical trial assessing treatment with LMWH resulted in a reduction in composite morbidity, including fetal death; however, it did not show a significant reduction in fetal death itself.[46] Subsequent trials have not demonstrated a mortality benefit, and thus, use of LMWH for stillbirth prevention is not recommended.[47] Additional medical treatments aimed at improving placental function have been considered, including phosphodiesterase inhibitors, hydroxychloroquine, and prednisolone. These treatments have primarily been studied in the setting of severe FGR, antiphospholipid syndrome, and severe placental pathologic condition, such as chronic histiocytic intervillositis.[48–50] There are no data to support their use for stillbirth prevention in an otherwise low-risk population without other clinical indications.

Antenatal Surveillance

Antenatal surveillance, such as nonstress tests (NSTs) and biophysical profiles (BPPs), is used as a clinical measure of fetal well-being. These tests rely on the premise that the fetal heart rate pattern and motor activity are influenced by fetal hypoxemia and acidemia.[51] Accordingly, these tests are best suited to identifying fetuses with an ongoing hypoxic insult owing to placental insufficiency rather than sudden or unexplained cases of fetal death. A reactive fetal heart rate tracing is defined as one having 2 fetal heart rate accelerations (increase by 15 beats per minute for 15 seconds) noted within a 20-minute period. The use of NSTs as a measure of fetal well-being depends on the neurologic development of the fetus, the presence of sleep-wake cycles, maternal medications, and other substances that cross the placenta. The reliability of NSTs improves with advancing gestational age, with nonreactive NSTs in up to 50% of patients tested between 24 and 28 weeks' gestation and 15% between 28 and 32 weeks' gestation. Hence, the criteria for a reactive NST before 32 weeks were adjusted to an acceleration threshold of 10 beats per minute for 10 seconds (rather than 15 beats per minute for 15 seconds), which improves the performance before 32 weeks.[51] The BPP builds on the NST with incorporation of fetal movement, tone, breathing, and amniotic fluid assessment. Each component is scored as 2 points, and a score of 8 or 10 is considered normal and reassuring. A score of 6 is equivocal, and a score ≤4 is abnormal. The stillbirth rate following a normal BPP is 0.8 per 1000. A modified BPP consists of an NST and amniotic fluid index and imparts a 0.8 per 1000 stillbirth risk in the following week.[52–54] The decision to proceed with

Condition	General Timing	Suggested Specific Timing
Placental/Uterine Conditions		
Placenta previa[b]	Late preterm/early term	36 0/7–37 6/7 weeks of gestation
Suspected accreta, increta, or percreta[b]	Late preterm	34 0/7–35 6/7 weeks of gestation
Vasa previa	Late preterm/early term	34 0/7–37 0/7 weeks of gestation
Prior classical cesarean	Late preterm/early term	36 0/7–37 0/7 weeks of gestation
Prior myomectomy requiring cesarean delivery[c]	Early term (individualize)	37 0/7–38 6/7 weeks of gestation
Previous uterine rupture	Late preterm/early term	36 0/7–37 0/7 weeks gestation
Fetal Conditions		
Oligohydramnios (isolated or otherwise uncomplicated [deepest vertical pocket less than 2 cm])	Late preterm/early term	36 0/7–37 6/7 weeks of gestation or at diagnosis if diagnosed later
Polyhydramnios (mild, idiopathic)[b]	Full term	39 0/7–39 6/7 weeks of gestation
Growth restriction (singleton)		
Otherwise uncomplicated, no concurrent findings, EFW between 3rd and 10th percentile	Early term/full term	38 0/7–39 0/7 weeks of gestation
Otherwise uncomplicated, no concurrent findings, EFW <3rd percentile	Early term	37 0/7 weeks of gestation or at diagnosis if diagnosed later
Abnormal umbilical artery dopplers: decreased end diastolic flow without absent end diastolic flow	Early term	37 0/7 weeks of gestation or at diagnosis if diagnosed later
Abnormal umbilical artery dopplers: absent end diastolic flow	Preterm/late preterm	33 0/7–34 0/7 weeks of gestation or at diagnosis if diagnosed later[d]
Abnormal umbilical artery dopplers: reversed end diastolic flow	Preterm	30 0/7–32 0/7 weeks of gestation[d] or at diagnosis if diagnosed later
Concurrent conditions (oligohydramnios, maternal co-morbidity [eg, preeclampsia, chronic hypertension])	Late preterm/early term	34 0/7–37 6/7 weeks of gestation
Multiple gestations—uncomplicated		
Dichorionic-diamniotic twins	Early term	38 0/7–38 6/7 weeks of gestation
Monochorionic-diamniotic twins	Late preterm/early term	34 0/7–37 6/7 weeks of gestation
Monochorionic-monoamniotic twins	Preterm/late preterm	32 0/7–34 weeks of gestation
Triplet and higher order multiples	Preterm/late preterm	Individualized
Alloimmunization		
At-risk pregnancy not requiring intrauterine transfusion	Early term	37 0/7–38 6/7 weeks of gestation
Requiring intrauterine transfusion	Late preterm or early term	Individualized
Maternal Conditions		
Hypertensive disorders of pregnancy		
Chronic hypertension: isolated, uncomplicated, controlled, not requiring medications	Early term/full term	38 0/7–39 6/7 weeks of gestation
Chronic hypertension: isolated, uncomplicated, controlled on medications	Early term/full term	37 0/7–39 6/7 weeks of gestation[e]
Chronic hypertension: difficult to control (requiring frequent medication adjustments)	Late preterm/early term	36 0/7–37 6/7 weeks of gestation
Gestational hypertension, without severe-range blood pressure	Early term	37 0/7 weeks or at diagnosis if diagnosed later
Gestational hypertension with severe-range blood pressures	Late preterm	34 0/7 weeks of gestation or at diagnosis if diagnosed later
Preeclampsia without severe features	Early term	37 0/7 weeks of gestation or at diagnosis if diagnosed later
Preeclampsia with severe features, stable maternal and fetal conditions, after fetal viability (includes superimposed)	Late preterm	34 0/7 weeks of gestation or at diagnosis if diagnosed later
Preeclampsia with severe features, unstable or complicated, after fetal viability (includes superimposed and HELLP)	Soon after maternal stabilization	Soon after maternal stabilization
Preeclampsia with severe features, before viability	Soon after maternal stabilization[f]	Soon after maternal stabilization[f]
Diabetes		
Pregestational diabetes well-controlled[b]	Full term	39 0/7–39 6/7 weeks of gestation
Pregestational diabetes with vascular complications, poor glucose control, or prior stillbirth	Late preterm/early term	36 0/7–38 6/7 weeks of gestation
Gestational: well controlled on diet and exercise	Full term	39 0/7–40 6/7 weeks of gestation
Gestational: well controlled on medications	Full term	39 0/7–39 6/7 weeks of gestation
Gestational: poorly controlled	Late preterm/early term	Individualized
HIV		
Intact membranes and viral load >1,000 copies/mL	Early-term cesarean delivery	38 0/7 weeks of gestation
Viral load ≤1,000 copies/mL with antiretroviral therapy	Full term (early term birth not indicated)	39 0/7 weeks of gestation or later
Intrahepatic cholestasis of pregnancy: total bile acid levels <100 micromol/L	Late preterm/early term	36 0/7–39 0/7 weeks of gestation[g] or at diagnosis if diagnosed later
Intrahepatic cholestasis of pregnancy: total bile acid levels ≥100 micromol/L	Late preterm	36 0/7 weeks of gestation or at[g] diagnosis if diagnosed later
Obstetric Conditions		
Preterm PROM	Late preterm	34 0/7 weeks of gestation or at diagnosis if diagnosed later
PROM (37 0/7 weeks of gestation and beyond)	Generally, at diagnosis	Generally, at diagnosis
Previous stillbirth	Full term (early term birth not routinely recommended)	Individualized[h]

Abbreviations: EFW, estimated fetal weight; HELLP, hemolysis, elevated liver enzymes, and low platelet count; PROM, prelabor rupture of membranes (also referred to as premature rupture of membranes).

[a]In situations in which there is a wide gestational age range for acceptable delivery thresholds, the lower range is not automatically preferable, and medical decision making for the upper or lower part of a range should depend on individual patient factors and risks and benefits.

[b]Uncomplicated, thus no fetal growth restriction, superimposed preeclampsia, or other complication. If these conditions are present, then the complicating conditions take precedence and earlier delivery may be indicated.

[c]Prior myomectomy may require earlier delivery similar to prior classical cesarean (36 0/7-37 0/7 weeks of gestation) in situations with more extensive or complicated myomectomy. Data are conflicting regarding specific timing of delivery. Furthermore, timing of delivery may be influenced by the degree and location of the prior uterine surgery, with the possibility of delivering as late as 38 6/7 weeks of gestation for a patient with a less extensive prior surgery. Timing of delivery should be individualized based on prior surgical details [it available and the clinical situation.

[d]Consultation with maternal-fetal medicine subspecialist is recommended.

[e]Expectant management beyond 39 0/7 weeks of gestation should only be done after careful consideration of the risks and benefits and with appropriate surveillance.

[f]Management individualized to particulars of maternal-fetal condition and gestational age.

[g]Measurement of serum bile acid levels and liver transaminase is recommended in patients with suspected intrahepatic cholestasis of pregnancy. Delivery before 36 weeks of gestation occasionally may be indicated depending on laboratory and clinical circumstances.

[h]Deliveries before 39 weeks of gestation are associated with an increased risk of admission to neonatal special care units for respiratory complications and other neonatal morbidities; however, maternal anxiety with a history of stillbirth should be considered and may warrant an early term delivery (37 0/7 weeks to 38 6/7 weeks) in women who are educated regarding, and accept, the associated neonatal risks.

antenatal surveillance using NSTs depends on clinical circumstance, gestational age, and intended use of clinical interventions such as delivery and cesarean.

Of course, the ultimate stillbirth prevention strategy is delivery. However, the decision to proceed with delivery must take into account the gestational age and the risks to the infant following delivery, particularly if preterm or early term delivery is considered. The point at which the fetal death risk exceeds the predicted infant mortality risk is a reasonable time to consider delivery and has been studied in multiple obstetric contexts.[10,55–57] The Society for Maternal-Fetal Medicine and American College of Obstetricians and Gynecologists have developed a guideline to assist physicians with timing and indications for late preterm and early delivery, and this is shown in **Fig. 1**.[29,58]

EVALUATION OF STILLBIRTHS IN THE SETTING OF FETAL GROWTH RESTRICTION

If a fetal death occurs, the maternal medical history and obstetric history should be carefully assessed to determine potential risk factors for placental insufficiency. The date that the fetus was last documented to have cardiac activity, last time at which fetal movement was known to the mother, and the criteria by which the pregnancy is dated should be obtained. Following this, providers can perform fetal biometry to estimate the fetal weight. Taken together, these data points can help to inform whether FGR is suspected before delivery.

Of utmost importance to the evaluation of fetal death are fetal autopsy and placental histopathology. The fetal autopsy has been shown to assist in identifying a cause of death in an unselected stillbirth population in 42% of cases. However, in cases in which FGR is suspected, this yield increases to 79%[59] This is due to the ability of the fetal autopsy to assist in determining a time interval from death, and thus confirming or ruling out FGR as well as detecting fetal changes secondary to growth restriction, such as evidence of chronic hypoxic stress. Obtaining placental pathology is of paramount importance following a stillbirth in the setting of suspected FGR.

In pregnancies complicated by FGR, placental evaluation by histopathology contributes to the clarification of the cause of death in 89% of cases.[59] There are numerous studies examining pathologic placental lesions in cases of stillbirth and FGR. In general, the mechanism of placental insufficiency and thus fetal death in these cases is thought to be due to impaired placental circulation and gas exchange. This may occur via maternal or fetal vascular changes or through inflammatory changes, which can result in fibrin deposition and infarction.[60] Among the most common lesions are villous infarction, maternal vascular changes, and villous morphologic changes.[61] These findings vary according to gestational age, with more severe findings in early-onset (before 28–32 weeks) FGR as compared with late-onset FGR. In addition, severe placental lesions, such as maternal floor infarction and massive chronic intervillositis, carry a high recurrence risk and thus inform counseling regarding future pregnancies.[62] As with other factors, they should not be relied on in isolation, as they may also occur in uncomplicated pregnancies, and up to 25% of placentas affected by FGR lack histopathologic evidence of placental insufficiency.[61] **Fig. 2** demonstrates severe placental lesions associated with placental insufficiency.

Fig. 1. Recommendations for the timing of delivery when conditions complicate pregnancy. (*Reprinted* with permission from American College of Obstetricians and Gynecologists. Medically indicated late-preterm and early-term deliveries. ACOG Committee Opinion No. 818. American College of Obstetricians and Gynecologists. Obstet Gynecol 2021;137:e29–33.)

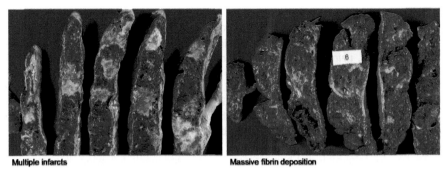

Multiple infarcts   **Massive fibrin deposition**

Fig. 2. Placental lesions associated with placental insufficiency and stillbirth.

Stillbirths in the setting of FGR should also have testing for antiphospholipid syndrome performed. Antiphospholipid antibodies are associated with thromboembolism and obstetric complications, including fetal death and early-onset (before 34 weeks) preeclampsia or placental insufficiency.[63-65] The antibodies most strongly associated with obstetric complications include lupus anticoagulant, anti-β2-glycoprotein-I, and anticardiolipin antibodies.[63,66] Adverse obstetric outcomes are suspected to be due to placental damage through either abnormal development or inflammation and thrombosis.[67] These placental insults increase the risk for FGR with a prevalence of 15% to 30% in most reports.[64,65,68,69] Antiphospholipid antibodies were assessed in a large cohort of stillbirths. There was a 3-fold increase in the chance of stillbirth when women tested positive for anticardiolipin or anti-β2-glycoprotein-I antibodies. Of these cases with positive antiphospholipid antibodies, 37% also were SGA.[70] In cases of FGR from the same cohort, testing for antiphospholipid antibodies helped to identify or refute a cause of death in 32% of cases.[59]

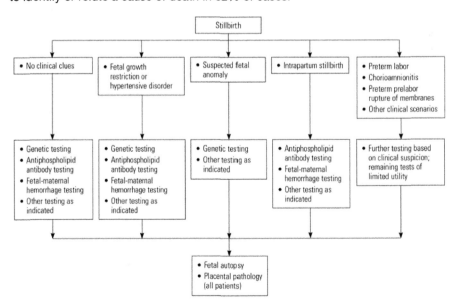

Fig. 3. Evaluation of stillbirth based on test utility in a variety of clinical scenarios. (*From* Management of Stillbirth: Obstetric Care Consensus No, 10. Obstet Gynecol. 2020 Mar;135(3):e110-e132, with permissions.)

Evaluating stillbirth cases affected by FGR for genetic abnormalities is also an important part of the stillbirth work-up. Genetic abnormalities in the placenta can lead to dysfunction resulting in placental insufficiency and FGR. While testing for genetic disorders, using chromosomal microarray is recommended following all stillbirths, as it confers increased diagnostic yield in FGR cases compared with cases without FGR (26% vs 12%, respectively).[40,59,71] In most cases, these abnormalities are coincident in the fetus and placenta but can also affect only the placenta as in confined placental mosaicism (CPM). Although CPM is an uncommon diagnosis in the general obstetric population, it has been identified in up to 15% of placentas from FGR pregnancies.[72]

Testing for fetal-maternal hemorrhage is also reasonable following diagnosis of a stillbirth, as this is a time-sensitive assay, and it is inexpensive.[71] Less common infection-related causes of placental insufficiency and stillbirth, such as cytomegalovirus and syphilis, should be tested for only when clinical evidence for infection is present. Stillbirth owing to these agents is rare, and if they are present with a severity to cause fetal death, there is typically evidence on placental pathology or fetal autopsy.[73] A suggested approach to evaluation of stillbirth in a variety of clinical circumstances, including suspected FGR, is shown in **Fig. 3**.

SUMMARY

FGR is one of the most readily identifiable clinical manifestations of placental insufficiency. Further work is needed to better risk stratify pregnancies at risk for placental insufficiency and thus stillbirth. The association of FGR with stillbirth has been demonstrated in many studies, but concern for an overestimated effect has been raised because of the possibility of a time lag from the time of death to diagnosis. Use of fetal autopsy and careful obstetric history can help to better estimate the gestational age at death and reduce the incorrect assignment of growth restriction. Studies have examined methods by which to account for this time lag, and when this is taken into account, the increased risk for stillbirth persists among FGR fetuses. For those pregnancies with recognized FGR, additional risk stratification by way of serial growth surveillance and umbilical artery Doppler monitoring is prudent. Antenatal testing in the form of NST or BPP and delivery timing should be tailored to the clinical circumstances. There is some benefit to medical treatment with low-dose aspirin in select populations, but other medical therapy for stillbirth prevention should be considered experimental. In stillbirths with FGR, evaluation with fetal autopsy, placental pathology, antiphospholipid antibodies, genetic evaluation, and fetal-maternal hemorrhage is recommended.

CLINICS CARE POINTS

- All pregnancies should undergo screening for fetal growth restriction by fundal height assessment, and when indicated, serial ultrasonographic examination.
- Fetal growth restriction is a major risk factor for stillbirth, and as such, pregnancies complicated by fetal growth restriction should undergo antenatal surveillance with delivery timed according to the clinical circumstance.
- In cases of fetal growth restriction and stillbirth, evaluation by fetal autopsy, placental pathology, antiphospholipid screening, genetic testing, and fetal-maternal hemorrhage testing are important to determining the underlying cause of the fetal death.

DISCLOSURE

The authors have nothing to disclose.

REFERENCES

1. MacDorman MF, Gregory EC. Fetal and perinatal mortality: United States, 2013. Natl Vital Stat Rep 2015;64(8):1–24.
2. Gregory EC, MacDorman MF, Martin JA. Trends in fetal and perinatal mortality in the United States, 2006-2012. NCHS Data Brief 2014;(169):1–8.
3. Lawn JE, Blencowe H, Waiswa P, et al. Stillbirths: rates, risk factors, and acceleration towards 2030. Lancet 2016;387(10018):587–603.
4. Page JM, Thorsten V, Reddy UM, et al. Potentially preventable stillbirth in a diverse U.S. cohort. Obstet Gynecol 2018;131(2):336–43.
5. Hoyert DL GE. Cause-of-death data from the fetal death file, 2015-2017. 2020; No. 4. Located at: National Vital Statistics Reports, Hyattsville, MD.
6. Stillbirth Collaborative Research Network Writing Group. Causes of death among stillbirths. JAMA 2011;306(22):2459–68.
7. Gardosi J, Mul T, Mongelli M, et al. Analysis of birthweight and gestational age in antepartum stillbirths. Br J Obstet Gynaecol 1998;105(5):524–30.
8. Cnattingius S, Haglund B, Kramer MS. Differences in late fetal death rates in association with determinants of small for gestational age fetuses: population based cohort study. BMJ 1998;316(7143):1483–7.
9. Frøen JF, Gardosi JO, Thurmann A, et al. Restricted fetal growth in sudden intrauterine unexplained death. Acta Obstet Gynecol Scand 2004;83(9):801–7.
10. Pilliod RA, Cheng YW, Snowden JM, et al. The risk of intrauterine fetal death in the small-for-gestational-age fetus. Am J Obstet Gynecol 2012;207(4):318.e1-6.
11. Hirst JE, Villar J, Victora CG, et al. The antepartum stillbirth syndrome: risk factors and pregnancy conditions identified from the INTERGROWTH-21(st) Project. BJOG 2018;125(9):1145–53.
12. Mendez-Figueroa H, Truong VT, Pedroza C, et al. Morbidity and mortality in small-for-gestational-age infants: a secondary analysis of nine MFMU network studies. Am J Perinatol 2017;34(4):323–32.
13. Mendez-Figueroa H, Truong VT, Pedroza C, et al. Small-for-gestational-age infants among uncomplicated pregnancies at term: a secondary analysis of 9 maternal-fetal medicine units network studies. Am J Obstet Gynecol 2016; 215(5):628.e1-e7.
14. Flenady V, Koopmans L, Middleton P, et al. Major risk factors for stillbirth in high-income countries: a systematic review and meta-analysis. Lancet 2011; 377(9774):1331–40.
15. Smith GC, Fretts RC. Stillbirth. Lancet 2007;370(9600):1715–25.
16. Conway DL, Hansen NI, Dudley DJ, et al. An algorithm for the estimation of gestational age at the time of fetal death. Paediatric Perinatal Epidemiol 2013;27(2): 145–57.
17. Drey EA, Kang MS, McFarland W, et al. Improving the accuracy of fetal foot length to confirm gestational duration. Obstet Gynecol 2005;105(4):773–8.
18. Man J, Hutchinson JC, Ashworth M, et al. Effects of intrauterine retention and postmortem interval on body weight following intrauterine death: implications for assessment of fetal growth restriction at autopsy. Ultrasound Obstet Gynecol 2016;48(5):574–8.
19. Bukowski R, Hansen NI, Willinger M, et al. Fetal growth and risk of stillbirth: a population-based case-control study. PLoS Med 2014;11(4):e1001633.

20. Practice Bulletin No. 175: Ultrasound in pregnancy. Obstet Gynecol 2016;128(6): e241–56.
21. Bricker L, Medley N, Pratt JJ. Routine ultrasound in late pregnancy (after 24 weeks' gestation). Cochrane Database Syst Rev 2015;(6):CD001451.
22. Henrichs J, Verfaille V, Jellema P, et al. Effectiveness of routine third trimester ultrasonography to reduce adverse perinatal outcomes in low risk pregnancy (the IRIS study): nationwide, pragmatic, multicentre, stepped wedge cluster randomised trial. BMJ 2019;367:l5517.
23. Smith GC. Screening and prevention of stillbirth. Best Pract Res Clin Obstet Gynaecol 2017;38:71–82.
24. Ott WJ. The diagnosis of altered fetal growth. Obstet Gynecol Clin North Am 1988;15(2):237–63.
25. Dudley NJ. A systematic review of the ultrasound estimation of fetal weight. Ultrasound Obstet Gynecol 2005;25(1):80–9.
26. Ott WJ. Diagnosis of intrauterine growth restriction: comparison of ultrasound parameters. Am J Perinatol 2002;19(3):133–7.
27. Unterscheider J, Daly S, Geary MP, et al. Optimizing the definition of intrauterine growth restriction: the multicenter prospective PORTO Study. Am J Obstet Gynecol 2013;208(4):290.e1-6.
28. Spong CY, Mercer BM, D'Alton M, et al. Timing of indicated late-preterm and early-term birth. Obstet Gynecol 2011;118(2 Pt 1):323–33.
29. Martins JG, Biggio JR, Abuhamad A. Society for Maternal-Fetal Medicine (SMFM) consult series #52: diagnosis and management of fetal growth restriction. Am J Obstet Gynecol 2020;223(4):B2–17.
30. Trudinger BJ. Doppler ultrasonography and fetal well-being. In: Albert Reece JCH E, Mahoney MJ, Petrie RH, editors. Medicine of the fetus & mother. Philadelphia (PA): JB Lippincott Co; 1992.
31. Alfirevic Z, Stampalija T, Dowswell T. Fetal and umbilical Doppler ultrasound in high-risk pregnancies. Cochrane Database Syst Rev 2017;6:CD007529.
32. McCowan LM, Harding JE, Roberts AB, et al. A pilot randomized controlled trial of two regimens of fetal surveillance for small-for-gestational-age fetuses with normal results of umbilical artery doppler velocimetry. Am J Obstet Gynecol 2000;182(1 Pt 1):81–6.
33. Caradeux J, Martinez-Portilla RJ, Basuki TR, et al. Risk of fetal death in growth-restricted fetuses with umbilical and/or ductus venosus absent or reversed end-diastolic velocities before 34 weeks of gestation: a systematic review and meta-analysis. Am J Obstet Gynecol 2018;218(2s):774–82.e1.
34. Lees C, Marlow N, Arabin B, et al. Perinatal morbidity and mortality in early-onset fetal growth restriction: cohort outcomes of the trial of randomized umbilical and fetal flow in Europe (TRUFFLE). Ultrasound Obstet Gynecol 2013;42(4):400–8.
35. Oros D, Figueras F, Cruz-Martinez R, et al. Longitudinal changes in uterine, umbilical and fetal cerebral Doppler indices in late-onset small-for-gestational age fetuses. Ultrasound Obstet Gynecol 2011;37(2):191–5.
36. Conde-Agudelo A, Bird S, Kennedy SH, et al. First- and second-trimester tests to predict stillbirth in unselected pregnant women: a systematic review and meta-analysis. BJOG 2015;122(1):41–55.
37. Lamont K, Scott NW, Jones GT, et al. Risk of recurrent stillbirth: systematic review and meta-analysis. BMJ 2015;350:h3080.
38. Dugoff L, Hobbins JC, Malone FD, et al. First-trimester maternal serum PAPP-A and free-beta subunit human chorionic gonadotropin concentrations and nuchal

translucency are associated with obstetric complications: a population-based screening study (the FASTER Trial). Am J Obstet Gynecol 2004;191(4):1446–51.

39. Heazell AE, Whitworth M, Duley L, et al. Use of biochemical tests of placental function for improving pregnancy outcome. Cochrane Database Syst Rev 2015;(11):Cd011202.

40. Reddy UM. Prediction and prevention of recurrent stillbirth. Obstet Gynecol 2007; 110(5):1151–64.

41. Cleaton MA, Dent CL, Howard M, et al. Fetus-derived DLK1 is required for maternal metabolic adaptations to pregnancy and is associated with fetal growth restriction. Nat Genet 2016;48(12):1473–80.

42. Duley L, Meher S, Hunter KE, et al. Antiplatelet agents for preventing pre-eclampsia and its complications. Cochrane Database Syst Rev 2019;2019(10).

43. ACOG Committee Opinion No. 743: low-dose aspirin use during pregnancy. Obstet Gynecol 2018;132(1):e44–52.

44. Jillian T, Henderson P, Vesco KK, et al. Draft of aspirin use to prevent preeclampsia and related morbidity and mortality: an evidence update for the U.S. Preventive Services Task Force. U.S. Preventive Services Task Force. 2021. Available at: file:///C:/Users/u6019768/Downloads/aspirin-preeclampsia-prevention-draft-evidence-review.pdf. Accessed February 25, 2021.

45. LeFevre ML, U.S. Preventive Services Task Force. Low-dose aspirin use for the prevention of morbidity and mortality from preeclampsia: U.S. Preventive Services Task Force recommendation statement. Ann Intern Med 2014;161(11): 819–26.

46. Rey E, Garneau P, David M, et al. Dalteparin for the prevention of recurrence of placental-mediated complications of pregnancy in women without thrombophilia: a pilot randomized controlled trial. J Thromb Haemost 2009;7(1):58–64.

47. Rodger MA, Gris J-C, De Vries JIP, et al. Low-molecular-weight heparin and recurrent placenta-mediated pregnancy complications: a meta-analysis of individual patient data from randomised controlled trials. Lancet 2016;388(10060): 2629–41.

48. Groom K, McCowan L, Mackay L, et al. STRIDER NZAus: a multicentre randomised controlled trial of sildenafil therapy in early-onset fetal growth restriction. BJOG 2019;126(8):997–1006.

49. Mekinian A, Costedoat-Chalumeau N, Masseau A, et al. Chronic histiocytic intervillositis: outcome, associated diseases and treatment in a multicenter prospective study. Autoimmunity 2015;48(1):40–5.

50. Pels A, Derks J, Elvan-Taspinar A, et al. Maternal sildenafil vs placebo in pregnant women with severe early-onset fetal growth restriction. JAMA Netw Open 2020;3(6):e205323.

51. Practice bulletin no. 145: antepartum fetal surveillance. Obstet Gynecol 2014; 124(1):182–92.

52. Freeman RK, Anderson G, Dorchester W. A prospective multi-institutional study of antepartum fetal heart rate monitoring. I. Risk of perinatal mortality and morbidity according to antepartum fetal heart rate test results. Am J Obstet Gynecol 1982; 143(7):771–7.

53. Manning FA, Morrison I, Harman CR, et al. Fetal assessment based on fetal biophysical profile scoring: experience in 19,221 referred high-risk pregnancies. II. An analysis of false-negative fetal deaths. Am J Obstet Gynecol 1987;157(4 Pt 1): 880–4.

54. Miller DA, Rabello YA, Paul RH. The modified biophysical profile: antepartum testing in the 1990s. Am J Obstet Gynecol 1996;174(3):812–7.

55. Page JM, Pilliod RA, Snowden JM, et al. The risk of stillbirth and infant death by each additional week of expectant management in twin pregnancies. Am J Obstet Gynecol 2015;212(5):630.e1-7.

56. Puljic A, Kim E, Page J, et al. The risk of infant and fetal death by each additional week of expectant management in intrahepatic cholestasis of pregnancy by gestational age. Am J Obstet Gynecol 2015;212(5):667.e1-5.

57. Rosenstein MG, Cheng YW, Snowden JM, et al. Risk of stillbirth and infant death stratified by gestational age. Obstet Gynecol 2012;120(1):76–82.

58. Medically indicated late-preterm and early-term deliveries: ACOG Committee Opinion, Number 818. Obstet Gynecol 2021;137(2):e29–33.

59. Page JM, Christiansen-Lindquist L, Thorsten V, et al. Diagnostic tests for evaluation of stillbirth: results from the stillbirth collaborative research network. Obstet Gynecol 2017;129(4):699–706.

60. Roberts JM. Pathophysiology of ischemic placental disease. Semin Perinatol 2014;38(3):139–45.

61. Mifsud W, Sebire NJ. Placental pathology in early-onset and late-onset fetal growth restriction. Fetal Diagn Ther 2014;36(2):117–28.

62. Roberts DJ. Placental pathology, a survival guide. Arch Pathol Lab Med 2008;132(4):641–51.

63. Practice Bulletin No. 132: antiphospholipid syndrome. Obstet Gynecol 2012;120(6):1514–21.

64. Branch DW, Silver RM, Blackwell JL, et al. Outcome of treated pregnancies in women with antiphospholipid syndrome: an update of the Utah experience. Obstet Gynecol 1992;80(4):614–20.

65. Lima F, Khamashta MA, Buchanan NM, et al. A study of sixty pregnancies in patients with the antiphospholipid syndrome. Clin Exp Rheumatol 1996;14(2):131–6.

66. Miyakis S, Lockshin MD, Atsumi T, et al. International consensus statement on an update of the classification criteria for definite antiphospholipid syndrome (APS). J Thromb Haemost 2006;4(2):295–306.

67. Meroni PL, Tedesco F, Locati M, et al. Anti-phospholipid antibody mediated fetal loss: still an open question from a pathogenic point of view. Lupus 2010;19(4):453–6.

68. Caruso A, De Carolis S, Ferrazzani S, et al. Pregnancy outcome in relation to uterine artery flow velocity waveforms and clinical characteristics in women with antiphospholipid syndrome. Obstet Gynecol 1993;82(6):970–7.

69. Kutteh WH. Antiphospholipid antibody-associated recurrent pregnancy loss: treatment with heparin and low-dose aspirin is superior to low-dose aspirin alone. Am J Obstet Gynecol 1996;174(5):1584–9.

70. Silver RM, Parker CB, Reddy UM, et al. Antiphospholipid antibodies in stillbirth. Obstet Gynecol 2013;122(3):641–57.

71. Metz TD, Berry RS, Fretts RC, et al. Obstetric care consensus #10: management of stillbirth: (replaces practice bulletin number 102, March 2009). Am J Obstet Gynecol 2020;222(3):B2–20.

72. Rajcan-Separovic E, Diego-Alvarez D, Robinson WP, et al. Identification of copy number variants in miscarriages from couples with idiopathic recurrent pregnancy loss. Hum Reprod 2010;25(11):2913–22.

73. Page JM, Bardsley T, Thorsten V, et al. Stillbirth associated with infection in a diverse U.S. cohort. Obstet Gynecol 2019;134(6):1187–96.

Short- and Long-Term Implications of Small for Gestational Age

Camille Fung, MD*, Erin Zinkhan, MD

KEYWORDS

- Fetal growth restriction • Intrauterine growth restriction • Small for gestational age
- Neurologic complications • Cardiometabolic complications • Epigenetics

KEY POINTS

- The short-term complications of fetal growth restriction are usually secondary to structural or biochemical changes.
- The long-term complications of fetal growth restriction are usually secondary to gene expression changes as a result of epigenetic changes.
- Neurologic and cardiometabolic consequences are the best described, but virtually every organ system is susceptible to fetal growth restriction–induced changes.

INTRODUCTION

Fetal growth restriction (FGR) describes a condition of failed fetal weight gain based on genetic potential and gestational age. FGR is often misquoted as being equivalent to small for gestational age (SGA), but distinctive conceptual differences exist. Although recent updated guidelines define FGR simply as an estimated fetal weight of less than the 10th percentile,[1] here we refer to the conceptual definition of FGR, which entails an inability to achieve one's growth potential and so can be present even when the fetal weight estimate is greater than the 10th percentile. This definition is in contrast with an SGA neonate, which is determined by a single weight measurement at birth as defined as less than the 10th percentile for weight, gestational age, and sex. An SGA fetus is additionally defined as less than the 10th percentile estimated fetal weight on ultrasound examination, adding another layer of uncertainty given imprecision in antenatal sonogram. Notably, the genetic contribution plays a significant role in determining SGA status. For example, if a fetus' genetic potential was destined to be at the 50th percentile but suffered FGR, she or he may be born SGA with a birth weight at less than the 10th percentile. In contrast, if a fetus' genetic potential was to be less than the 10th percentile and remained so throughout gestation,

Division of Neonatology, Department of Pediatrics, University of Utah, 295 Chipeta Way, Salt Lake City, UT 84108, USA
* Corresponding author.
E-mail address: camille.fung@hsc.utah.edu

Obstet Gynecol Clin N Am 48 (2021) 311–323
https://doi.org/10.1016/j.ogc.2021.02.004
0889-8545/21/© 2021 Elsevier Inc. All rights reserved.

that fetus would not be considered to have FGR, but would still be classified as SGA after delivery. This distinction is important in understanding risks for short- and/or long-term complications as described in this article.

COMPLICATIONS OF FETAL GROWTH RESTRICTION

Barker's hypothesis of the fetal origins of health and disease describes a mechanism through which a fetus adapts to an adverse prenatal environment, such as FGR. This adaptation is crucial for short-term survival, but results in specific fetal gene expression changes that persist after birth when the fetus is no longer in a hostile environment. In other words, these genes and their corresponding proteins have an altered expression that results in abnormal function in postnatal life. Persistently altered gene expression becomes the basis for FGR-induced childhood and adulthood diseases.

Before we delve further into these childhood and adulthood diseases, many of the immediate postnatal complications of FGR are secondary to structural or biochemical changes rather than gene expression changes (**Fig. 1**). For example, FGR infants are more prone to heat loss because of decreased subcutaneous adipose stores and increased body surface area and to hypoglycemia because of decreased glycogen stores in the liver and poor oral feeding. However, with support, many of these immediate complications of FGR resolve with minimal long-term health impact.[2]

Unfortunately, many of the adult diseases and medical problems associated with FGR begin in childhood and persist into adulthood. These include an impaired immune system owing to decreased neutrophils and response to infectious stimuli; renal

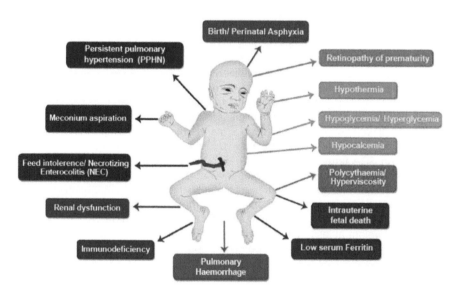

Fig. 1. Immediate postnatal complications of FGR. A baby born at preterm or term gestation with FGR is at greater risks for birth/perinatal asphyxia, retinopathy of prematurity, hypothermia, hypoglycemia or hyperglycemia, hypocalcemia, polycythemia/hyperviscosity, intrauterine death, low serum ferritin, pulmonary hemorrhage, immunodeficiency, renal dysfunction, feeding intolerance, necrotizing enterocolitis (NEC), meconium aspiration, and pulmonary hypertension. (*From* Sharma D, Shastri S, Sharma P. Intrauterine growth restriction: Antenatal and postnatal aspects. *Clin Med Insights Pediatr.* 2016;10:67-83.)

dysfunction owing to decreased nephrogenesis; pancreatic dysfunction and decreased insulin secretion; endocrine dysfunction; cardiometabolic disorders including diabetes, obesity, hyperlipidemia, hypertension, myocardial infarction, and stroke; and neurologic disorders including developmental delays and psychiatric and behavioral disorders (**Fig. 2**). The neurologic and cardiometabolic sequelae are the most well described in the literature and therefore are the focus of the rest of this article.

Neurologic Sequelae of Fetal Growth Restriction

Epidemiologic studies have increasingly documented the association between an adverse in utero environment and an offspring's poor neurologic outcome. In fact, suboptimal fetal growth in the form of FGR resulting in SGA is now a well-recognized risk factor for motor and sensory neurodevelopmental deficits, cognitive and learning impairments, and cerebral palsy.[3–8] Before we discuss the human and animal data behind FGR-induced altered brain structure and function, we must be aware that the inconsistent clinical definition of FGR likely contributes to an underestimation of the true prevalence of these neurologic sequelae. This inconsistency arose because of an inaccurate distinction between poor fetal weight gain owing to a pathologic compromise, that is, true FGR, and a constitutionally SGA infant who is healthy. Traditionally, the diagnosis of FGR referred to an infant with a birth weight of less than the 10th percentile for gestational age and sex.[9] More recently, incorporating measures of placental insufficiency such as with abnormal umbilical artery Doppler flow velocimetry during pregnancy have attempted to distinguish offspring with true FGR

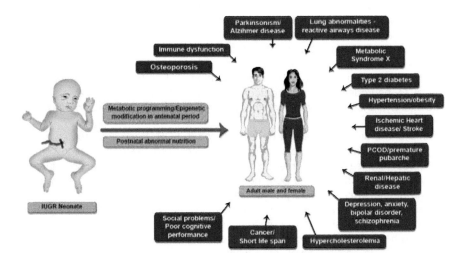

Fig. 2. Short- and long-term postnatal complications of FGR. A neonate who has suffered FGR experiences metabolic programming/epigenetic modification in the antenatal period coupled with postnatal abnormal nutrition is at greater risks for osteoporosis, immune dysfunction, Parkinsonism, Alzheimer disease, lung abnormalities including bronchopulmonary dysplasia and reactive airway disease, metabolic syndrome, type 2 diabetes, hypertension, obesity, ischemic heart disease, stroke, polycystic ovary disease (PCOD), premature pubarche, renal disease, hepatic disease, psychiatric derangements, hypercholesterolemia, cancer, shortened life span, social problems, and poor cognitive performance. Both males and females are susceptible, but sexual dimorphism exists in the presentation of these diseases. (*From* Sharma D, Shastri S, Sharma P. Intrauterine growth restriction: Antenatal and postnatal aspects. *Clin Med Insights Pediatr.* 2016;10:67-83.)

from those who are constitutionally small.[1] It is our opinion that, to counsel families about their offspring's future neurologic outcome risk, epidemiologic studies must continue to make this important distinction.

Altered brain blood flow after fetal growth restriction

As mentioned elsewhere in this article, placental insufficiency is the greatest contributor to FGR in high-income countries.[10] The etiologies of placental insufficiency are many, but include hypertensive disease of pregnancy, tobacco smoking, and diabetes mellitus. Placental insufficiency results in chronic fetal hypoxemia, decreased fetal nutrient availability, and decreased fetal nutrient use, culminating in fetal growth deceleration. The growth-restricted fetus responds by redistributing blood flow to favor essential organs such as the brain, heart, and adrenal glands.[11] However, this redistribution of cardiac output to protect brain growth ("brain sparing"), previously termed asymmetric growth restriction, does not ensure normal brain development.[11,12] Recent studies in FGR fetuses suggest that a decreased middle cerebral artery (MCA) Doppler pulsatility index, which is commonly used to assess the severity of placental insufficiency, may only detect an advanced stage of blood flow redistribution because vasodilatation in the anterior cerebral artery comes before vasodilation in the MCA.[13,14] This preferential perfusion to the frontal region is the earliest adaptive response to chronic hypoxemia. As the chronicity of hypoxemia intensifies, perfusion to the MCA changes to favor the basal ganglia at the expense of the frontal lobe, and the decreased MCA pulsatility index becomes apparent.[15]

Altered brain structure after fetal growth restriction

Regardless of the status of blood flow redistribution, the neuropathologic consequences of FGR on the developing brain are heterogeneous and often unpredictable. They depend on the timing and severity of the in utero compromise, on whether the infant is born at a preterm or term gestation, and on whether other coexisting complications affect the trajectory of brain development.[16] Two broad factors seem to be critical to neurodevelopmental outcome in general, namely, the severity of the placental dysfunction together with the gestational age at onset, plus the gestational age at delivery.[17]

Deficits in brain structure can be widespread in FGR. Decreased total white and gray matter volume in multiple brain regions including the cortex, hippocampus, and cerebellum lead to a decreased head circumference. Small head size during infancy is a strong predictor for poor neurodevelopmental outcome.[18,19] White matter volume decrease is secondary to decreased myelin content, delayed myelination, and/or decreased connectivity. One useful imaging advancement in neonatal medicine has been diffusion tensor imaging assessment of fractional anisotropy via MRI, which provides details on microstructural organization and integrity of the white matter tracts. In healthy, myelinated white matter, fractional anisotropy values are high and radial diffusivity is low, showing that water molecules preferentially diffuse in the direction of fiber tracts. Diffusion tensor imaging of the white matter in 12-month-old infants with FGR has shown altered fractional anisotropy in various large white matter tracts of the corpus callosum and internal capsule.[20] Additionally, whole brain connectome analysis has shown decreased global and local network efficiency using graph model measures, as well as decreased connectivity in long-range corticobasal ganglia connections in the prefrontal and limbic networks in preterm infants born with FGR.[21,22]

Gray matter volume pathology is due to a total decreased in the number of neural cells, cell migration defects resulting in simplified gyrification, and/or altered synaptic formation.[16] Experimental models of FGR in rodents, guinea pigs, rabbits, and sheep have shed significant insight into the brain's developmental adaptations that contribute to brain injury particularly in the gray matter. Similar to human FGR brain imaging, morphologic alterations in FGR animals have included a decreased volume of the motor and visual cortices, hippocampus, basal ganglia, and cerebellum.[23–25] Volume loss is explained by neuronal loss across a number of brain regions, including the hippocampus[26,27] and surviving neurons show selective changes in the morphology of the hippocampal neuronal dendrites.[28] In addition, developmental maturation of oligodendrocytes and myelination of axons are altered causing axonal injury and nerve conduction defects.[29,30] Overall, there seems to be an imbalance in the regulation of cellular proliferation, differentiation, and apoptosis within the developing brain of fetuses with growth restriction.

Altered brain function after fetal growth restriction

It follows that FGR significantly affects brain function given the aforementioned changes in neural cells and cell morphologies. Reiterating an important concept, the neurodevelopmental consequences of FGR are dictated by the severity, timing (early vs late onset), and the gestational age at delivery. Depending on the brain regions involved, these sequelae can also have varied and wide manifestations. One study cites that infants with FGR are 4 to 6 times more likely to develop cerebral palsy than infants without FGR.[31] A recent systematic review of early childhood neurodevelopmental outcomes after FGR reviewed 731 studies, of which 16 were included.[32] Eleven studies found poorer neurodevelopmental outcomes after FGR. Ten studies found motor, 8 studies found cognitive, and 7 studies found language delays. Other delays included social development, attention, and adaptive behavior. Of note, only 8 studies included abnormal Doppler parameters in their FGR definition.

The highest risk for neurologic deficits is conferred by FGR with absent or reversed end diastolic velocity in the umbilical artery. Indeed, at school age, these children perform worse on assessment tasks for cognition, motor function, behavior, and educational achievements than children who had mild to moderate FGR.[33] Preterm birth is also likely to be an exacerbating factor when combined with FGR. Some investigators would argue that preterm birth overrides the neurologic impact of FGR.[4] A large, prospective French study examined the neurologic outcomes in school-age children who were born with an appropriate weight versus SGA at 24 to 28 weeks or 29 to 32 weeks. They showed that cognitive deficits, inattention, hyperactivity, and school difficulties were similar in the 24 to 28 weeks cohort regardless of birth weight and to those infants who were SGA at 29 to 32 weeks. The appropriately grown 29 to 32 weeks fared better, but still had mild cognitive and behavioral issues.[5] The child's sex also seems to play a role in outcomes. Preterm male infants born at 24 to 29 weeks with early onset FGR had poorer school achievement and more behavioral problems compared with preterm female or appropriately grown male infants.[34,35] In female infants, more severe growth restriction is a strong predictor for impaired cognition, whereas less severe FGR is not.[36] Depression, schizophrenia, and mood disorders are other adverse outcomes associated with FGR. As children grow into early adulthood, a study that followed FGR term infants through 16 to 26 years of age in England showed that they had relatively lower academic achievement test scores, lower teacher rating of school success, and were less likely to have professional employment.[37] Therefore, it seems that brain changes in fetal life significantly affect neurologic function for the life of the individual born with FGR.

It is worth mentioning 2 large prospective studies published this year in Norway and Finland that examined the associations of maternal hypertensive disease of pregnancy with offspring neurologic outcomes.[38,39] Lahti-Pulkkinen and associates[39] found that maternal gestational hypertension, chronic hypertension, and preeclampsia and its severity increased the offspring hazard of any childhood mental disorders at ages 6.4 to 10.8 years. Maternal hypertensive disorders, diabetes mellitus, and overweight/obesity additively increased offspring hazard of mental disorders. Interestingly in this study, preterm births only partially mediated the effects of any mental disorder. The second study by Sun and colleagues[38] examined the associations between preeclampsia in term pregnancies and neurologic outcomes at a mean follow-up of 14 years. Children exposed to preeclampsia were at increased risks for attention deficit hyperactivity disorder (adjusted odds ratio [AOR], 1.18; 95% confidence interval [CI], 1.05–1.33), autism spectrum disorder (AOR, 1.29; 95% CI, 1.08–1.54), epilepsy (AOR, 1.50; 95% CI, 1.16–1.93), intellectual disability (AOR, 1.50; 95% CI, 1.13–1.97), and cerebral palsy (AOR, 1.30; 95% CI, 0.94–1.80). These 2 studies are important to consider because they provide evidence that childhood neurologic outcomes are associated with pregnancy complications, independent of gestational age at birth.

Having reviewed the neurologic sequelae of FGR, the section on the Cardiometabolic Sequelae of Fetal Growth Restriction discusses the cardiometabolic consequences of FGR. It is worth mentioning that the attainment of good neurologic outcome often means good catch up growth in postnatal life, particularly good brain growth. However, because the FGR offspring's gene expression profile has adapted to a "starved" environment in utero, the provision of normal nutrition based on current nutritional guidelines may be excessive for their maladapted metabolic system, placing these infants at increased risk for overfeeding and promoting an earlier onset of cardiometabolic diseases. Unfortunately, we lack evidence to know how optimal nutrition and catch up growth are defined for FGR infants. Rapid crossover of percentiles in all growth parameters is likely not beneficial to the cardiovascular health in the long term.[40]

Cardiometabolic Sequelae of Fetal Growth Restriction

Cardiovascular disease remains the leading cause of mortality in the United States despite the widespread use of medications to control modifiable cardiovascular risk factors.[41] The financial cost of cardiovascular disease is in excess of $200 billion each year.[42] The chance of developing cardiovascular disease increases with increasing numbers of cardiovascular risk factors, including hypertension, hyperlipidemia, insulin resistance, obesity, genetic factors, and lifestyle factors such as smoking.

Stroke and ischemic heart disease

In the past 30 to 40 years, the impact of birth weight on cardiometabolic disease development has become well-recognized. Dr David Barker and coworkers[43] first showed an inverse relationship between birth weight with ischemic heart disease and stroke in 1989. Mortality from ischemic heart disease and stroke nearly doubled between infants born at the lowest and the highest percentiles. Multiple studies have since corroborated Dr Barker's findings with either an inverse relationship or a U-shaped relationship between birth weight and cardiovascular disease.[44–47] The increased risk in cardiovascular disease associated with low birth weight was due to failure to achieve growth potential and not due to low birth weight from prematurity.[48,49] Importantly the impact of birth weight on cardiovascular complications was independent of socioeconomic status, confirming intrauterine growth as a marker of life-long cardiovascular health.[46]

Suboptimal intrauterine growth not only increases cardiovascular disease incidence, but also increases risk factors for cardiovascular disease including hypertension, hyperlipidemia, diabetes, and obesity.[50–57] The cardiometabolic risk from growth restriction is amplified if an individual with FGR subsequently develops diabetes, obesity, or other cardiovascular risk factors.[58]

Hypertension

Hypertension is defined as either elevated systolic or diastolic blood pressure. An inverse relationship exists between birth weight and both systolic and diastolic blood pressures. The association between birth weight and hypertension remains true for multiple populations in both developed and developing countries.[53,55] This effect is estimated to be between 0.6 and 9.1 mm Hg for systolic blood pressure in adulthood. Individuals with FGR also have an increase in diastolic blood pressure of approximately 4 mm Hg.[51,56] Although the impact of birth weight on blood pressure seems modest, its effect on increasing blood pressure begins in childhood.[52]

Further compounding the impact of FGR on blood pressure and cardiovascular disease, cardiac dysfunction also increases in an inverse relationship to birth weight.[50,54] Even in utero, vascular and cardiac adaptation to an adverse intrauterine environment occurs with diminished cardiac output and compliance and an increased intraventricular pressure.[57] The impact of birth weight on blood pressure and cardiac function starting in childhood and lasting through adult life highlights the life-long impact of intrauterine growth on childhood and adult blood pressure and cardiovascular health.

Animal studies demonstrate FGR-induced altered extracellular matrix deposition and vascular function throughout life in multiple animal models.[59–61] These findings suggest that the development of the heart and vasculature is set on an altered and at least partially irreversible trajectory in utero that predisposes to hypertension and cardiovascular disease throughout life.

Metabolic syndrome

The metabolic syndrome is defined most commonly as the combination of hyperlipidemia, insulin resistance, and obesity.[62] Hypertension is sometimes included in the diagnoses of the metabolic syndrome.[62] The metabolic syndrome increases the risk of cardiovascular disease, myocardial infarction, stroke, and mortality.[62] The impact of the intrauterine environment on the development of the metabolic syndrome cannot be overstated. Up to one-half of metabolic syndrome cases can be attributed to an adverse intrauterine environment.[58] For example, 1 study noted the risk of developing metabolic syndrome in adulthood was 10-fold greater for infants whose birthweight was in the lowest percentiles compared with the highest.[44]

Hyperlipidemia

High serum cholesterol and triglyceride levels are independent clinical risk factors for atherosclerosis, cardiovascular disease, myocardial infarction, and stroke.[63,64] Adults who were born with the smallest abdominal girths, an indicator of poor fetal growth, had increased total cholesterol by an average of 23 mg/dL and low-density lipoprotein cholesterol by an average of 19 mg/dL.[65] Growth restriction also increases apolipoprotein B by 1.5-fold when measured by cordocentesis.[66] Elevated apolipoprotein B is associated with the development of atherosclerosis in adulthood. Low-density lipoproteins were 1.9-fold more susceptible to oxidation in SGA newborns, another finding that predisposes to atherosclerosis.[67]

At birth, infants with growth restriction had an average of a 9 mg/dL increase in serum triglyceride levels.[68] Another study showed a 2-fold increase in plasma triglyceride levels at birth in SGA infants.[67] Further, infants born at the lowest percentiles of birth weight had an increase in serum triglyceride levels by approximately 27 mmol/dL.[69] The impact of growth restriction on hypertriglyceridemia is theorized to originate from altered hepatic lipid metabolism and decreased triglyceride use in peripheral tissues.

Insulin resistance

Insulin resistance is a condition of insufficient response of peripheral tissues to circulating insulin levels, often resulting in increased serum glucose concentrations and an eventual diagnosis of type 2 diabetes mellitus. Low birth weight increases the risk of insulin resistance.[70] A more than 2-fold increase in insulin resistance was seen in adults who were born in the lowest birthweight percentiles.[71] The risk of insulin resistance in adulthood decreases by an odds of 0.75 for each kilogram increase in birth weight.[72] Adults who were in the lowest percentiles for birth weight had a 5% increase in fasting glucose and 6% increase in fasting insulin levels.[73] A diagnosis of insulin resistance was 3 times more likely in adults born at the lowest birth weight percentiles.[74] The increased risk of insulin resistance is thought to be due to the impact of growth restriction on pancreatic function; abnormal accumulation of lipids in nonphysiologic storage depots such as the muscle, liver, and visceral adipose tissue; and on peripheral tissue insulin resistance.

Obesity

Growth restriction is often associated with obesity, particularly central or visceral obesity, and decreased lean muscle mass.[75] Lean muscle mass in adulthood is positively correlated with birth weight, and an increased waist:hip ratio, an indicator of increased visceral adiposity, is negatively correlated with birth weight.[76] Although obesity is an important component of developing insulin resistance, obesity often only leads to disease in predisposed people, such as those with growth restriction.[74] Another important distinction is that although a growth-restricted individual is predisposed to obesity, she or he may not necessarily have increased body weight owing to decreased lean muscle mass. Therefore, other measures such as waist:hip ratios may be more indicative of abnormal adipose deposition than weight or body mass index alone.

Epigenetics

We began this article by mentioning gene expression changes that occur during FGR as an adaptation to the adverse in utero environment. These gene expression changes occur not because of a change in the genetic code, such as with a gene mutation, but rather a result of gene transcription success to produce more or less messenger RNA (mRNA) for protein production. This gene transcription success is due to epigenetics, which relies on accessibility of the transcriptional machinery to the DNA sequence. Modifications such as methylation to the DNA sequence itself or acetylation to the histone proteins that the DNA sequence wraps around will result in a more closed or open chromatin respectively for transcriptional access. The post-transcriptional modification of mRNA levels also can occur by binding of inhibitory microRNA to a specific mRNA sequence, resulting in degradation of that mRNA molecule. A detailed description of epigenetics is beyond the scope of this article, but this process is what drives fetal gene expression changes for in utero adaptation. We refer readers to several of these references for more detailed explanation.[77–79]

SUMMARY

FGR clearly poses significant neurologic and cardiometabolic risks to the offspring. Many questions remain, however, both on the clinical and basic science fronts. There is a need to determine the timing of delivery when placental insufficiency and fetal growth deceleration are observed, develop noninvasive tools to accurately monitor fetal brain growth in face of FGR, and clarify the prenatal epigenetic mechanisms responsible for adaptation and their postnatal manifestations. We must continue to challenge ourselves with these questions if we are to provide protective strategies to maximize our children's future neurodevelopmental and cardiometabolic health.

CLINICS CARE POINTS

- There is a need for improved clarity and consistency in the terminology of fetal and neonatal growth status.
- Poor fetal growth is associated with adverse effects on neurologic structure, function, and development into adulthood. This is independent of gestational age at delivery.
- Poor fetal growth is associated with childhood cardiometabolic deviations as well as mortality from cardiovascular disease in adulthood.
- Effective strategies for the prevention of FGR's many sequelae are urgently needed.

DISCLOSURE

The authors have nothing to disclose. Dr Zinkhan has left the University of Utah since the initial invitation and her current employer is Mednax Company. She maintains an adjunct position at the University of Utah, however.

REFERENCES

1. Society for Maternal-Fetal Medicine. Electronic address pso, Martins JG, Biggio JR, Abuhamad A. Society for Maternal-Fetal Medicine Consult Series #52: diagnosis and management of fetal growth restriction: (Replaces Clinical Guideline Number 3, April 2012). Am J Obstet Gynecol 2020;223(4):B2–17.
2. Sharma D, Shastri S, Sharma P. Intrauterine growth restriction: antenatal and postnatal aspects. Clin Med Insights Pediatr 2016;10:67–83.
3. Gagnon R. Placental insufficiency and its consequences. Eur J Obstet Gynecol Reprod Biol 2003;110(Suppl 1):S99–107.
4. Yanney M, Marlow N. Paediatric consequences of fetal growth restriction. Semin Fetal Neonatal Med 2004;9(5):411–8.
5. Guellec I, Lapillonne A, Renolleau S, et al. Neurologic outcomes at school age in very preterm infants born with severe or mild growth restriction. Pediatrics 2011; 127(4):e883–91.
6. von Beckerath AK, Kollmann M, Rotky-Fast C, et al. Perinatal complications and long-term neurodevelopmental outcome of infants with intrauterine growth restriction. Am J Obstet Gynecol 2013;208(2):130.e1–6.
7. Blair EM, Nelson KB. Fetal growth restriction and risk of cerebral palsy in singletons born after at least 35 weeks' gestation. Am J Obstet Gynecol 2015;212(4): 520.e1–7.
8. Gilchrist C, Cumberland A, Walker D, et al. Intrauterine growth restriction and development of the hippocampus: implications for learning and memory in children and adolescents. Lancet Child Adolesc Health 2018;2(10):755–64.
9. Kingdom J, Smith G. Diagnosis and management of IUGR. In: Kingdom P, editor. In: intrauterine growth restriction aetiology and management. London: Springer; 2000. p. 257–73.

10. Figueras F, Gratacos E. Update on the diagnosis and classification of fetal growth restriction and proposal of a stage-based management protocol. Fetal Diagn Ther 2014;36(2):86–98.

11. Poudel R, McMillen IC, Dunn SL, et al. Impact of chronic hypoxemia on blood flow to the brain, heart, and adrenal gland in the late-gestation IUGR sheep fetus. Am J Physiol Regul Integr Comp Physiol 2015;308(3):R151–62.

12. McMillen IC, Adams MB, Ross JT, et al. Fetal growth restriction: adaptations and consequences. Reproduction 2001;122(2):195–204.

13. Figueroa-Diesel H, Hernandez-Andrade E, Acosta-Rojas R, et al. Doppler changes in the main fetal brain arteries at different stages of hemodynamic adaptation in severe intrauterine growth restriction. Ultrasound Obstet Gynecol 2007; 30(3):297–302.

14. Rossi A, Romanello I, Forzano L, et al. Evaluation of fetal cerebral blood flow perfusion using power Doppler ultrasound angiography (3D-PDA) in growth-restricted fetuses. Facts Views Vis Obgyn 2011;3(3):175–80.

15. Hernandez-Andrade E, Serralde JA, Cruz-Martinez R. Can anomalies of fetal brain circulation be useful in the management of growth restricted fetuses? Prenat Diagn 2012;32(2):103–12.

16. Miller SL, Huppi PS, Mallard C. The consequences of fetal growth restriction on brain structure and neurodevelopmental outcome. J Physiol 2016;594(4):807–23.

17. Baschat AA. Neurodevelopment following fetal growth restriction and its relationship with antepartum parameters of placental dysfunction. Ultrasound Obstet Gynecol 2011;37(5):501–14.

18. Gale CR, O'Callaghan FJ, Bredow M, et al, Avon longitudinal Study of P, Children Study T. The influence of head growth in fetal life, infancy, and childhood on intelligence at the ages of 4 and 8 years. Pediatrics 2006;118(4):1486–92.

19. Ochiai M, Nakayama H, Sato K, et al. Head circumference and long-term outcome in small-for-gestational age infants. J Perinat Med 2008;36(4):341–7.

20. Padilla N, Junque C, Figueras F, et al. Differential vulnerability of gray matter and white matter to intrauterine growth restriction in preterm infants at 12 months corrected age. Brain Res 2014;1545:1–11.

21. Batalle D, Eixarch E, Figueras F, et al. Altered small-world topology of structural brain networks in infants with intrauterine growth restriction and its association with later neurodevelopmental outcome. Neuroimage 2012;60(2):1352–66.

22. Fischi-Gomez E, Vasung L, Meskaldji DE, et al. Structural brain connectivity in school-age preterm infants provides evidence for impaired networks relevant for higher order cognitive skills and social cognition. Cereb Cortex 2015;25(9): 2793–805.

23. Mallard EC, Rees S, Stringer M, et al. Effects of chronic placental insufficiency on brain development in fetal sheep. Pediatr Res 1998;43(2):262–70.

24. Rees S, Harding R. Brain development during fetal life: influences of the intrauterine environment. Neurosci Lett 2004;361(1–3):111–4.

25. Lodygensky GA, Seghier ML, Warfield SK, et al. Intrauterine growth restriction affects the preterm infant's hippocampus. Pediatr Res 2008;63(4):438–43.

26. Fung C, Ke X, Brown AS, et al. Uteroplacental insufficiency alters rat hippocampal cellular phenotype in conjunction with ErbB receptor expression. Pediatr Res 2012;72(1):2–9.

27. Miller SL, Yawno T, Alers NO, et al. Antenatal antioxidant treatment with melatonin to decrease newborn neurodevelopmental deficits and brain injury caused by fetal growth restriction. J Pineal Res 2014;56(3):283–94.

28. Dieni S, Rees S. Dendritic morphology is altered in hippocampal neurons following prenatal compromise. J Neurobiol 2003;55(1):41–52.
29. Olivier P, Baud O, Bouslama M, et al. Moderate growth restriction: deleterious and protective effects on white matter damage. Neurobiol Dis 2007;26(1):253–63.
30. Chang JL, Bashir M, Santiago C, et al. Intrauterine growth restriction and hyperoxia as a cause of white matter injury. Dev Neurosci 2018;40(4):344–57.
31. Jarvis S, Glinianaia SV, Torrioli MG, et al. Cerebral palsy and intrauterine growth in single births: European collaborative study. Lancet 2003;362(9390):1106–11.
32. Levine TA, Grunau RE, McAuliffe FM, et al. Early childhood neurodevelopment after intrauterine growth restriction: a systematic review. Pediatrics 2015;135(1): 126–41.
33. Schreuder AM, McDonnell M, Gaffney G, et al. Outcome at school age following antenatal detection of absent or reversed end diastolic flow velocity in the umbilical artery. Arch Dis Child Fetal Neonatal Ed 2002;86(2):F108–14.
34. Parkinson CE, Wallis S, Harvey D. School achievement and behaviour of children who were small-for-dates at birth. Dev Med Child Neurol 1981;23(1):41–50.
35. Morsing E, Asard M, Ley D, et al. Cognitive function after intrauterine growth restriction and very preterm birth. Pediatrics 2011;127(4):e874–82.
36. Streimish IG, Ehrenkranz RA, Allred EN, et al. Birth weight- and fetal weight-growth restriction: impact on neurodevelopment. Early Hum Dev 2012;88(9): 765–71.
37. Strauss RS. Adult functional outcome of those born small for gestational age: twenty-six-year follow-up of the 1970 British Birth Cohort. JAMA 2000;283(5): 625–32.
38. Sun BZ, Moster D, Harmon QE, et al. Association of preeclampsia in term births with neurodevelopmental disorders in offspring. JAMA Psychiatry 2020;77(8):823–9.
39. Lahti-Pulkkinen M, Girchenko P, Tuovinen S, et al. Maternal hypertensive pregnancy disorders and mental disorders in children. Hypertension 2020;75(6): 1429–38.
40. Cho WK, Suh BK. Catch-up growth and catch-up fat in children born small for gestational age. Korean J Pediatr 2016;59(1):1–7.
41. Heron M. Deaths: leading causes for 2017. Natl Vital Stat Rep 2019;68(6):1–77.
42. Fryar CD, Chen TC, Li X. Prevalence of uncontrolled risk factors for cardiovascular disease: United States, 1999-2010. NCHS Data Brief 2012;(103):1–8.
43. Barker DJ, Winter PD, Osmond C, et al. Weight in infancy and death from ischaemic heart disease. Lancet 1989;2(8663):577–80.
44. Barker DJ, Hales CN, Fall CH, et al. Type 2 (non-insulin-dependent) diabetes mellitus, hypertension and hyperlipidaemia (syndrome X): relation to reduced fetal growth. Diabtologia 1993;36(1):62–7.
45. Rich-Edwards JW, Stampfer MJ, Manson JE, et al. Birth weight and risk of cardiovascular disease in a cohort of women followed up since 1976. BMJ 1997; 315(7105):396–400.
46. Leon DA, Lithell HO, Vagero D, et al. Reduced fetal growth rate and increased risk of death from ischaemic heart disease: cohort study of 15 000 Swedish men and women born 1915-29. BMJ 1998;317(7153):241–5.
47. Andersen LG, Angquist L, Eriksson JG, et al. Birth weight, childhood body mass index and risk of coronary heart disease in adults: combined historical cohort studies. PLoS One 2010;5(11):e14126.
48. Osmond C, Barker DJ, Winter PD, et al. Early growth and death from cardiovascular disease in women. BMJ 1993;307(6918):1519–24.

49. Barker DJ, Osmond C, Simmonds SJ, et al. The relation of small head circumference and thinness at birth to death from cardiovascular disease in adult life. BMJ 1993;306(6875):422–6.

50. Martyn CN, Barker DJ, Jespersen S, et al. Growth in utero, adult blood pressure, and arterial compliance. Br Heart J 1995;73(2):116–21.

51. Leon DA, Koupilova I, Lithell HO, et al. Failure to realise growth potential in utero and adult obesity in relation to blood pressure in 50 year old Swedish men. BMJ 1996;312(7028):401–6.

52. Nilsson PM, Ostergren PO, Nyberg P, et al. Low birth weight is associated with elevated systolic blood pressure in adolescence: a prospective study of a birth cohort of 149378 Swedish boys. J Hypertens 1997;15(12 Pt 2):1627–31.

53. Huxley RR, Shiell AW, Law CM. The role of size at birth and postnatal catch-up growth in determining systolic blood pressure: a systematic review of the literature. J Hypertens 2000;18(7):815–31.

54. Lamont D, Parker L, White M, et al. Risk of cardiovascular disease measured by carotid intima-media thickness at age 49-51: lifecourse study. BMJ 2000; 320(7230):273–8.

55. Huxley R, Neil A, Collins R. Unravelling the fetal origins hypothesis: is there really an inverse association between birthweight and subsequent blood pressure? Lancet 2002;360(9334):659–65.

56. Hemachandra AH, Klebanoff MA, Duggan AK, et al. The association between intrauterine growth restriction in the full-term infant and high blood pressure at age 7 years: results from the Collaborative Perinatal Project. Int J Epidemiol 2006; 35(4):871–7.

57. Verburg BO, Jaddoe VW, Wladimiroff JW, et al. Fetal hemodynamic adaptive changes related to intrauterine growth: the Generation R Study. Circulation 2008;117(5):649–59.

58. Sohi G, Revesz A, Hardy DB. Permanent implications of intrauterine growth restriction on cholesterol homeostasis. Semin Reprod Med 2011;29(3):246–56.

59. Dodson RB, Rozance PJ, Fleenor BS, et al. Increased arterial stiffness and extracellular matrix reorganization in intrauterine growth-restricted fetal sheep. Pediatr Res 2013;73(2):147–54.

60. Demicheva E, Crispi F. Long-term follow-up of intrauterine growth restriction: cardiovascular disorders. Fetal Diagn Ther 2014;36(2):143–53.

61. Dodson RB, Miller TA, Powers K, et al. Intrauterine growth restriction influences vascular remodeling and stiffening in the weanling rat more than sex or diet. Am J Physiol Heart Circ Physiol 2017;312(2):H250–64.

62. Huang PL. A comprehensive definition for metabolic syndrome. Dis Model Mech 2009;2(5–6):231–7.

63. Nobili A, D'Avanzo B, Santoro L, et al. Serum cholesterol and acute myocardial infarction: a case-control study from the GISSI-2 trial. Gruppo Italiano per lo Studio della Sopravvivenza nell'Infarto-Epidemiologia dei Fattori di Rischio dell'Infarto Miocardico Investigators. Br Heart J 1994;71(5):468–73.

64. Stavenow L, Kjellstrom T. Influence of serum triglyceride levels on the risk for myocardial infarction in 12,510 middle aged males: interaction with serum cholesterol. Atherosclerosis 1999;147(2):243–7.

65. Barker DJ, Martyn CN, Osmond C, et al. Growth in utero and serum cholesterol concentrations in adult life. BMJ 1993;307(6918):1524–7.

66. Radunovic N, Kuczynski E, Rosen T, et al. Plasma apolipoprotein A-I and B concentrations in growth-retarded fetuses: a link between low birth weight and adult atherosclerosis. J Clin Endocrinol Metab 2000;85(1):85–8.

67. Kim SM, Lee SM, Kim SJ, et al. Cord and maternal sera from small neonates share dysfunctional lipoproteins with proatherogenic properties: evidence for Barker's hypothesis. J Clin Lipidol 2017;11(6):1318–28.e3.
68. Molina M, Casanueva V, Cid X, et al. [Lipid profile in newborns with intrauterine growth retardation]. Rev Med Chil 2000;128(7):741–8.
69. Fall CH, Osmond C, Barker DJ, et al. Fetal and infant growth and cardiovascular risk factors in women. BMJ 1995;310(6977):428–32.
70. Phillips DI. Relation of fetal growth to adult muscle mass and glucose tolerance. Diabet Med 1995;12(8):686–90.
71. Raghupathy P, Antonisamy B, Geethanjali FS, et al. Glucose tolerance, insulin resistance and insulin secretion in young south Indian adults: relationships to parental size, neonatal size and childhood body mass index. Diabetes Res Clin Pract 2010;87(2):283–92.
72. Owen CG, Whincup PH, Kaye SJ, et al. Does initial breastfeeding lead to lower blood cholesterol in adult life? A quantitative review of the evidence. Am J Clin Nutr 2008;88(2):305–14.
73. Barker DJ, Osmond C, Forsen TJ, et al. Trajectories of growth among children who have coronary events as adults. N Engl J Med 2005;353(17):1802–9.
74. Osmond C, Barker DJ. Fetal, infant, and childhood growth are predictors of coronary heart disease, diabetes, and hypertension in adult men and women. Environ Health Perspect 2000;108(Suppl 3):545–53.
75. Law CM, Barker DJ, Osmond C, et al. Early growth and abdominal fatness in adult life. J Epidemiol Community Health 1992;46(3):184–6.
76. Wells JC, Chomtho S, Fewtrell MS. Programming of body composition by early growth and nutrition. Proc Nutr Soc 2007;66(3):423–34.
77. Fu Q, McKnight RA, Yu X, et al. Uteroplacental insufficiency induces site-specific changes in histone H3 covalent modifications and affects DNA-histone H3 positioning in day 0 IUGR rat liver. Physiol Genomics 2004;20(1):108–16.
78. Fung C, McKnight RA, Lane RH. Environmental influences on epigenetic gene regulation. Neoreviews 2013;14:e121–7.
79. Fung CM, Yang Y, Fu Q, et al. IUGR prevents IGF-1 upregulation in juvenile male mice by perturbing postnatal IGF-1 chromatin remodeling. Pediatr Res 2015; 78(1):14–23.

Short- and Long-Term Outcomes Associated with Large for Gestational Age Birth Weight

Christina M. Scifres, MD

KEYWORDS

- Large for gestational age birth weight • Macrosomia • Diabetes • Obesity
- Cardiovascular disease • Birth trauma • Shoulder dystocia • Hypoglycemia

KEY POINTS

- Large for gestational age birth weight (LGA) is associated with short-term risk for birth trauma and newborn morbidity.
- LGA birth weight is associated with long-term risk for morbidities such as overweight/obesity, diabetes, and cardiovascular disease.
- Prevention of LGA birth weight may decrease the risk for multiple complications.

INTRODUCTION

Large for gestational age (LGA) birth weight is associated with an increased risk for perinatal morbidity and long-term metabolic complications. This review summarizes the impact of LGA birth weight on both short- and long-term offspring outcomes. One challenge associated with evaluating the risks associated with higher birth weight is that varying definitions have been used to describe excess fetal growth. In many studies, LGA is defined as a birth weight greater than the 90th percentile for gestational age.[1,2] However, other investigators have suggested that the definition of LGA should be restricted to infants with birth weight greater than the 97th percentile (2 standard deviations above the mean), because it is this group of infants who are at the greatest risk for perinatal morbidity and mortality.[3,4] In this review, use of the term LGA refers to a birth weight greater than the 90th percentile unless otherwise specified, because this is the most common definition used. Among singleton live births in the United States, infants born at 40 weeks' gestation at the 90th percentile had birth weight of greater than 4000 g, and those born at the 97th percentile had a birth weight of greater than 4400 g.[2] Another commonly used term to describe excess fetal growth is macrosomia, which implies growth beyond an absolute birth weight,

Department of Obstetrics and Gynecology, Indiana University School of Medicine, 550 N. University Boulevard, UH 2440, Indianapolis, IN 46202, USA
E-mail address: cmscifre@iu.edu

Obstet Gynecol Clin N Am 48 (2021) 325–337
https://doi.org/10.1016/j.ogc.2021.02.005

obgyn.theclinics.com

typically 4000 or 4500 g, regardless of gestational age. Regardless of the definition used, excess fetal growth is common. In 2018, data from the National Center for Health Statistics showed that 7.8% of all live-born infants in the United States weighed 4000 g or more, 1% weighed more than 4500 g, and 0.1% weighed more than 5000 g.[5]

The short- and long-term health outcomes associated with LGA birth weight may depend on the underlying etiology, but there is a paucity of data to provide clarity. Genetic causes of early excessive fetal growth include Beckwith–Wiedeman syndrome, Simpson–Golabi–Behmel syndrome, Sotos syndrome, Weaver syndrome, and Berardinelli lipodystrophy. In these instances, the prognosis associated with the underlying syndrome is the most significant influence on outcomes. However, in most cases of LGA birth weight there is likely an interplay of fetal genetic growth potential and excess delivery of nutrients to the fetus, although the mechanisms that control fetal weight gain and growth are incompletely understood.

RISK FACTORS FOR LARGE FOR GESTATIONAL AGE BIRTH WEIGHT

Maternal factors associated with LGA birth weight include diabetes, overweight and obesity, and excess gestational weight gain. LGA birth weight is common in infants of mothers with diabetes, particularly in the setting of suboptimal glycemic control.[6] Excess delivery of glucose to the fetus results in fetal hyperglycemia, hyperinsulinemia, and increased growth.[7] This excess fetal growth is also associated with increased body fat and thicker skinfolds compared with the offspring of women without diabetes.[8] Recent data suggest that fetal genotype and maternal glucose levels have an additive effect on fetal growth.[9] Higher maternal triglycerides have also been associated with excess fetal growth.[10,11]

The risk of an LGA offspring increases in a linear fashion as the prepregnancy maternal weight increases , and obese women have the highest risk for delivery of an LGA birth weight infant.[12] This relationship between maternal body mass index (BMI) and fetal growth is independent of maternal glucose levels.[13] Finally, excess maternal weight gain during pregnancy is associated with LGA birth weight.[14] Women across the spectrum of prepregnancy BMI categories with excess gestational weight gain are 1.85 times more likely to deliver an infant with LGA birth weight than women with weight gain within recommendations.[14]

NEONATAL COMPLICATIONS ASSOCIATED WITH LARGE FOR GESTATIONAL AGE BIRTH WEIGHT
Severity of Fetal Overgrowth and the Risk for Neonatal Complications

Multiple studies have demonstrated that neonatal morbidity for term infants is greater in infants with birth weight greater than 4000 g compared with those with birth weight between 2500 and 3999 g[4,15] The risk for both infant and maternal morbidity is increased when birth weight is either LGA or between 4000 and 4500 g, and it increases sharply when the birth weight is more than 4500 g[4,16–18] Because of this, macrosomia is commonly divided into 3 categories, each with differing types and levels of risk: (1) 4000 to 4499 g, (2) 4500 to 4999 g, and (3) more than 5000 g.[19]

The risk for morbidity based on increasing levels of macrosomia was highlighted using data that included all singleton live births in the United States from 1995 to 1997 with a gestational age between 37 and 44 weeks of gestation. The authors clearly demonstrated progressively increasing morbidity that occurs as the birth weight increases above 4000 g.[4] As shown in **Table 1**, the risk for adverse outcomes including birth injury, an Apgar score of 3 or less at 5 minutes of life, assisted ventilation for more than 30 minutes, and meconium aspiration increased progressively from normal

Table 1 Neonatal outcomes by macrosomia class				
	Control (3000–3999 g) Percent with Outcome aOR (95% CI)	Grade 1 (4000–4499 g) Percent with Outcome aOR (95% CI)	Grade 2 (4500–4999 g) Percent with Outcome aOR (95% CI)	Grade 3 (≥5000 g) Percent with Outcome aOR (95% CI)
Birth Injury	0.3 Ref	0.5 1.99 (1.92–2.05)	0.8 3.14 (2.96–3.32)	1.3 4.53 (3.95–5.19)
Apgar score ≤3 (5 min)	0.1 Ref	0.1 1.30 (1.21–1.39)	0.2 2.01 (1.76–2.29)	0.5 5.20 (4.09–6.62)
Assisted ventilation ≥30 min	0.3 Ref	0.3 1.19 (1.14–1.23)	0.5 1.85 (1.73–1.99)	1.3 3.96 (3.45–4.55)
Meconium aspiration	0.2 Ref	0.3 1.28 (1.23–1.34)	0.4 1.65 (1.52–1.79)	0.6 2.61 (2.15–3.16)
Neonatal mortality rate (<28 d)	0.07 Ref	0.06 0.87 (0.80–0.96)	0.07 1.0 (0.83–1.21)	.19 2.69 (1.91–3.80)
Infant mortality rate (<1 y)	0.22 Ref	0.16 0.82 (0.78–0.86)	0.18 0.91 (0.80–1.02)	0.40 2.01 (1.58–2.55)

Abbreviation: aOR, adjusted odds ratio.
  All logistic regression models include measures of maternal race, age, education, marital status, prenatal care use, parity, previous macrosomic birth, previous pregnancy loss, maternal diabetes mellitus, hypertension, smoking, alcohol use, and gestational age; the reference group was 3000–3999 g.
  Data from Boulet SL, Alexander GR, Salihu HM, Pass M. Macrosomic births in the United States: determinants, outcomes, and proposed grades of risk. Am J Obstet Gynecol 2003; 188:1372-8.

weight (birth weight 3000–3999 g) to grade 1 (birth weight 400–4499 g), grade 2 (4500–4999 g), and grade 3 (birth weight ≥5000 g) macrosomia. Both neonatal and infant mortality were increased only in those infants with grade 3 macrosomia. Not all data are consistent; a large cohort study of more than 6 million birth and infant death records from the United States demonstrated that infants with birth weights from 4000 to 4499 g were not at an increased risk of morbidity or mortality compared with those with a birth weight of 3500 to 3999 g. However, infants with birth weights of 4500 to 4999 g were at significantly increased risk of stillbirth, neonatal mortality (especially because of birth asphyxia), birth injury, neonatal asphyxia, meconium aspiration, and cesarean delivery. A birth weight of 5000 g or greater was associated with even higher risks, including an increased risk of sudden infant death syndrome.[17]

  Although much of these data focused on infants with a birth weight greater than 4000 g, a retrospective cohort study using US Vital Statistics from 2011 to 2013 found that infants delivered between 37 and 39 weeks of gestation who were LGA (>90th percentile) but less than 4000 g were at an increased risk for composite neonatal morbidity that included any of the following: Apgar score of less than 5 at 5 minutes, assisted ventilation for more than 6 hours, seizure or serious neurologic dysfunction, significant birth injury, or neonatal mortality. In this same cohort, composite maternal mortality, including maternal transfusion, ruptured uterus, unplanned hysterectomy, admission to the intensive care unit, or unplanned procedures, was also higher in pregnancies complicated by LGA birth weight.[18] King and colleagues[20] also found that an ultrasound examination estimated fetal weight greater than 4000 or 4500 g in laboring women at term was associated with a higher risk for composite perinatal morbidity that included shoulder dystocia, third- or fourth-degree perineal laceration, postpartum hemorrhage, maternal hospitalization for 5 or more days, neonatal birth trauma, meconium aspiration syndrome, perinatal infection, and neonatal length of stay of 5 or more days.[20]

Large for Gestational Age Birth Weight and Preterm Birth

LGA birth weight (birth weight >97th percentile) may be associated with an increased risk of preterm birth. Using a Dutch perinatal registry of singleton births in nulliparous women from 1999 to 2010, van Zijl and colleagues[21] found that the risk of preterm birth between 25 and less than 37 weeks of gestation was greater in LGA (birth weight >97th percentile for age) birth weight infants compared with those with a birth weight that is appropriate for gestational age (AGA) (11.3% vs 7.3%, odds ratio [OR], 1.8; 95% confidence interval [CI], 1.7–1.9).

Unlike term LGA infants who are at increased risk for morbidity, there are some data to suggest that, among infants born preterm, LGA birth weight is associated with lower morbidity and mortality when compared with AGA birth weight infants matched for gestational age. These findings were illustrated by a retrospective review of data from the Vermont Oxford Network of preterm infants at 22 to 29 weeks of gestation born between 2006 and 2014.[22] Compared with AGA infants, LGA preterm infants had decreased risks of mortality, respiratory distress syndrome, patent ductus arteriosus, necrotizing enterocolitis, late-onset sepsis, severe retinopathy of prematurity, and chronic lung disease. LGA infants were more likely to have early onset sepsis and severe intraventricular hemorrhage, but these findings were not consistent across gestational ages. These data suggest that, for preterm infants, higher birth weight may be a protective factor, resulting in better outcomes. However, these findings are limited by a lack of information regarding maternal medical comorbidities such as diabetes that may impact neonatal outcomes. These results were unchanged when the authors excluded infants born above the 97th percentile of birth weight for gestational age, but it is still possible that these findings may have been impacted by misdating of LGA infants.

Large for Gestational Age GA Birth Weight and Birth Defects

Fetal overgrowth may be associated with increased risk for minor congenital anomalies. A retrospective case control study of more than 2 million births in Latin America found that, after adjusting for covariates including maternal diabetes, LGA was associated with the following anomalies: talipes calcaneovalgus (OR, 4.82), hip subluxation caused by intrauterine deformation (OR, 1.63), hydrocephaly (OR, 3.1), combined angiomatoses (OR, 2.77), and nonbrown pigmented nevi (OR, 1.46).[23] The authors of a separate report from the Texas Birth Defects Monitoring Division found that infants with congenital anomalies were more likely than infants without birth defects to have a birth weight of 4500 g or greater (OR, 1.65; 95% CI, 1.39–1.96).[24]

Large for Gestational Age Birth Weight and Neonatal Metabolic Abnormalities

LGA infants may have increased intrauterine exposure to excessive nutrients, especially glucose, which may result in hyperinsulinemia, increased use of oxygen and glucose, and oxidative stress.[25,26] Compared with their AGA counterparts, infants with LGA birth weight may also have increased levels of cord blood leptin and insulin as well as decreased levels of adiponectin and soluble leptin receptor.[27,28] Ahlsson and colleagues also found that infants with LGA birth weight demonstrate increased lipolysis and a propensity[26] for decreased insulin sensitivity at birth. Although the mechanisms are incompletely understood, metabolic abnormalities seen in LGA infants may lead to complications including hypoglycemia, polycythemia, and asphyxia.

Hypoglycemia can occur in LGA infants when the placental supply of glucose is interrupted at birth, even in the absence of maternal diabetes. Groenedaal and colleagues used the Netherlands Perinatal Registry data from 1997 to 2002 to evaluate the relationship between LGA birth weight (>90th percentile) and neonatal hypoglycemia in infants without other risk factors for hypoglycemia. Among LGA infants of women without diabetes, hypoglycemia occurred in 10.5% and seizures possibly related to hypoglycemia occurred in 0.2% of these infants.[29] In another large case series of 887 LGA infants (birth weight of >90th percentile) born to women without diabetes, 16% had hypoglycemia (blood glucose level of <40 mg/dL) during the first 24 hours of life.[30] These data highlight the importance of routine postdelivery glucose monitoring in infants with LGA birth weight.

Polycythemia also occurs more frequently in LGA infants born to women both with and without diabetes when compared with AGA infants.[31,32] Although the precise mechanism of LGA-associated polycythemia is unknown, it is thought to be due to an increased production of erythropoietin, which results from the fetal hypoxia caused by the increased oxidative demands associated with hyperglycemia and hyperinsulinemia.

Large for Gestational Age Birth Weight and Neonatal Intensive Care Admission

LGA infants are often admitted to the neonatal intensive care unit (NICU) for indications beyond hypoglycemia. This finding was demonstrated by a study from the Arizona Neonatal Intensive Care Program for infants born between 1994 and 1998.[33] In this study, the characteristics of infants with a birth weight greater than 4000 g who were enrolled in the Arizona Neonatal Intensive Care Program (criteria included prolonged NICU stay [>72 hours], readmission to a NICU, or transport to a NICU) were described. The 4 most common diagnoses in LGA infants (accounting for 53% of the admission diagnoses) were respiratory distress (19%), transient tachypnea of the newborn (16%), hypoglycemia (9%), and meconium aspiration (9%).[33] In a separate analysis, Tolosa and colleagues[34] found that 11.7% of infants with a birth weight of greater than 4000 g were admitted to the NICU. The most common diagnoses leading to NICU admission included respiratory distress, suspected sepsis, hypoglycemia, and perinatal depression. The average length of stay for all macrocosmic infants admitted to the NICU was 8 ± 6 days, and this stay was increased to 22 ± 13 days for infants with grade 3 macrosomia.

LGA infants are more likely to develop respiratory distress than AGA infants.[4,33] There are several potential causes for the increased risk for respiratory complications. Some data have suggested that there is an increased risk for respiratory distress syndrome in newborns of women with diabetes.[35] The higher incidence of cesarean deliveries in LGA infants likely also increases the risk of respiratory complications in the newborn.[36] In addition, meconium aspiration may be more common in LGA infants.[4]

Large for Gestational Age Birth Weight and Shoulder Dystocia

Larger infants, especially those with macrosomia, are at an increased risk for shoulder dystocia, brachial plexus injury, and clavicular fracture,[4,37,38] and the risk of birth injury increases with the severity of macrosomia.[4] Shoulder dystocia occurs in 0.2% to 3.0% of all vaginal deliveries,[39] but this risk increases to 9% to 14% the when birth weight is more than 4500 g.[16,40,41] Maternal diabetes further increases the risk for shoulder dystocia. Among pregnancies complicated by diabetes, a birth weight of 4500 g or more has been associated with a 20% to 50% risk for shoulder dystocia.[16,40]

Shoulder dystocia is associated with increased risk for birth injury, and the risk for birth injury among LGA infants is higher for vaginal compared with cesarean delivery. In one large case series, birth injury was 3 times more likely when LGA infants (birth weight 4500–5000 g) were delivered vaginally compared with cesarean delivery (9.3% vs 2.6%; P<.003).[37] Macrosomic newborns also have a 10-fold increased risk for clavicular fracture.[33] In addition to fractures, brachial plexus injuries are more common in macrosomic infants. In the United States, transient and persistent neonatal brachial plexus injuries complicate 1.5 per 1000 total births.[42] A meta-analysis found that the odds for brachial plexus injury was increased by 11-fold among infants who weigh more than 4000 g and by 20-fold among infants weighing more than 4500 g, although mode of delivery was not accounted for.[43] Case control studies demonstrate that the odds of brachial plexus palsy among newborns delivered vaginally is 18-fold to 21-fold higher when birth weights exceed 4500 g,[44–46] with absolute rates between 2.6% and 7.0%.[47,48] Brachial plexus palsy also can occur in the absence of shoulder dystocia or with cesarean birth.[42] Large case series confirm that 80% to 90% of brachial plexus palsy will resolve by 1 year of age,[49,50] indicating that most cases of brachial plexus palsy will resolve without permanent disability. However, birth weights of more than 4500 g are associated with a higher risk for persistent injury.[51,52]

Large for Gestational Age Birth Weight and Stillbirth or Neonatal Death

Macrosomic infants are at an increased risk for perinatal asphyxia, and this risk may be greatest in offspring of women with diabetes.[3,4,37,53] The higher frequency of low Apgar scores in LGA infants compared with AGA infants provides indirect evidence of the increased risk for perinatal asphyxia in LGA infants. Contributing factors are thought to include increased oxygen use owing to fetal hyperglycemia and hyperinsulinemia, and complications of delivery related to shoulder dystocia.

Although neonatal mortality is higher in LGA than in AGA term infants, it is only substantially higher in only the most severe grade of macrosomia. In a study of all singleton, term live births between 1995 and 1997, the neonatal mortality rate was only higher in infants born with grade 3 macrosomia (birth weight of >5000 g) compared with normal birth weight (<4000 g) infants (adjusted OR, 2.69; 95% CI, 1.91–3.8).[4] Similar results were noted in a Canadian study that reported more than a 2-fold increased risk of deaths in term infants with birth weight of greater than the 97th percentile compared with AGA term infants.[53] Recent data also indicate that the risk for stillbirth may be increased in the setting of fetal macrosomia when the birth weight exceeds 4500 g (OR, 1.27; 95% CI, 1.22–1.32) or 5000 g (OR, 5.69; 95% CI, 5.69–6.22).[54]

LONG-TERM OUTCOMES ASSOCIATED WITH LARGE FOR GESTATIONAL AGE BIRTH WEIGHT
Childhood Development and Outcomes Associated with Large for Gestational Age Birth Weight

It is of utmost importance to understand how LGA birth weight affects long-term growth and development. Data increasingly show that the origins of obesity begin very early in life, with multiple risk factors present before 2 years of age.[55] Multiple studies have found an association between birth weight and BMI or overweight/obesity in childhood and young adulthood.[56–58] Traditionally it was thought that LGA birth weight was followed by a decreasing growth trajectory in infancy.[59] However, more recent data suggest that this may not be the case. Hediger and colleagues[60] used data from the Third National Health and Nutrition Examination Survey to compare early childhood growth patterns of LGA newborns compared with AGA newborns. They found that infants with LGA birth weight were heavier, taller, and had a larger head circumference through 47 months of age. These same investigators also used the Third National Health and Nutrition Examination Survey data to assess the impact of LGA birth weight on muscularity and "fatness" in childhood.[61] They found that, from the ages of 2 to 47 months, infants with LGA birth weight had higher levels of muscularity and less excess fatness. This finding was particularly true at the youngest gestational ages. Hediger and colleagues[62] also found that children born LGA remain longer and heavier from 36 to 83 months of age, and that children born LGA may be prone to increasing accumulation of fat in early childhood. However, they were unable to account for maternal characteristics such as diabetes in their analyses. Kapral and colleagues[63] found that infants who either had a birth weight at term of greater than 4500 g or those who were born preterm with a birth weight z-score of more than the 90th percentile for gestational age subsequently had higher BMI z-scores from kindergarten to second grade when compared with normal birthweight controls. Data from the Identification and Prevention of Dietary- and Lifestyle-Induced Health Effects in Children and Infants Study demonstrated that a birth weight of greater than the 90th percentile in the absence of maternal diabetes was associated with increased odds of overweight/obesity in both boys (OR, 1.7; 95% CI, 1.3–2.2) and girls (OR, 1.6; 95% CI, 1.3–2.0), whereas a birth weight of greater than the 90th percentile in the setting of maternal diabetes demonstrated a significant association with childhood weight only in girls (OR, 2.6; 95% CI, 1.1–6.4).[64]

Several studies have examined infant and early childhood factors that are associated with growth in infancy. In a Norwegian cohort, Lande and colleagues[65] compared feeding practices between infants with a high ponderal index (PI; calculated using the formula mass [kg]/height [m^3]) at birth (a PI of >90th percentile) and normal PI at birth (a PI between the 10th and 90th percentiles) and examined how birth size and infant feeding practices were related to BMI at 12 months. They found that infants with a higher PI at birth had a shorter duration of exclusive breastfeeding. In addition, both high PI at birth and short-term exclusive breastfeeding were associated with a higher BMI at 12 months, highlighting the complex interplay between birth weight and infant feeding practices on infant growth. Although prior cross-sectional work found that, compared with normal weight infants, larger infants have similar parent-reported eating behaviors and feeding practices, infants with a birth weight of greater than 4000 g who maintained a high weight for length at 7 to 8 months of age had lower maternal-reported satiety responsiveness and maternal social interactions during feeding.[66] Sleep may also play an important role in the growth and development of infants who are macrosomic at birth. Goetz and colleagues[67] examined sleep practices during infancy and toddlerhood among children with a birth weight of greater than 4000 g. They found that a longer sleep duration in the first several years of life is associated with the development of a normal BMI among macrosomic infants. However, there is a paucity of interventional trials designed to improve health outcomes specifically targeting infants with LGA birth weight.

Data suggest that LGA birth weight may also be associated with metabolic disturbances in childhood that portend the development of later diabetes and insulin resistance. A cross-sectional study of prepubertal children found that LGA birth weight was associated with increased insulin resistance and oxidative stress, even in normal weight children.[68] Several additional studies show that a history of LGA birth weight is associated with increased insulin resistance among prepubertal children. However, data are conflicting regarding the magnitude and direction of alterations in adiponectin that accompany these changes in insulin resistance.[69,70] Both heavier birth weight and greater weight gain after birth are associated with increased risk for hypertension during childhood.[71]

There is also strong interest in the impact of fetal overgrowth on long-term neuro-developmental outcomes, but the available data are limited. In a study of 2930 children from the Early Childhood Longitudinal Study, Birth Cohort (ECLS-B), the cognitive function of 271 children with birth weights greater than or equal to the 90th percentile did not differ from that of children with normal birth weight (defined as a birth weight between the 5th and 89th percentiles) at 9 months, and 2.0, 3.5, and 5.5 years of age.[72] Although these data are reassuring, observational studies have suggested that maternal gestational diabetes and type 2 diabetes (both of which are associated with an increased risk for fetal overgrowth) may be associated with an increased risk for autism and other adverse neurodevelopmental outcomes.[73,74]

Fetal overgrowth has also been associated with several additional adverse outcomes that may be less intuitive but warrant mention. Although the mechanism is uncertain, LGA birth weight has been associated with an increased risk for dental caries in early childhood.[75] Fetal overgrowth has also been linked to several childhood leukemias as well as tumors of the central nervous system, renal tumors, soft tissue sarcomas, neuroblastoma, lymphoma, and germ cell tumors.[76–78] Further work is needed to clarify the nature of these relationships.

Longer Term Outcomes Associated with Large for Gestational Age Birth Weight

LGA birth weight has also been linked to obesity in later life. Studies from both the Netherlands and Israel found that higher birth weight was associated with an increased risk for overweight and obesity at 17 to 26 years of age.[79,80] In a study from Sweden, mothers born LGA were more likely to be overweight or obese than their AGA counterparts. Those overweight women were also more likely to give birth to LGA infants, propagating a vicious cycle.[81] LGA birth weight has also been linked to later medical comorbidities including type 2 diabetes[82,83] and cardiovascular disease.[84]

SUMMARY

Fetal overgrowth is associated with multiple adverse short- and long-term adverse outcomes, and we still have much to learn regarding how to optimize outcomes for these infants. Birth weight is distinct from body composition, and more robust studies are needed to clarify the pattern of fat and lean body mass distribution of infants with LGA birth weight to assess whether we can accurately identify babies at highest risk for later-life metabolic complications. We know that treating maternal diabetes can decrease the risk for LGA birth weight. However, the majority of LGA infants are born to women without diabetes, and there are few consistently successful interventions targeting maternal obesity and excess gestational weight gain. Nutrition before conception and during pregnancy plays a fundamental role in influencing maternal weight gain, fetal growth, and neonatal outcomes,[85,86] but there is a paucity of data regarding optimal maternal nutrition in pregnancies complicated by LGA fetal growth. Once an LGA infant is born, there is also much to learn about how to optimize health and alter the trajectory toward obesity and metabolic disease. The early postnatal nutritional environment, and in particular breastfeeding, may modulate the long-term risks of obesity.[87] However, many available epidemiologic studies do not report information on infant feeding practices. Detailed information on pregnancy factors associated with excess fetal growth and infancy/early childhood factors associated with later obesity will be critical to develop evidence-based interventions to improve the health of infants with LGA birth weight.

CLINICS CARE POINTS

- LGA birth weight is associated with multiple adverse short- and long-term outcomes.
- The prevention of LGA birth weight may decrease the risk for multiple complications including NICU admission, respiratory distress, neonatal metabolic abnormalities, including hypoglycemia, birth trauma, and possibly even stillbirth or neonatal death.
- LGA birth weight is associated with a long-term risk for overweight/obesity, diabetes, cardiovascular disease, and even some childhood cancers, highlighting the need for interventions to prevent long-term complications.

DISCLOSURE

The author reports no conflicts of interest.

REFERENCES

1. Talge NM, Mudd LM, Sikorskii A, et al. United States birth weight reference corrected for implausible gestational age estimates. Pediatrics 2014;133(5):844–53.
2. Alexander GR, Himes JH, Kaufman RB, et al. A United States national reference for fetal growth. Obstet Gynecol 1996;87(2):163–8.
3. Xu H, Simonet F, Luo ZC. Optimal birth weight percentile cut-offs in defining small- or large-for-gestational-age. Acta Paediatr 2010;99(4):550–5.
4. Boulet SL, Alexander GR, Salihu HM, et al. Macrosomic births in the United States: determinants, outcomes, and proposed grades of risk. Am J Obstet Gynecol 2003;188(5):1372–8.
5. Martin JA, Hamilton BE, Osterman MJK, et al. Births: final data for 2018. Natl Vital Stat Rep 2019;68(13):1–47.
6. Hartling L, Dryden DM, Guthrie A, et al. Benefits and harms of treating gestational diabetes mellitus: a systematic review and meta-analysis for the U.S. Preventive Services Task Force and the National Institutes of Health Office of Medical Applications of Research. Ann Intern Med 2013;159(2):123–9.
7. Barbour LA. Metabolic culprits in obese pregnancies and gestational diabetes mellitus: big babies, big twists, big picture: the 2018 Norbert Freinkel Award Lecture. Diabetes Care 2019;42(5):718–26.
8. Catalano PM, Thomas A, Huston-Presley L, et al. Increased fetal adiposity: a very sensitive marker of abnormal in utero development. Am J Obstet Gynecol 2003; 189(6):1698–704.
9. Hughes AE, Nodzenski M, Beaumont RN, et al. Fetal genotype and maternal glucose have independent and additive effects on birth weight. Diabetes 2018; 67(5):1024–9.
10. Schaefer-Graf UM, Graf K, Kulbacka I, et al. Maternal lipids as strong determinants of fetal environment and growth in pregnancies with gestational diabetes mellitus. Diabetes Care 2008;31(9):1858–63.
11. Barbour LA, Hernandez TL. Maternal lipids and fetal overgrowth: making fat from fat. Clin Ther 2018;40(10):1638–47.
12. Catalano PM, Shankar K. Obesity and pregnancy: mechanisms of short term and long term adverse consequences for mother and child. BMJ 2017; 356:j1.
13. Group HSCR. Hyperglycaemia and Adverse Pregnancy Outcome (HAPO) Study: associations with maternal body mass index. BJOG 2010;117(5):575–84.

14. Goldstein RF, Abell SK, Ranasinha S, et al. Association of gestational weight gain with maternal and infant outcomes: a systematic review and meta-analysis. JAMA 2017;317(21):2207–25.
15. Linder N, Lahat Y, Kogan A, et al. Macrosomic newborns of non-diabetic mothers: anthropometric measurements and neonatal complications. Arch Dis Child Fetal Neonatal Ed 2014;99(5):F353–8.
16. Nesbitt TS, Gilbert WM, Herrchen B. Shoulder dystocia and associated risk factors with macrosomic infants born in California. Am J Obstet Gynecol 1998; 179(2):476–80.
17. Zhang X, Decker A, Platt RW, et al. How big is too big? The perinatal consequences of fetal macrosomia. Am J Obstet Gynecol 2008;198(5):517.e1–6.
18. Doty MS, Chen HY, Sibai BM, et al. Maternal and Neonatal morbidity associated with early term delivery of large-for-gestational-age but nonmacrosomic neonates. Obstet Gynecol 2019;133(6):1160–6.
19. American College of Obstetricians and Gynecologists' Committee on Practice Bulletins—Obstetrics. Practice Bulletin No. 173: fetal macrosomia. Obstet Gynecol 2016;128(5):e195–209.
20. King JR, Korst LM, Miller DA, et al. Increased composite maternal and neonatal morbidity associated with ultrasonographically suspected fetal macrosomia. J Matern Fetal Neonatal Med 2012;25(10):1953–9.
21. van Zijl MD, Oudijk MA, Ravelli ACJ, et al. Large-for-gestational-age fetuses have an increased risk for spontaneous preterm birth. J Perinatol 2019;39(8):1050–6.
22. Boghossian NS, Geraci M, Edwards EM, et al. In-hospital outcomes in large for gestational age infants at 22-29 weeks of gestation. J Pediatr 2018;198: 174–80.e13.
23. Lapunzina P, Camelo JS, Rittler M, et al. Risks of congenital anomalies in large for gestational age infants. J Pediatr 2002;140(2):200–4.
24. Waller DK, Keddie AM, Canfield MA, et al. Do infants with major congenital anomalies have an excess of macrosomia? Teratology 2001;64(6):311–7.
25. Akinbi HT, Gerdes JS. Macrosomic infants of nondiabetic mothers and elevated C-peptide levels in cord blood. J Pediatr 1995;127(3):481–4.
26. Ahlsson FS, Diderholm B, Ewald U, et al. Lipolysis and insulin sensitivity at birth in infants who are large for gestational age. Pediatrics 2007;120(5):958–65.
27. Mazaki-Tovi S, Kanety H, Pariente C, et al. Cord blood adiponectin in large-for-gestational age newborns. Am J Obstet Gynecol 2005;193(3 Pt 2):1238–42.
28. Lausten-Thomsen U, Christiansen M, Hedley PL, et al. Adipokines in umbilical cord blood from children born large for gestational age. J Pediatr Endocrinol Metab 2016;29(1):33–7.
29. Groenendaal F, Elferink-Stinkens PM, Netherlands Perinatal R. Hypoglycaemia and seizures in large-for-gestational-age (LGA) full-term neonates. Acta Paediatr 2006;95(7):874–6.
30. Schaefer-Graf UM, Rossi R, Buhrer C, et al. Rate and risk factors of hypoglycemia in large-for-gestational-age newborn infants of nondiabetic mothers. Am J Obstet Gynecol 2002;187(4):913–7.
31. Dollberg S, Marom R, Mimouni FB, et al. Normoblasts in large for gestational age infants. Arch Dis Child Fetal Neonatal Ed 2000;83(2):F148–9.
32. Mimouni F, Miodovnik M, Siddiqi TA, et al. Perinatal asphyxia in infants of insulin-dependent diabetic mothers. J Pediatr 1988;113(2):345–53.
33. Gillean JR, Coonrod DV, Russ R, et al. Big infants in the neonatal intensive care unit. Am J Obstet Gynecol 2005;192(6):1948–53, discussion 53-5.

34. Tolosa JN, Calhoun DA. Maternal and neonatal demographics of macrosomic infants admitted to the neonatal intensive care unit. J Perinatol 2017;37(12):1292–6.

35. Robert MF, Neff RK, Hubbell JP, et al. Association between maternal diabetes and the respiratory-distress syndrome in the newborn. N Engl J Med 1976;294(7): 357–60.

36. Plunkett BA, Sandoval G, Bailit JL, et al. Association of labor with neonatal respiratory outcomes at 36-40 weeks of gestation. Obstet Gynecol 2019;134(3): 495–501.

37. Spellacy WN, Miller S, Winegar A, et al. Macrosomia–maternal characteristics and infant complications. Obstet Gynecol 1985;66(2):158–61.

38. Ju H, Chadha Y, Donovan T, et al. Fetal macrosomia and pregnancy outcomes. Aust N Z J Obstet Gynaecol 2009;49(5):504–9.

39. Gherman RB, Chauhan S, Ouzounian JG, et al. Shoulder dystocia: the unpreventable obstetric emergency with empiric management guidelines. Am J Obstet Gynecol 2006;195(3):657–72.

40. Lipscomb KR, Gregory K, Shaw K. The outcome of macrosomic infants weighing at least 4500 grams: Los Angeles County + University of Southern California experience. Obstet Gynecol 1995;85(4):558–64.

41. Raio L, Ghezzi F, Di Naro E, et al. Perinatal outcome of fetuses with a birth weight greater than 4500 g: an analysis of 3356 cases. Eur J Obstet Gynecol Reprod Biol 2003;109(2):160–5.

42. Executive summary: neonatal brachial plexus palsy. Report of the American College of Obstetricians and Gynecologists' Task Force on Neonatal Brachial Plexus Palsy. Obstet Gynecol 2014;123(4):902–4.

43. Beta J, Khan N, Khalil A, et al. Maternal and neonatal complications of fetal macrosomia: systematic review and meta-analysis. Ultrasound Obstet Gynecol 2019; 54(3):308–18.

44. Ecker JL, Greenberg JA, Norwitz ER, et al. Birth weight as a predictor of brachial plexus injury. Obstet Gynecol 1997;89(5 Pt 1):643–7.

45. Perlow JH, Wigton T, Hart J, et al. Birth trauma. A five-year review of incidence and associated perinatal factors. J Reprod Med 1996;41(10):754–60.

46. McFarland LV, Raskin M, Daling JR, et al. Erb/Duchenne's palsy: a consequence of fetal macrosomia and method of delivery. Obstet Gynecol 1986;68(6):784–8.

47. Bryant DR, Leonardi MR, Landwehr JB, et al. Limited usefulness of fetal weight in predicting neonatal brachial plexus injury. Am J Obstet Gynecol 1998;179(3 Pt 1): 686–9.

48. Esakoff TF, Cheng YW, Sparks TN, et al. The association between birthweight 4000 g or greater and perinatal outcomes in patients with and without gestational diabetes mellitus. Am J Obstet Gynecol 2009;200(6):672.e1–4.

49. Morrison JC, Sanders JR, Magann EF, et al. The diagnosis and management of dystocia of the shoulder. Surg Gynecol Obstet 1992;175(6):515–22.

50. Hardy AE. Birth injuries of the brachial plexus: incidence and prognosis. J Bone Joint Surg Br 1981;63-B(1):98–101.

51. Gherman RB, Ouzounian JG, Satin AJ, et al. A comparison of shoulder dystocia-associated transient and permanent brachial plexus palsies. Obstet Gynecol 2003;102(3):544–8.

52. Kolderup LB, Laros RK Jr, Musci TJ. Incidence of persistent birth injury in macrosomic infants: association with mode of delivery. Am J Obstet Gynecol 1997; 177(1):37–41.

53. Lackman F, Capewell V, Richardson B, et al. The risks of spontaneous preterm delivery and perinatal mortality in relation to size at birth according to fetal versus neonatal growth standards. Am J Obstet Gynecol 2001;184(5):946–53.

54. Salihu HM, Dongarwar D, King LM, et al. Phenotypes of fetal macrosomia and risk of stillbirth among term deliveries over the previous four decades. Birth 2020; 47(2):202–10.

55. Woo Baidal JA, Locks LM, Cheng ER, et al. Risk factors for childhood obesity in the first 1,000 days: a systematic review. Am J Prev Med 2016;50(6):761–79.

56. Rogers I, Group E-BS. The influence of birthweight and intrauterine environment on adiposity and fat distribution in later life. Int J Obes Relat Metab Disord 2003; 27(7):755–77.

57. Schellong K, Schulz S, Harder T, et al. Birth weight and long-term overweight risk: systematic review and a meta-analysis including 643,902 persons from 66 studies and 26 countries globally. PLoS One 2012;7(10):e47776.

58. Yu ZB, Han SP, Zhu GZ, et al. Birth weight and subsequent risk of obesity: a systematic review and meta-analysis. Obes Rev 2011;12(7):525–42.

59. Smith DW, Truog W, Rogers JE, et al. Shifting linear growth during infancy: illustration of genetic factors in growth from fetal life through infancy. J Pediatr 1976; 89(2):225–30.

60. Hediger ML, Overpeck MD, Maurer KR, et al. Growth of infants and young children born small or large for gestational age: findings from the Third National Health and Nutrition Examination Survey. Arch Pediatr Adolesc Med 1998; 152(12):1225–31.

61. Hediger ML, Overpeck MD, Kuczmarski RJ, et al. Muscularity and fatness of infants and young children born small- or large-for-gestational-age. Pediatrics 1998;102(5):E60.

62. Hediger ML, Overpeck MD, McGlynn A, et al. Growth and fatness at three to six years of age of children born small- or large-for-gestational age. Pediatrics 1999; 104(3):e33.

63. Kapral N, Miller SE, Scharf RJ, et al. Associations between birthweight and overweight and obesity in school-age children. Pediatr Obes 2018;13(6):333–41.

64. Sparano S, Ahrens W, De Henauw S, et al. Being macrosomic at birth is an independent predictor of overweight in children: results from the IDEFICS study. Matern Child Health J 2013;17(8):1373–81.

65. Lande B, Andersen LF, Henriksen T, et al. Relations between high ponderal index at birth, feeding practices and body mass index in infancy. Eur J Clin Nutr 2005; 59(11):1241–9.

66. Odar Stough C, Bolling C, Zion C, et al. Comparison of high and normal birth weight infants on eating, feeding practices, and subsequent weight. Matern Child Health J 2018;22(12):1805–14.

67. Goetz AR, Beebe DW, Peugh JL, et al. Longer sleep duration during infancy and toddlerhood predicts weight normalization among high birth weight infants. Sleep 2019;42(2):zsy214.

68. Chiavaroli V, Giannini C, D'Adamo E, et al. Insulin resistance and oxidative stress in children born small and large for gestational age. Pediatrics 2009;124(2): 695–702.

69. Darendeliler F, Poyrazoglu S, Sancakli O, et al. Adiponectin is an indicator of insulin resistance in non-obese prepubertal children born large for gestational age (LGA) and is affected by birth weight. Clin Endocrinol (Oxf) 2009;70(5):710–6.

70. Giapros V, Evagelidou E, Challa A, et al. Serum adiponectin and leptin levels and insulin resistance in children born large for gestational age are affected by the degree of overweight. Clin Endocrinol (Oxf) 2007;66(3):353–9.
71. Bowers K, Liu G, Wang P, et al. Birth weight, postnatal weight change, and risk for high blood pressure among Chinese children. Pediatrics 2011;127(5):e1272–9.
72. Paulson JF, Mehta SH, Sokol RJ, et al. Large for gestational age and long-term cognitive function. Am J Obstet Gynecol 2014;210(4):343.e1–4.
73. Xiang AH, Wang X, Martinez MP, et al. Association of maternal diabetes with autism in offspring. JAMA 2015;313(14):1425–34.
74. Xu G, Jing J, Bowers K, et al. Maternal diabetes and the risk of autism spectrum disorders in the offspring: a systematic review and meta-analysis. J Autism Dev Disord 2014;44(4):766–75.
75. Yokomichi H, Tanaka T, Suzuki K, et al. Macrosomic neonates carry increased risk of dental caries in early childhood: findings from a cohort study, the Okinawa Child Health Study, Japan. PLoS One 2015;10(7):e0133872.
76. Okcu MF, Goodman KJ, Carozza SE, et al. Birth weight, ethnicity, and occurrence of cancer in children: a population-based, incident case-control study in the State of Texas, USA. Cancer Causes Control 2002;13(7):595–602.
77. Caughey RW, Michels KB. Birth weight and childhood leukemia: a meta-analysis and review of the current evidence. Int J Cancer 2009;124(11):2658–70.
78. O'Neill KA, Murphy MF, Bunch KJ, et al. Infant birthweight and risk of childhood cancer: international population-based case control studies of 40 000 cases. Int J Epidemiol 2015;44(1):153–68.
79. Sorensen HT, Sabroe S, Rothman KJ, et al. Relation between weight and length at birth and body mass index in young adulthood: cohort study. BMJ 1997; 315(7116):1137.
80. Seidman DS, Laor A, Gale R, et al. A longitudinal study of birth weight and being overweight in late adolescence. Am J Dis Child 1991;145(7):782–5.
81. Cnattingius S, Villamor E, Lagerros YT, et al. High birth weight and obesity–a vicious circle across generations. Int J Obes (Lond) 2012;36(10):1320–4.
82. Harder T, Rodekamp E, Schellong K, et al. Birth weight and subsequent risk of type 2 diabetes: a meta-analysis. Am J Epidemiol 2007;165(8):849–57.
83. Johnsson IW, Haglund B, Ahlsson F, et al. A high birth weight is associated with increased risk of type 2 diabetes and obesity. Pediatr Obes 2015;10(2):77–83.
84. Skilton MR, Siitonen N, Wurtz P, et al. High birth weight is associated with obesity and increased carotid wall thickness in young adults: the cardiovascular risk in young Finns study. Arterioscler Thromb Vasc Biol 2014;34(5):1064–8.
85. Gresham E, Byles JE, Bisquera A, et al. Effects of dietary interventions on neonatal and infant outcomes: a systematic review and meta-analysis. Am J Clin Nutr 2014;100(5):1298–321.
86. Muhlhausler BS, Gugusheff JR, Ong ZY, et al. Nutritional approaches to breaking the intergenerational cycle of obesity. Can J Physiol Pharmacol 2013;91(6): 421–8.
87. Arenz S, Ruckerl R, Koletzko B, et al. Breast-feeding and childhood obesity–a systematic review. Int J Obes Relat Metab Disord 2004;28(10):1247–56.

Ultrasound Diagnosis of the Small and Large Fetus

Alice Self, MD, Aris T. Papageorghiou, MD*

KEYWORDS

- Antenatal imaging • Ultrasound • Doppler • High-risk pregnancy

KEY POINTS

- Accurate dating is essential for the correct identification of the SGA and LGA fetus.
- Internationally recommended guidelines should be followed for the measurement of fetal biometry and Dopplers.
- A comprehensive assessment of fetal growth over time better detects the compromised fetus than assessing fetal size alone.
- Reproducibility and quality assurance of ultrasound measurements is a key part of good fetal assessment.
- Maternal access to ultrasound and significant infrastructure improvements are needed for the WHO recommendation of universal ultrasound before 24 weeks gestation to be of clinical benefit.

INTRODUCTION

It is well recognized that suboptimal fetal growth increases the risk of still birth, fetal distress, and neonatal complications. Macrosomia also is associated with increased morbidity to both fetus and mother, although to a lesser extent than fetal growth restriction (FGR). Clinical palpation or the measurement of the symphysis-fundal height provided the only means of estimating fetal growth until the advent of ultrasound. Since then, the accuracy of fetal biometry has significantly improved and for many years has been a pillar of antenatal care—from the assessment of gestational age (GA) to the detection of fetal abnormalities and the monitoring of fetal growth. The use of Doppler technology now is well established in assessing fetal well-being, and there is increasing interest in the role of 3-dimensional (3-D) ultrasound and magnetic resonance technology (MRI) technology for evaluating fetal growth.

This article looks at the role of antenatal imaging in the diagnosis of FGR and the large-for-gestational-age (LGA) fetus with a focus on how to obtain the required measurements using 2-dimensional (2-D) ultrasound; how to assess fetal growth; the role of ultrasound to help differentiate FGR from the small-for-gestational-age (SGA) fetus;

Nuffield Department of Women's and Reproductive Health, University of Oxford, Oxford, UK
* Corresponding author. Nuffield Department of Women's and Reproductive Health, University of Oxford, Level 3, Women's Centre, John Radcliffe Hospital, Oxford OX3 9DU, UK.
E-mail address: aris.papageorghiou@wrh.ox.ac.uk

Obstet Gynecol Clin N Am 48 (2021) 339–357
https://doi.org/10.1016/j.ogc.2021.03.003
0889-8545/21/© 2021 Elsevier Inc. All rights reserved.

the role of imaging to diagnose an LGA fetus; and some of the global health challenges in making ultrasound technology more widely available in low-income and middle-income countries (LMICs).

ASSESSING GESTATIONAL AGE

It is impossible to assess the appropriateness of fetal size without an accurate estimate of GA. Far from being limited to helping diagnose and guide the management of fetal growth disorders, the GA underpins the majority of decision making during antenatal care. Many women are unsure of their last menstrual period (LMP), and the LMP has been shown an unreliable parameter from which to date a pregnancy.[1,2]

Ultrasound-based measurement of the fetal crown-rump length (CRL) appears to be the most accurate method to estimate of GA. This assumes that all fetuses at a given GA are equal in size; although this is biologically implausible, it seems this makes little difference practically, with the accuracy being ±8% of the known GA (equating to ±4–8 d) when the CRL is between 10-80mm.[3] Overall, when dating on ultrasound, first-trimester CRL is the most accurate, and, once established, the estimated date of delivery must not be changed according to the biometry of later scans.

FIRST TRIMESTER: CROWN-RUMP LENGTH MEASUREMENT

The CRL should be measured from a midsagittal (or median) section, demonstrating (**Fig. 1**) the following:

- The crown and rump, midline facial profile, and fetal spine should be clearly defined in a single view.
- The head should be in a neutral position with a pocket of amniotic fluid between the fetal chin and the chest that approximates the width of the bright echo of the palate.
- The fetus should be lying horizontally across the screen with moderate curvature of lower spine, ensuring the sacrum is below the level of the chin.
- Magnify the image to ensure the fetus fills more than two-thirds of the window.

A CRL measurement is taken by placing the calipers across the longest distance from the outer borders of the skin over the skull to that over the rump. A review of the methodology of studies estimating GA from the CRL recommends high-quality charts for such dating.[4]

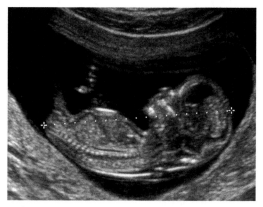

Fig. 1. First trimester: CRL measurement.

SECOND TRIMESTER

Although improving access to first trimester dating is the gold standard, optimizing GA estimation in later pregnancy should not be neglected, because globally many women do not have an ultrasound scan until later in the second and third trimesters. The accuracy of GA from fetal biometry diminishes with advancing gestation. In general, once the CRL exceeds 84 mm, fetal curling makes the measurement less reliable and estimation from head circumference (HC) is recommended; this has been found more robust than dating based on the biparietal diameter (BPD).[1,5,6] Guidance to obtain these measurements is discussed later; however, because the BPD is dependent on head shape, it is more susceptible to underestimating the GA in a dolichocephalic fetus. The authors, therefore, recommend the use of the HC for fetal dating in accordance with international recommendations[6,7]; adding femur length (FL) measurement slightly improves the prediction interval of GA further.[6]

GESTATIONAL AGE ASSESSMENT IN LATE PREGNANCY

The accuracy of measurements to determine GA, such as the HC, diminish significantly with advancing gestation both as a result of natural variation and as a result of maternal and fetal disorders. It is questionable as to whether HC should be used to estimate GA beyond 24 weeks. Some recommendations are to use HC only to 25 weeks[7] whereas the Society of Obstetricians and Gynecologists of Canada and the American College of Obstetricians and Gynecologists guidance discuss the potential for using a multiple-parameter approach or considering ultrasound signs of fetal maturity and nonstandard parameters, such as the transcerebellar diameter instead of HC alone.[5,8] Recent advances also have been made in using machine learning–based approaches for GA estimation in late pregnancy.[9] More research needs to be done to clarify the best approach.

FETAL BIOMETRY: MEASURING TECHNIQUES

HC, BPD, abdominal circumference (AC), and FL are the most common parameters used for assessment of fetal size and growth.[7,10] Combinations of these parameters then can be combined to calculate an estimated fetal weight (EFW).

BIPARIETAL DIAMETER

The BPD should be measured at the thalamic level with an angle of insonation of 90° to the midline echo (**Fig. 2**). The following criteria should be met:

- The head should fill at least 30% of the monitor and be oval-shaped and symmetrical.
- The cavum septum pellucidum should be identified anteriorly, one-third along the length of the falx cerebri (midline echo).
- The thalami should be located symmetrically on each side of the midline.
- The cerebellum should not be visible.

The BPD is measured by placing calipers across the widest diameter of the skull perpendicular to the midline. Historically, measurements were made from the outer edge of the near skull echo to the inner edge of the far echo; however, as ultrasound equipment has developed, it has made increasing sense to measure from 1 outer edge to the other outer edge because this better approximates neonatal measurements. In reality, neither measurement is more reproducible than the other.[11] Although consistency with neonatal measurements suggests use of the outer to outer technique,

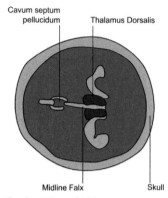
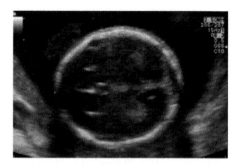

Cavum septum pellucidum   Thalamus Dorsalis

Midline Falx   Skull

Fig. 2. BPD and HC.

international standards have used both methods,[12,13] and the most important thing is that the method used for measuring is consistent with the reference charts being used.

HEAD CIRCUMFERENCE

The HC should be measured from the same image as the BPD using a cross-sectional, horizontal image at the transthalamic level. The transventricular level also can be used for measurement of the HC because it is no less reproducible than the transthalamic plane.[11] The ellipse function is recommended because it allows for a more reproducible measurement.[11] Using the ellipse function, the HC is measured by positioning the ellipse directly around the outer skull bone echoes. Alternatively the HC can be calculated from measurements of the BPD and occipitofrontal diameter (OFD) using the formula $HC_{(calculated)} = 1.62 \times (BPD + OFD)$. Using this method, the International Society of Ultrasound in Obstetrics and Gynecology (ISUOG) recommends the BPD should be measured from the outer border of the proximal edge to the inner border of the distal edge and the OFD by placing calipers in the middle of the bone echo of the occipital and frontal bones.[10]

ABDOMINAL CIRCUMFERENCE

AC is measured from a transverse section of the fetal abdomen (**Fig. 3**). The section should be magnified to fill at least 30% of the monitor and should meet the following criteria:

- Stomach bubble visible
- Umbilical vein in its anterior third or at the level of the portal sinus
- Single rib
- Kidneys and bladder should not be visible
- As close as possible to circular by avoiding distortion from applying too much pressure with the transducer

As with the HC, the AC can be measured directly using an ellipse function, or it can be calculated from the anteroposterior abdominal diameter (APAD) and transverse abdominal diameter (TAD). With both, the measurement is made around the skin line. If the AC is calculated from APAD and TAD, the APAD is measured from the skin edge covering the spine through to the anterior abdominal wall and the TAD is measured at the widest point perpendicular to the APAD. These measures are inserted into the formula $AC = \pi (APAD + TAD)/2 = 1.57 \times (APAD + TAD)$.[10]

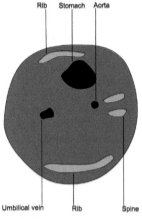
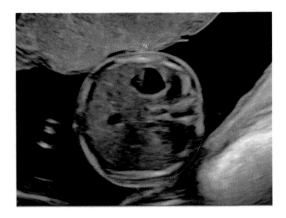

Fig. 3. AC.

FEMUR LENGTH

The femur closest to the probe is measured and should be imaged as close as possible to the horizontal plane, under magnification, so that it fills at least 30% of the monitor (**Fig. 4**). The full length of the femur should be visualized with clearly defined ends of the ossified diaphysis that can be best attained by the angle of insonation being slightly offset from 90°. The calipers are placed at either end of the diaphysis taking care to not include the distal femoral epiphysis or any artifact that could falsely extend the length.

ASSESSING FETAL GROWTH

It is conceptually important to differentiate between fetal size and fetal growth. Fetal size, measured at a singular time point during pregnancy, may identify a fetus that is SGA or LGA but says nothing about whether the fetus is meeting or exceeding its growth potential. In contrast, fetal growth is a dynamic process assessing change over time and better identifies those at risk of adverse pregnancy outcome, based on the identification of abnormal growth patterns. Assessing fetal growth is essential for the diagnosis of FGR and clearly requires maternal access to ultrasound on more than 1 occasion during pregnancy and appropriate management based on the findings.

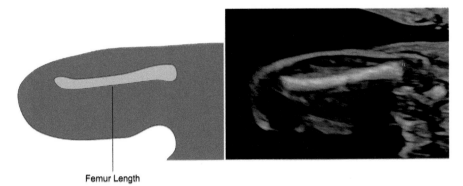

Fig. 4. FL.

The World Health Organization (WHO) Multicentre Growth Reference Study produced charts for childhood growth in 2004, which now are used routinely worldwide. Their charts are based on the principal that childhood growth is impacted predominantly by environmental and socioeconomic factors rather than genetic ones, so growth charts can be standardized across populations.[14] The INTERGROWTH-21st followed the same methodology to produce fetal growth standards so that, for the first time, it is possible to consistently compare an infant's growth and nutritional status with those of their contemporaries around the world, from in utero until the age of 5.[15] EFW as a summary measure commonly is used but this comes from a composite calculation of ultrasound measures, including errors; and it includes fat-based indicators that may be impacted by excessive nutrition.[15] A focus on a preferred measure—such as EFW—for fetal growth is unhelpful because ultrasound provides an armory of tools with which to assess fetal size and growth.[16] Therefore, individual biometric parameters as well as the calculation of the EFW should be monitored over time to assist with decision making.

CALCULATING ESTIMATED FETAL WEIGHT

There are 2 distinct steps involved in using EFW clinically. The first is calculating the EFW from ultrasound parameters. Here, it appears that the formula by Hadlock and colleagues, in 1985, remains the most accurate in estimating weight.[17–19] The second step is assessing this EFW at a given GA to calculate a percentile and to compare size (and growth over time) to standards. For this purpose, ultrasonographically estimated EFW should be used in preference to charts derived from the birth weight of premature infants[20] (**Fig. 5**).

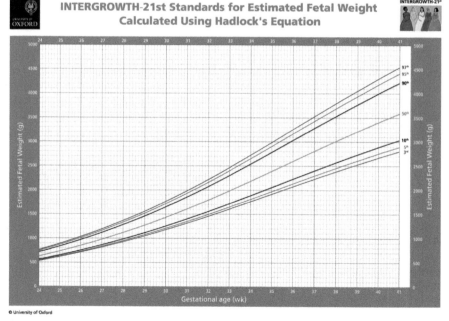

Fig. 5. INTERGROWTH-21st standards for EFW. Calculated using Hadlock's equation. (*Courtesy of* Aris T. Papageorghiou, MD, Oxford, UK.)

The formula with most widespread use for EFW (in grams)[21] is
$$EFW = 10^{(1.326 + 0.0107 \times HC + 0.0438 \times AC + 0.158 \times FL - 0.00326 \times AC \times FL)}$$

The random error of this formula is between 4.3% and 14.8%,[17] which means that at term, EFW could differ by 400 g from the actual weight. These errors reportedly are greater at the extremes of weight, such as FGR and macrosomia,[22] so interpretation in isolation should be made with caution. Although EFW constitutes a summary assessment of fetal size, it is important to comprehensively assess growth using individual parameters as well. Thus, the same EFW can be calculated from very different fetal growth phenotypes, so the extra detail provided by monitoring patterns of growth within individual parameters must not be ignored. For this reason, ISUOG recommends that EFW should not be calculated more often than every 3 weeks, although this should not preclude fetal biometry being measured more frequently as clinically indicated.[20]

There are numerous other permutations of EFW formulas available for use, but the AC is ubiquitous. Although it can be tempting to use formulas with more parameters, due to their marginally greater accuracy, it is worth remembering that the AC becomes increasingly difficult to accurately and reliably measure with advancing fetal maturity and that any errors are amplified when multiplied together, so ensuring AC measurements are more accurate is likely the best focus.[23] This again reinforces why quality assurance and audit are so important in ultrasound departments.

MODALITIES FOR DIAGNOSIS OF SMALL FOR GESTATIONAL AGE AND FETAL GROWTH RESTRICTION

Ultrasound plays an important role in the diagnosis and monitoring of the SGA fetus. Furthermore, it helps identify the etiology of FGR, for example, whether this is placenta- or nonplacenta-mediated. The ultrasound stigmata of structural and genetic anomalies or congenital infections should be assessed with a thorough fetal anatomy survey in addition to an assessment of fetal size. The assessment of size is particularly important because fetuses with EFW less than third centile are at greater risk of adverse outcome[24] and survival improves with increments in birthweight.[25] When FGR is suspected or growth surveillance is indicated, fetal growth should be monitored with serial scans and evidence of placental dysfunction and fetal redistribution identified using Doppler ultrasound.

SGA is defined by a statistical deviation of fetal size from a reference standard, with the typical threshold at the tenth centile. This differs from FGR principally because the former also encompasses many constitutionally small but healthy fetuses and because FGR may include fetuses with biometry greater than tenth centile that do not meet their growth potential. Some investigators recommend using FGR as a prenatal designation and SGA as a postnatal designation of size-for-GA in order to simplify terminology for clinical use.[8] However, defining FGR and SGA based on suspicion for compromised growth rather than size alone, as discussed in this article, provides an important conceptual distinction that can be useful to guide management.

Given the difficulties in defining FGR, an international consensus project was undertaken in 2016 to try to move the field forward, with the aims of identifying fetuses at risk, assisting future research projects, and allowing comparisons of different FGR studies. This consensus made clear that fetal size alone is insufficient for the diagnosis of FGR (unless the AC or EFW is below the third centile).[26] It also highlighted that reduced growth velocity should alert the physician to possible growth restriction.[26,27] This consensus definition moved away from defining FGR purely on size and toward including functional assessment, such as Doppler and growth over time (**Table 1**).

Table 1 Consensus-based definitions for early (<32-week) and late (≥32-week) fetal growth restriction, in the absence of congenital anomalies	
Early Fetal Growth Restriction	**Late Fetal Growth Restriction**
AC or EFW < third centile or UA-AEDF	AC or EFW < third centile
Or	*Or at least 2 out of 3 of*
1. AC or EFW < tenth centile plus	1. AC or EFW < tenth centile
2. UtA-PI > 95th centile and/or	2. AC or EFW crossing >2 quartiles on fetal growth chart[a]
3. UA-PI >95th centile	3. CPR < 5th centile or UA-PI > 95th centile

[a] This is specified as a noncustomized chart.

Data from Gordijn SJ, Beune IM, Thilaganathan B, et al. Consensus definition of fetal growth restriction: a Delphi procedure. Ultrasound in Obstetrics & Gynecology. 2016;48(3):333-339.

DOPPLER EVALUATION OF THE FETOPLACENTAL CIRCULATION

Placental insufficiency results in decreases in blood flow to the fetus that can be detected by Doppler ultrasound and that advances in a mostly predictable manner. There is likely to be a latency from the detection of any abnormality to any effect on fetal size or decompensation, which makes Doppler useful for fetal monitoring and an important area for research.[26] A better understanding of this latent period can help time the administration of corticosteroids, magnesium sulfate, referral, and delivery in a unit equipped to manage any prematurity and to determine the safest mode of delivery.

As early as the first trimester, and certainly by 21 weeks to 23 weeks, uterine artery (UtA) Doppler can be used to predict pregnancies at risk of preeclampsia and FGR. As pregnancy advances, umbilical artery (UA) Doppler demonstrates high impedance to flow between the fetus and the placenta. Fetal compensation results in preferential shunting of blood to the brain, myocardium, and adrenal glands to the cost of peripheral organs and the kidneys. The ISUOG Practice Guideline: Use of Doppler Ultrasonography in Obstetrics[28] is an excellent source of information pertaining to the safe and accurate use of Doppler.

Uterine Artery Doppler

Under normal circumstances, trophoblastic invasion results in a gradual reduction of impedance through the UtAs. This usually causes the loss of any diastolic notch (present in approximately 50% of first-trimester scans) and a reducing pulsatility index (PI) as gestation advances. There has been a move away from notching as a marker of abnormal vascular tone toward the more reliable measure of PI in predicting adverse outcomes.[29] Evidence from the SPREE and ASPRE trials demonstrated that combined first-trimester screening for preeclampsia, which includes measuring first-trimester UtA Doppler, detects approximately 50% of SGA deliveries before 37 weeks and approximately 60% of deliveries less than 32 weeks, although it is not good at detecting SGA born after 37 weeks.[30] UtA Dopplers are also measured in second and third trimesters as screening for growth restriction and preeclampsia and as part of the assessment of a fetus with suspected growth restriction.[31,32]

UtA Doppler can be measured transabdominally and transvaginally and should be quantified bilaterally. In the first trimester, the paracervical vascular plexus should be visualized lateral to the cervical canal and the artery measured at the point where it turns cranially to ascend into the uterine body. In the second trimester, using the transabdominal route, the arteries are identified where they cross the external iliac artery and measured 1 cm downstream from this point or before any bifurcation. For a second-trimester transvaginal assessment, the probe is placed into the lateral fornix and color Doppler identifies the UtA at the level of the internal cervical os. References ranges are specific to the scanning route used and should be used accordingly.[28]

Umbilical Artery Doppler

UA Doppler is the only Doppler measurement providing diagnostic and prognostic information for management of FGR.[33] Impedance to uteroplacental perfusion can be identified by an increasing PI in the UAs which may cascade to absent end-diastolic flow (AEDF) and latterly reversed end-diastolic flow (REDF). The PORTO study showed that both an EFW less than third centile and an abnormal UA Doppler (PI >95th centile or AEDF/REDF) were associated strongly with adverse perinatal outcome in SGA fetuses.[24] A Cochrane review calculated that monitoring UA Doppler in high risk pregnancies may reduce perinatal deaths by 29%,[34] although UA Dopplers are not a good marker of milder placental disease, such as in many late-onset FGR fetuses. In late FGR, a normal UA Doppler may give false reassurance because 20% of fetuses showed evidence of brain sparing despite normal UA Doppler.[32]

Impedance is highest at the fetal end and of the UA and AEDF/REDF is likely to be first seen at this site.[28] A free loop of cord is recommended for obtaining UA Doppler waveforms. If Doppler flow is away from the probe, it is not necessary to invert the Doppler display,[28] but the baseline should be adjusted to see the complete waveform; effort should be made to avoid pick up of venous flow from the neighboring umbilical vein.

Middle Cerebral Artery Doppler

The middle cerebral artery (MCA) Doppler is obtained from an axial section of the brain showing the thalami and sphenoid bone wings. Color flow mapping should be used to identify the circle of Willis into which the pulsed wave Doppler gate should be positioned over the proximal third of the MCA close to its origin with the internal carotid artery. The angle of insonation should be as close to $0°$ as possible. The sampling location and angle are significant because the velocity decreases with distance from the point of origin and increasing angles increase the error. This is important particularly when using raw velocity measurements, such as when using MCA-peak systolic velocity to detect fetal anemia.[28]

A reduction in MCA-PI is an indicator of brain sparing but the detection of changes is less sensitive than when calculating the cerebroplacental ratio (CPR), which is the MCA-PI divided by the UA-PI, or umbilicocerebral ratio (UCR), the opposite calculation of CPR. MCA-PI less than fifth centile and an increased UCR both have been shown to be associated with poorer outcomes.[35] A progressive reduction of the CPR has been shown in late SGA fetuses approaching delivery[32] and is a good predictor for perinatal death, whereas a normal CPR can differentiate fetuses accurately with suspected growth restriction who are not at increased risk of death.[36] Contrary to previous thought that CPR was useful only for monitoring late-onset FGR, a meta-analysis by Conde-Agudelo and colleagues[36] also showed that CPR may have higher predictive accuracy for adverse outcome among early-onset FGR rather than late-onset FGR. More research is needed to better understand the role of MCA Doppler in screening and monitoring for FGR, and randomized controlled trials currently are under way to ascertain whether MCA Doppler can be used to time delivery.[35]

Ductus Venosus Doppler

The TRUFFLE trial sought to differentiate between whether delivery triggered by reduced short-term variability during cardiotocograph (CTG) monitoring; a ductus venosus (DV)-PI greater than 95th centile; or the loss or reversal of the a-wave in the DV waveform was associated with better outcomes in early-onset FGR. Neurodevelopmental outcome at 2 years among surviving infants was significantly better in the group randomized to delivery with a-wave changes.[37] Whether these a-wave changes are due to venous dilatation to increase blood flow to the heart or because of high cardiac afterload from increased vascular placental resistance cannot be certain,[27] but DV Doppler is the strongest single parameter to predict fetal death in early-onset FGR.[33]

The DV connects the intra-abdominal portion of the umbilical vein to the inferior vena cava just below the diaphragm. It is identified from a midsagittal longitudinal plane or an oblique transverse plane through the upper abdomen. Color flow should be used to demonstrate the higher velocity flow at the narrowed entrance to the DV from whence the Doppler measurement should be sampled; velocities usually are between 55 cm/s and 90 cm/s.

Summary of Key Points in Obtaining Adequate Doppler

Of utmost importance is to remember the as low as reasonably achievable (ALARA) principle. Doppler, especially color Doppler, increases the total power emitted and increases the thermal index, potentially exposing the fetus to harmful levels of ultrasound energy.[28] The TI should be kept less than or equal to 1.0 with exposure time as short as possible and certainly under an hour.[28]

- Obtain measurements during fetal quiescence in the absence of fetal breathing wherever possible.
- The optimal angle of insonation is complete alignment with the blood flow as small deviations can cause significant velocity errors that angle correction may not adequately correct for. Power Doppler is less impacted by this than pulsed wave Doppler.
- Doppler horizontal sweep speed should display 4 to 6 and no more than 10 waveforms.
- The peak velocity of the waveform should fit at least 75% of the Doppler screen.
- Wider sampling gates are preferable to ensure maximum velocities are recorded, but, if interference from other vessels is experienced, then the gate can be narrowed.
- PI shows a linear correlation with vascular resistance and does not approach infinity in AEDF/REDF, so is used most commonly in practice.
- Caution should be exercised using wall motion filters to eliminate low frequency noise because they can spuriously create an impression of AEDF.
- If color is used, the frame rate is reduced with increasing box size so the smallest boxes possible should be used. The velocity scale or pulse repetition frequency should be adjusted to the real color velocity of the vessels of interest so that low velocity vessels are visible and high-velocity vessels are not impacted by aliasing.

AMNIOTIC FLUID ASSESSMENT

A reduction in amniotic fluid can be indicative of reduced blood flow to the fetal kidneys and chronic hypoxia as part of the brain-sparing effect of reduced placental perfusion. Although oligohydramnios is associated with adverse fetal outcome, studies have not shown that it is significantly beneficial in classifying SGA fetuses as having a higher incidence of adverse outcome; but fetuses with oligohydramnios did have a higher incidence of neonatal intensive care unit admission if EFW was less than third centile or fifth centile.[24] Assessment of liquor (fluid) volume also constitutes part of the biophysical profile (BPP).

Although the abnormalities in amniotic fluid are strongly associated with poor outcome,[38] they do not accurately predict outcome risk for individuals; the most likely reason is the poor reproducibility of measurement.[39] Amniotic fluid levels can be assessed using a measurement of the maximum vertical pocket (MVP) of amniotic fluid or from the calculation of the amniotic fluid index (AFI). There is a range of definitions, but most commonly oligohydramnios is defined as a MVP of less than 2 cm or an AFI less than 5 cm. In order to measure a pocket of liquor:

- Hold the probe at 90° to the floor.
- Scan over abdomen to find the deepest pocket of amniotic fluid.
- Ensure that there is no cord within the pocket to be measured.
- Measure deepest pocket depth from the edge of the uterus or placenta straight down to the fetal part.

If the AFI is being measured, the maternal abdomen is divided into 4 quadrants and the total of the deepest pockets in each of the 4 quadrants is calculated.

At term, use of MVP less than 2 cm to define oligohydramnios is favored over AFI less than 5 cm becuase AFI led to more labor inductions without any improvement in outcomes over MVP in 1 multicenter RCT of 1052 women in Germany.[40]

BIOPHYSICAL PROFILE

The BPP score is calculated from an ultrasound evaluation of fetal breathing, limb or body movements, tone, and the deepest pocket of amniotic fluid plus a nonstress CTG test. At least 30 seconds of breathing movements should be seen during a 30-minute time frame as well as 3 or more body movements and at least 1 episode of flexion and extension of a fetal limb or the hand. These findings should be accompanied by a single vertical pool depth of 2 cm or more to score maximum points for the ultrasound part of the test. It can be a useful assessment in late FGR and carries the same weight for recommended delivery as AEDF/REDF delivery if BPP is less than or equal to 4.[27]

OTHER MODALITIES

In medicine it is rare for a single investigation to suffice for both diagnosis and management; the same can be said for the use of ultrasound in the prediction, diagnosis, and management of FGR. The TRUFFLE trial had a computerized CTG safety net for all arms of the trial, triggering delivery for 23% and 33% of fetuses in the 2 DV arms.[37] The transferability of the trial's findings is limited to units with access to computerized CTG unless evidence can be gathered to show that standard CTG and/or BPP could be beneficial. Biomarkers are of considerable interest, particularly to screen for FGR, such as work from the Fetal Medicine Foundation looking at placental growth factor in combination with UtA Doppler to predict preeclampsia and FGR.[30]

DIAGNOSIS OF LARGE FOR GESTATIONAL AGE

Antenatal prediction of macrosomia is notoriously poor and is not helped by the lack of consensus regarding a definition of LGA: EFW greater than 90th centile for GA, greater than 4 kg, or greater than 4.5 kg, or something else entirely? A birthweight over 4.5 kg clearly is associated with an increase in both maternal and neonatal morbidity and mortality, but this increase also has been demonstrated for fetuses weighing over 4 kg in diabetic mothers. Furthermore controversy remains as to whether fetuses should be screened for macrosomia because (1) ultrasound diagnosis is unreliable, (2) 90% of LGA fetuses do not have any complications, and (3) prevention by earlier induction of labor or cesarean section may or may not be of benefit.[23] A recent meta-analysis[41] suggested that induction of labor at 37 weeks to 40 weeks in fetuses identified as macrosomic after 37 weeks' gestation would reduce the rates of shoulder dystocia and fractures. It did not, however, find a reduction in the more concerning outcomes of brachial plexus injury and intraventricular hemorrhage, and an important conclusion was made that there is a need for further research on induction of labor for suspected fetal macrosomia, including on improving the accuracy of the diagnosis.

It seems intuitive that a LGA EFW should correlate well with an LGA birthweight and also that the AC is a logical marker for increased adiposity. A recent review sought to identify which definition of LGA was better associated with fetal macrosomia and associated complications in low and mixed-risk populations.[42] Suspected LGA was defined as EFW greater than 4 kg or greater than 90th centile or an AC greater than 36 cm or greater than 90th centile. The most commonly used formula only had a 55.2% sensitivity for a birthweight greater than 4 kg, and AC greater than 36 cm or greater than 90th centile had a sensitivity of 57.8%. Using any of the formulas tested, an EFW greater than 4 kg or greater than 90th centile had a 67.5% sensitivity for an outcome of birthweight greater than 4.5 kg or greater than 97th centile and only 22% for shoulder dystocia. The meta-analysis was impacted by significant heterogeneity, and there were insufficient data to assess other adverse outcomes.[42] Another study showed that the best performing EFW formula for predicting birthweight greater than 4 kg in diabetic mothers only had a sensitivity of 45%.[43]

As with the distinction between SGA fetuses and those with growth restriction, it also has been suggested that there may need to be better differentiators between LGA fetuses at greater risk of complications and those that are not.[42] A review by Robinson and colleagues[44] has suggested that other markers, such as AC to HC difference greater than 50 mm and AD minus BPD greater than or equal to 2.6 cm, may have higher positive predictive value for adverse outcomes in fetuses with suspected macrosomia. The measurement of fetal limb volumes and other soft tissue markers, such as abdominal adiposity, may assist with this distinction but as yet have not been substantiated. LGA is associated with polyhydramnios (which again has numerous definitions), especially in the case of maternal diabetes, but raised amniotic fluid volume is not predictive of LGA; rather it is the combination of oligohydramnios and an EFW less than 90th centile that can almost exclude the possibility of LGA.[45]

THREE-DIMENSIONAL ULTRASONOGRAPHY AND MAGNETIC RESONANCE IMAGING

Technological advances mean that 3-D ultrasound and MRI use is more commonplace. Fractional limb volumes can be obtained using 3-D, and an equation combining 2-D biometry of the BPD, AC, and thigh volume has been demonstrated to be a better predictor of EFW greater than 4 kg than Hadlock's 1985 formula[21] in fetuses of women with gestational diabetes.

The use of MRI is an emerging field but without evidence to substantiate MRI-based EFW as more sensitive than ultrasonography for detecting macrosomia.[46] Perhaps of greater significance will be the role of functional MRI in assessing placental function, but this is very much an area under research.[47]

REPRODUCIBILITY AND QUALITY ASSURANCE OF ULTRASOUND MEASUREMENTS

The quality and reproducibility of fetal measurements rely on

1. Well maintained and accurate machines and measurement software
2. Appropriate selection of measurement charts
3. The quality of image plane acquisition and measurement[48]

It is likely that the significant methodological heterogeneity between different studies contributes significantly to the wide variation in centiles for both biometry and Doppler measurements.[4,49,50] It is recommended that ultrasound departments have robust procedures in place for image storage, review, and scoring and have a process for assessing the intraobserver and interobserver variability as a means to assess reproducibility.[51] Image scoring systems for fetal biometry are now used to assess the quality of images acquired[52] rather than subjective assessment alone. These scoring systems and quantitative assessment, comparing z-score distributions between measured and expected biometry measurements, are a useful means of assessing quality. They have been demonstrated to assist training and to improve the consistency of measurements by even experienced sonographers in standardization exercises.[53] Similar scoring systems have been developed for Doppler assessment,[54,55] but only the scoring systems for UA and UtA Doppler demonstrated significantly greater agreement between reviewers than subjective assessment alone.[54]

KEY CONSIDERATIONS IN A GLOBAL CONTEXT: CHALLENGES FOR WIDESPREAD ULTRASOUND USE

The greatest burden of neonatal morbidity and mortality is shouldered by LMICs, and significant efforts need to be made in these countries to achieve the WHO Sustainable Development Goal to reduce neonatal mortality to under 12 per 1000 by 2030. To help meet this target, the WHO published antenatal care recommendations, which included the recommendation that all women have an ultrasound before 24 weeks' gestation.[56] The implementation of this recommendation is not without significant challenges, added to which the assessment of fetal growth in LMICs must be considered carefully within a global context.

International standards for fetal and childhood growth can facilitate better population-level comparisons between countries and identify key areas for targeted interventions to optimize fetal growth and reduce under 5 morbidity and mortality.[13,14] The INTERGROWTH-21st project followed the same methodology as the WHO Multicentre Growth Reference Study to create an international fetal growth standard, believing that it is an injustice if local reference charts misclassify any SGA fetus as normally grown because this would normalize impaired growth due to maternal malnutrition and disease.[15] The prevalence of SGA can be seen to vary enormously from one country to the next (**Fig. 6**) and would be concealed if local reference charts simply classified the smallest 10% of fetuses as SGA, thus potentially depriving many of the world's estimated 23.3 million SGA neonates access to better health care.[15]

Although routine ultrasound use has not been shown to improve pregnancy outcomes,[57] there remains hope that it may have a greater role in LMICs in diagnosing and guiding the management of fetal problems if its use can be more widely implemented in conjunction with improvements to health care provision. There are many barriers to more widespread use of ultrasound in LMICs. These were investigated in a survey spanning 44 different countries, which identified a lack of training, lack and cost of equipment (both obtaining and maintenance), lack of maintenance, and lack of power as some of the major issues.[58]

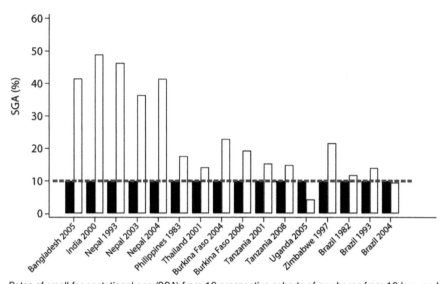

Rates of small for gestational age (SGA) from 16 prospective cohorts of newborns from 10 low- and middle-income countries. Empty columns show prevalence of SGA using INTERGROWTH-21st standards,[47] compared with effect of using fixed cut-off SGA rate of 10% that would result from using local reference charts (black columns). Data from Kozuki et al.[56]

Fig. 6. Rates of SGA from 16 prospective cohorts of newborns from 10 LMICs using INTER-GROWTH-21st standards. (*From* Papageorghiou AT, Kennedy SH, Salomon LJ, Altman DG, Ohuma EO, et. al; International Fetal and Newborn Growth Consortium for the 21(st) Century (INTERGROWTH-21(st)). The INTERGROWTH-21st fetal growth standards: toward the global integration of pregnancy and pediatric care. Am J Obstet Gynecol. 2018 Feb;218(2S):S630-S640. https://doi.org/10.1016/j.ajog.2018.01.011. PMID: 29422205.)

In recent years, the cost of portable devices has reduced significantly; however, their use is impeded in countries like India where sex determination is illegal and ultrasound machine use is highly regulated. Notwithstanding this limitation, less expensive and more portable probes, that can be synced with a mobile phone or tablet, are likely to be most efficacious in improving access to ultrasound, but their usage needs to be combined with the ability to acquire and interpret images.

Training of personnel to perform ultrasound scans is vital if the WHO recommendation is to be realized. A review by Kim and colleagues[59] identified several studies, which demonstrated that task-shifting and intensive training programs can equip community health professionals, who usually would not have training in ultrasound, with the skills needed to provide ultrasound services that improved clinical management. There has also been growing interest in the use of simplified obstetric sweep protocols in conjunction with telemedicine services[60] and automation technology[61] to reduce the training required to acquire useful information. Nevertheless, with the current diagnostic recommendations for FGR,[26] it will be impossible to distinguish between SGA and FGR unless women can access providers trained to measure fetal Dopplers.

Achieving universal access to early ultrasound dating and the identification of multiple pregnancy is most likely the goal that could have the greatest impact on pregnancy outcomes. Many women in sub-Saharan Africa do not have any antenatal care until late in the second trimester or even third trimester, and ultrasound dating is inherently unreliable for GA determination at this stage.[5] For the 30% to 40% of women who are unsure of their LMP, SFH measurements are unlikely to be an effective screening tool because it is all too tempting to readjust expected delivery dates based on significant deviations from what is expected. But the lack of an early ultrasound has many implications that are not limited to problems regarding the smaller-than-expected uterus. As seen by 1 of the authors (AS) in a setting where no ultrasound was available, a woman was relatively sure of her dates, clinically measured LGA at term, and was delivered by cesarean section, only for premature twins to be delivered and die several days later. These 2 very preventable deaths could have had a different outcome had an ultrasound scan provided a correct GA, had the twins been identified, and had steroids been given in preparation for a preterm delivery if still indicated.

Inevitably the diagnosis of in utero problems can prove of benefit only if the surrounding infrastructure can enable optimal management of the identified problem; premature delivery to prevent a stillbirth is no help if there is inadequate provision of neonatal care to optimize the chance of intact survival. In Goldenberg and colleagues'[57] words: "We conclude that without improvement in the quality of care at health facilities in LMIC, there appears to be limited impact of routine ANC use of US alone."

SUMMARY

Antenatal imaging plays a crucial role in the management of high-risk pregnancies. Accurate dating is a core pillar of antenatal care and relies on the acquisition of reliable and reproducible ultrasound images and measurements. The same principle of quality image acquisition is necessary for assessing fetal growth and performing Doppler measurements to help diagnose pregnancy complications, stratify risk, and guide management. Regular quality assessment within ultrasound departments is necessary to achieve these aims. Further research is needed in order to ascertain whether current methods for estimating fetal weight can be improved with 3-D ultrasound or MRI; optimize dating of those with late initiation of prenatal care to minimize underdiagnosis of FGR; and identify the best strategies to make ultrasound more available in LMICs.

CLINICS CARE POINTS

- CRL should be used to date pregnancies until the fetus is 84 mm in length; thereafter, HC is recommended until 24 weeks.[6,7]
- Measurement techniques should be the same as those for the charts used to assess size.[20]
- All Doppler measurements should be taken with the angle of insonation as close to 0° as possible to minimize error.[28]
- Practitioners performing biometry and Doppler measurements should undergo regular quality control checks and undergo retraining if images of insufficient quality or measurements persistently outside acceptable levels of agreement.[20]
- Global health ultrasound initiatives must be developed in conjunction with improvements to medical infrastructures.[57]

DISCLOSURE

A.T. Papageorghiou is a Senior Advisor of Intelligent Ultrasound. No other competing interests are declared. A.T. Papageorghiou is supported by the Oxford Partnership

Comprehensive Biomedical Research Centre with funding from the NIHR Biomedical Research Centre (BRC) funding scheme. The funding sources had no involvement at any stage of research from design, conduct, to writing.

REFERENCES

1. Taipale P, Hiilesmaa V. Predicting delivery date by ultrasound and last menstrual period in early gestation. Obstet Gynecol 2001;97(2):189–94.
2. Høgberg U, Larsson N. Early dating by ultrasound and perinatal outcome. A cohort study. Acta Obstet Gynecol Scand 1997;76(10):907–12.
3. Hadlock FP, Shah YP, Kanon DJ, et al. Fetal crown-rump length: reevaluation of relation to menstrual age (5-18 weeks) with high-resolution real-time US. Radiology 1992;182(2):501–5.
4. Napolitano R, Dhami J, Ohuma EO, et al. Pregnancy dating by fetal crown-rump length: a systematic review of charts. BJOG 2014;121(5):556–65.
5. Butt K, Lim KI. Guideline No. 388-determination of gestational age by ultrasound. J Obstet Gynaecol Can 2019;41(10):1497–507.
6. Salomon LJ, Alfirevic Z, Bilardo CM, et al. ISUOG practice guidelines: performance of first-trimester fetal ultrasound scan. Ultrasound Obstet Gynecol 2013; 41(1):102–13.
7. Loughna P, Chitty L, Evans T, et al. Fetal size and dating: charts recommended for clinical obstetric practice. Ultrasound 2009;17(3):160–6.
8. Committee Opinion No 700: methods for estimating the due date. Obstet Gynecol 2017;129(5):e150–4.
9. Fung R, Villar J, Dashti A, et al. Achieving accurate estimates of fetal gestational age and personalised predictions of fetal growth based on data from an international prospective cohort study: a population-based machine learning study. Lancet Digit Health 2020;2(7):e368–75.
10. Salomon LJ, Alfirevic Z, Berghella V, et al. Practice guidelines for performance of the routine mid-trimester fetal ultrasound scan. Ultrasound Obstet Gynecol 2011; 37(1):116–26.
11. Napolitano R, Donadono V, Ohuma EO, et al. Scientific basis for standardization of fetal head measurements by ultrasound: a reproducibility study. Ultrasound Obstet Gynecol 2016;48(1):80–5.
12. Papageorghiou AT, Ohuma EO, Altman DG, et al. International standards for fetal growth based on serial ultrasound measurements: the Fetal Growth Longitudinal Study of the INTERGROWTH-21st Project. Lancet 2014;384(9946):869–79.
13. Kiserud T, Piaggio G, Carroli G, et al. The World Health Organization fetal growth charts: a multinational longitudinal study of ultrasound biometric measurements and estimated fetal weight. PLoS Med 2017;14(1):e1002220.
14. Who Multicentre Growth Reference Study G, de Onis M. WHO Child Growth Standards based on length/height, weight and age. Acta Paediatr 2006;95(S450): 76–85.
15. Papageorghiou AT, Kennedy SH, Salomon LJ, et al. The INTERGROWTH-21(st) fetal growth standards: toward the global integration of pregnancy and pediatric care. Am J Obstet Gynecol 2018;218(2s):S630–40.
16. Stirnemann J, Villar J, Salomon LJ, et al. International estimated fetal weight standards of the INTERGROWTH-21(st) Project. Ultrasound Obstet Gynecol 2017; 49(4):478–86.
17. Milner J, Arezina J. The accuracy of ultrasound estimation of fetal weight in comparison to birth weight: a systematic review. Ultrasound 2018;26(1):32–41.

18. Dudley NJ. A systematic review of the ultrasound estimation of fetal weight. Ultrasound Obstet Gynecol 2005;25(1):80–9.
19. Monier I, Ego A, Benachi A, et al. Comparison of the Hadlock and INTERGROWTH formulas for calculating estimated fetal weight in a preterm population in France. Am J Obstet Gynecol 2018;219(5):476.e471.
20. Salomon LJ, Alfirevic Z, Da Silva Costa F, et al. ISUOG Practice Guidelines: ultrasound assessment of fetal biometry and growth. Ultrasound Obstet Gynecol 2019;53(6):715–23.
21. Hadlock FP, Harrist RB, Sharman RS, et al. Estimation of fetal weight with the use of head, body, and femur measurements–a prospective study. Am J Obstet Gynecol 1985;151(3):333–7.
22. Ben-Haroush A, Yogev Y, Bar J, et al. Accuracy of sonographically estimated fetal weight in 840 women with different pregnancy complications prior to induction of labor. Ultrasound Obstet Gynecol 2004;23(2):172–6.
23. Nyberg DA, Abuhamad A, Ville Y. Ultrasound assessment of abnormal fetal growth. Semin Perinatol 2004;28(1):3–22.
24. Unterscheider J, Daly S, Geary MP, et al. Optimizing the definition of intrauterine growth restriction: the multicenter prospective PORTO Study. Am J Obstet Gynecol 2013;208(4):290, e291-296.
25. Hack M, Horbar JD, Malloy MH, et al. Very low birth weight outcomes of the National Institute of Child Health and Human Development Neonatal Network. Pediatrics 1991;87(5):587–97.
26. Gordijn SJ, Beune IM, Thilaganathan B, et al. Consensus definition of fetal growth restriction: a Delphi procedure. Ultrasound Obstet Gynecol 2016;48(3):333–9.
27. Lees CC, Stampalija T, Baschat A, et al. ISUOG Practice Guidelines: diagnosis and management of small-for-gestational-age fetus and fetal growth restriction. Ultrasound Obstet Gynecol 2020;56(2):298–312.
28. Bhide A, Acharya G, Bilardo CM, et al. ISUOG practice guidelines: use of Doppler ultrasonography in obstetrics. Ultrasound Obstet Gynecol 2013;41(2):233–9.
29. Khong SL, Kane SC, Brennecke SP, et al. First-trimester uterine artery Doppler analysis in the prediction of later pregnancy complications. Dis Markers 2015;2015:679730.
30. Tan MY, Poon LC, Rolnik DL, et al. Prediction and prevention of small-for-gestational-age neonates: evidence from SPREE and ASPRE. Ultrasound Obstet Gynecol 2018;52(1):52–9.
31. Vergani P, Roncaglia N, Andreotti C, et al. Prognostic value of uterine artery Doppler velocimetry in growth-restricted fetuses delivered near term. Am J Obstet Gynecol 2002;187(4):932–6.
32. Oros D, Figueras F, Cruz-Martinez R, et al. Longitudinal changes in uterine, umbilical and fetal cerebral Doppler indices in late-onset small-for-gestational age fetuses. Ultrasound Obstet Gynecol 2011;37(2):191–5.
33. Figueras F, Gratacós E. Update on the diagnosis and classification of fetal growth restriction and proposal of a stage-based management protocol. Fetal Diagn Ther 2014;36(2):86–98.
34. Alfirevic Z, Stampalija T, Dowswell T. Fetal and umbilical Doppler ultrasound in high-risk pregnancies. Cochrane Database Syst Rev 2017;6(6):Cd007529.
35. Stampalija T, Thornton J, Marlow N, et al. Fetal cerebral Doppler changes and outcome in late preterm fetal growth restriction: prospective cohort study. Ultrasound Obstet Gynecol 2020;56(2):173–81.

36. Conde-Agudelo A, Villar J, Kennedy SH, et al. Predictive accuracy of cerebropla-cental ratio for adverse perinatal and neurodevelopmental outcomes in sus-pected fetal growth restriction: systematic review and meta-analysis. Ultrasound Obstet Gynecol 2018;52(4):430–41.

37. Bilardo CM, Hecher K, Visser GHA, et al. Severe fetal growth restriction at 26-32 weeks: key messages from the TRUFFLE study. Ultrasound Obstet Gynecol 2017;50(3):285–90.

38. Morris RK, Meller CH, Tamblyn J, et al. Association and prediction of amniotic fluid measurements for adverse pregnancy outcome: systematic review and meta-analysis. BJOG 2014;121(6):686–99.

39. Sande JA, Ioannou C, Sarris I, et al. Reproducibility of measuring amniotic fluid index and single deepest vertical pool throughout gestation. Prenat Diagn 2015;35(5):434–9.

40. Kehl S, Schelkle A, Thomas A, et al. Single deepest vertical pocket or amniotic fluid index as evaluation test for predicting adverse pregnancy outcome (SAFE trial): a multicenter, open-label, randomized controlled trial. Ultrasound Obstet Gynecol 2016;47(6):674–9.

41. Boulvain M, Irion O, Dowswell T, et al. Induction of labour at or near term for sus-pected fetal macrosomia. Cochrane Database Syst Rev 2016;2016(5):Cd000938.

42. Moraitis AA, Shreeve N, Sovio U, et al. Universal third-trimester ultrasonic screening using fetal macrosomia in the prediction of adverse perinatal outcome: a systematic review and meta-analysis of diagnostic test accuracy. PLoS Med 2020;17(10):e1003190.

43. Combs CA, Rosenn B, Miodovnik M, et al. Sonographic EFW and macrosomia: is there an optimum formula to predict diabetic fetal macrosomia? J Maternal-Fetal Med 2000;9(1):55–61.

44. Robinson R, Walker KF, White VA, et al. The test accuracy of antenatal ultrasound definitions of fetal macrosomia to predict birth injury: a systematic review. Eur J Obstet Gynecol Reprod Biol 2020;246:79–85.

45. Benson CB, Coughlin BF, Doubilet PM. Amniotic fluid volume in large-for-gestational-age fetuses of nondiabetic mothers. J Ultrasound Med 1991;10(3):149–51.

46. Malin GL, Bugg GJ, Takwoingi Y, et al. Antenatal magnetic resonance imaging versus ultrasound for predicting neonatal macrosomia: a systematic review and meta-analysis. BJOG 2016;123(1):77–88.

47. Siauve N, Chalouhi GE, Deloison B, et al. Functional imaging of the human placenta with magnetic resonance. Am J Obstet Gynecol 2015;213(4 Suppl):S103–14.

48. O'Gorman N, Salomon LJ. Fetal biometry to assess the size and growth of the fetus. Best Pract Res Clin Obstet Gynaecol 2018;49:3–15.

49. Ioannou C, Talbot K, Ohuma E, et al. Systematic review of methodology used in ultrasound studies aimed at creating charts of fetal size. BJOG 2012;119(12):1425–39.

50. Oros D, Ruiz-Martinez S, Staines-Urias E, et al. Reference ranges for Doppler indices of umbilical and fetal middle cerebral arteries and cerebroplacental ratio: systematic review. Ultrasound Obstet Gynecol 2019;53(4):454–64.

51. Sarris I, Ioannou C, Ohuma EO, et al. Standardisation and quality control of ultra-sound measurements taken in the INTERGROWTH-21st Project. BJOG 2013;120(Suppl 2):33–7, v.

52. Salomon LJ, Bernard JP, Duyme M, et al. Feasibility and reproducibility of an image-scoring method for quality control of fetal biometry in the second trimester. Ultrasound Obstet Gynecol 2006;27(1):34–40.
53. Sarris I, Ioannou C, Dighe M, et al. Standardization of fetal ultrasound biometry measurements: improving the quality and consistency of measurements. Ultrasound Obstet Gynecol 2011;38(6):681–7.
54. Molloholli M, Napolitano R, Ohuma EO, et al. Image-scoring system for umbilical and uterine artery pulsed-wave Doppler ultrasound measurement. Ultrasound Obstet Gynecol 2019;53(2):251–5.
55. Ruiz-Martinez S, Volpe G, Vannuccini S, et al. An objective scoring method to evaluate image quality of middle cerebral artery Doppler. J Matern Fetal Neonatal Med 2020;33(3):421–6.
56. WHO. WHO Guidelines Approved by the Guidelines Review Committee. In: WHO recommendations on antenatal care for a positive pregnancy experience. Geneva: World Health Organization; 2016.
57. Goldenberg RL, Nathan RO, Swanson D, et al. Routine antenatal ultrasound in low- and middle-income countries: first look - a cluster randomised trial. BJOG 2018;125(12):1591–9.
58. Shah S, Bellows BA, Adedipe AA, et al. Perceived barriers in the use of ultrasound in developing countries. Crit Ultrasound J 2015;7(1):28.
59. Kim ET, Singh K, Moran A, et al. Obstetric ultrasound use in low and middle income countries: a narrative review. Reprod Health 2018;15(1):129.
60. Marini TJ, Oppenheimer DC, Baran TM, et al. New ultrasound telediagnostic system for low-resource areas. J Ultrasound Med 2020;40(3):583–95.
61. van den Heuvel TLA, Petros H, Santini S, et al. Automated fetal head detection and circumference estimation from free-hand ultrasound sweeps using deep learning in resource-limited countries. Ultrasound Med Biol 2019;45(3):773–85.

Routine Third Trimester Sonogram: Friend or Foe

Katie Stephens, MBChB, Alexandros Moraitis, MD,
Gordon C.S. Smith, DSc*

KEYWORDS

- Ultrasound • Stillbirth • Fetal growth restriction • Doppler • Screening
- Fetal presentation • Large for gestational age • Small for gestational age

KEY POINTS

- Universal ultrasound could increase prenatal diagnosis of some conditions, such as small and large for gestational age fetuses (SGA and LGA respectively).
- Implementation of screening has the potential to cause harm through unnecessary intervention in women who screen false positive.
- The evidence around screening and intervening on the basis of ultrasonic SGA or LGA is weak, but combining ultrasound with other markers, such as blood biomarkers, may result in clinically effective screening and intervention.
- Consideration should be given to the immediate implementation of universal screening for breech presentation near term and this could be achieved using point-of-care ultrasound.

BACKGROUND

Ultrasound scans are widely used in the third trimester to identify and manage pregnancy complications with the aim of optimizing pregnancy outcomes. The 2 main strategies currently used are routine and selective ultrasonography. A routine third trimester ultrasound screening policy means all women are offered an obstetric ultrasound scan at a defined gestation in the third trimester. When a selective strategy is adopted, ultrasound scans are offered in the third trimester in a targeted manner, based on clinical indications, such as previous pregnancy history, current symptoms, or examination findings in the third trimester.[1]

Many different parameters can be measured during a third trimester ultrasound scan. In this review, we consider the parameters most frequently reported, which include the estimated fetal weight (EFW), fetal presentation, amniotic fluid volume,

Funding: none.
Department of Obstetrics and Gynaecology, University of Cambridge, Box 223, The Rosie Hospital, Robinson Way, Cambridge CB2 0SW, United Kingdom
* Corresponding author.
E-mail address: gcss2@cam.ac.uk

Obstet Gynecol Clin N Am 48 (2021) 359–369
https://doi.org/10.1016/j.ogc.2021.02.006
0889-8545/21/© 2021 Elsevier Inc. All rights reserved.

obgyn.theclinics.com

and Doppler measurements, which estimate downstream resistance to blood flow, for example, in the umbilical artery and middle cerebral artery.

Before considering the use of routine third trimester ultrasound, it is vital to consider the elements of an effective screening test. An effective screening test ideally has a high sensitivity, where the test correctly identifies a high proportion of the affected population. Screening tests need to have high specificity to ensure low-risk women are not incorrectly classified as high risk. Incorrect classification as high risk may result in unnecessary intervention in an uncomplicated pregnancy. Finally, for a screening test to have a benefit to a population, there needs to be a proven disease-modifying intervention. A trial of a screening test may not demonstrate benefits either because the test does not identify truly high-risk women, or because there is no effective intervention to mitigate the risk.

Meta-analyses focusing on the use of routine third trimester ultrasonography have demonstrated no benefit to mother or baby.[2,3] The largest Cochrane review to date, included 13 randomized control trials and 35,000 women.[2] A meta-analysis is generally considered the highest level of evidence; however, it is important to interpret the conclusions of this meta-analysis with caution due to multiple limitations.[4] The meta-analysis included studies with different definitions of screen positive. For example, many studies analyzed a variant of estimated fetal size, whereas one study only considered assessment of placental calcification. Combining these studies in a single analysis assumes comparable effectiveness of all methods to predict the given outcome, which is unlikely to be the case. Moreover, none of the trials coupled a positive result to a disease-modifying intervention; a requirement to see a benefit of screening. The Cochrane review included all studies in which routine ultrasound scanning was completed after 24 weeks. The systematic review and meta-analysis undertaken by Al-Hafez and colleagues[3] has begun to address this issue by only including those studies in which an ultrasound was completed in the third trimester, but the timing and number of ultrasound scans remains varied. The specific timing of the ultrasound scan in the third trimester is likely to be important to maximize sensitivity and specificity and to ensure that the benefits of intervention outweigh possible harm, largely due to complications associated with preterm delivery. Finally, current meta-analyses are underpowered to detect an effect of routine ultrasound on perinatal mortality; there will be a tendency for all underpowered studies to report a negative result.[2,3]

FRIEND
Prevention of Undiagnosed Breech Presentation

Breech presentation affects 2% to 4% of all term pregnancies.[5,6] The clearest benefit of routine third trimester ultrasonography is unambiguously to determine fetal presentation at the time of ultrasound scan. In a prospective cohort study of women in Cambridge, UK, the Pregnancy Outcome Prediction study (POPs), all participants had a presentation scan reported at 36 weeks of gestational age. In this study no women presented in labor with an undiagnosed breech presentation following a late third trimester ultrasound scan.[7] When a breech presentation is identified, there is a chance of spontaneous version to a cephalic presentation in the interval between the ultrasound scan and delivery; however, this reduces with advancing gestation and when an ultrasound scan is completed at term, 97% will remain breech until the time of delivery.[8]

When a selective ultrasound policy is followed, the initial screening test for a noncephalic presentation is abdominal palpation close to term.[9] Where there is a suspicion of a noncephalic presentation, an ultrasound scan is offered. Abdominal palpation has a 57% to 70% sensitivity for identifying a breech presentation.[10,11] Determining the presentation before the onset of labor is important, given that when a breech presentation is identified in labor the only options for delivery are a vaginal breech delivery or an emergency cesarean delivery (**Fig. 1**). A vaginal breech delivery is associated with an increased risk of severe complications including umbilical cord compression and fetal head entrapment following delivery of the fetal body.[8,12] Given these risks, most women with an undiagnosed breech presentation in labor would be delivered by an emergency cesarean. However, this is not a risk-free approach, as an emergency cesarean delivery results in increased morbidity and mortality for the mother and infant and increased costs compared with an elective cesarean delivery.[7,13] For women identified as having a breech presentation before the onset of labor, there are clearly defined interventions to reduce the associated risks (summarized in **Fig. 1**).[9] First, external cephalic version can be offered, wherein the clinician attempts to manipulate the fetus manually to achieve a cephalic presentation. If this is unsuccessful and the fetus remains breech, a cesarean delivery is offered and usually done. A planned cesarean delivery reduces the risk of perinatal/neonatal death by fourfold compared with a vaginal breech delivery.[8]

A cost analysis based on data from the English National Health Service (NHS) reported that a routine ultrasound scanning policy to determine fetal presentation is likely to be cost-effective if an ultrasound scan can be completed for less than £19.80 (~$26) per woman.[7] It is unlikely that a routine ultrasound for fetal presentation

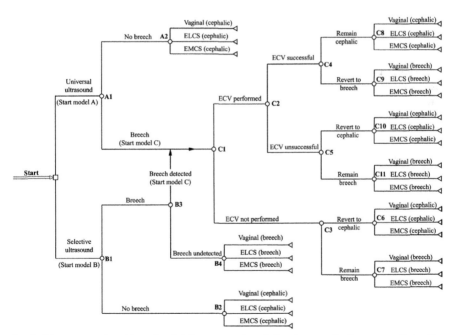

Fig. 1. Management options for fetal presentation following a selective or routine ultrasound screening policy. (*From* Wastlund D, Moraitis AA, Dacey A, Sovio U, Wilson ECF, Smith GCS. Screening for breech presentation using universal late-pregnancy ultrasonography: A prospective cohort study and cost effectiveness analysis. *PLoS Med.* Jun 2019;16(4):e1002778. https://doi.org/10.1371/journal.pmed.1002778)

could be completed for this cost if undertaken by an ultrasonographer using a high-specification machine. However, to make the introduction of a presentation scan cost-effective, the ultrasound scan could be completed during a routine antenatal appointment as, due to its simplicity, the test could be performed by a doctor or midwife with basic training in the technique, using an inexpensive point-of-care ultrasound system.

Prevention of Stillbirth

The benefits of routine third trimester ultrasound become more difficult to delineate when the aim is to prevent stillbirth. In high-risk women, many ultrasound parameters are associated with an increased risk of stillbirth, including a small for gestational age (SGA) (defined as EFW <10th percentile) fetus, reduced amniotic fluid volume, raised umbilical artery Doppler pulsatility index, and low cerebroplacental ratio (CPR),[14–18] that is, the ratio of the pulsatility index in the middle cerebral artery to the pulsatility index in the umbilical artery. Fetal growth restriction (FGR) is associated with a low CPR, due to increased resistance within the umbilical artery and reduced resistance within the middle cerebral artery, the latter due the chemoreceptor reflex stimulated by arterial hypoxemia, a consequence of placental insufficiency.[19] Emphasis has therefore been placed by some on performing these tests to identify fetuses at higher risk of stillbirth to allow intervention before fetal demise. For these women, delivery is the only highly effective intervention to prevent stillbirth.[20]

Because of the rarity of stillbirth at term in a low-risk population, we have minimal direct information on the relationship between different ultrasound parameters and the risk of stillbirth. Therefore, studies often focus on ultrasound parameters to predict groups at higher risk of stillbirth such as SGA. This is justified by the observation that being SGA is associated with a fourfold increased risk of stillbirth.[14] The POP study demonstrated that a routine screening policy compared with a selective policy increased the sensitivity of identifying SGA fetuses from 20% to 57%.[21]

It is important to recognize that infants can be SGA because they are constitutionally small rather than small due to FGR. Furthermore, not all growth-restricted fetuses will have an EFW less than 10th percentile. To try to improve the diagnosis of true FGR, a Delphi consensus surveyed a large number of maternal-fetal medicine specialists to derive a better definition of ultrasonic diagnosis of FGR. Their definition of FGR includes a combination of biometric markers (EFW or abdominal circumference) and functional parameters (umbilical artery Doppler pulsatility index or the CPR).[22]

There is quantitative evidence that ultrasonic measurements other than biometry are associated with fetal outcome, including SGA and neonatal morbidity. It is reasonable to assume that such associations might reflect a relationship between the given measure and FGR. Reduced amniotic fluid volume, raised umbilical artery Doppler and reduced CPR are all associated with an increased risk of delivering an SGA fetus in a low-risk or unselected population.[23,24] Despite being associated with an infant being SGA, a raised umbilical artery Doppler measurement did not predict neonatal morbidity in a meta-analysis including 67,764 women.[24] More severe changes to blood flow within the umbilical artery Doppler including absent or reversed diastolic flow are predictive of adverse outcomes including stillbirth and neonatal morbidity in high-risk populations.[25] However, the incidence of identifying more extreme blood flow abnormalities would be extremely low when a routine third trimester scan was completed in a low-risk population. Other ultrasound parameters including an EFW less than 10th percentile, low CPR, and oligohydramnios are associated with an increased risk of neonatal morbidity and are, therefore, more likely to be of benefit as a screening test.[21,24]

Preventing Birth Complications Associated with Large for Gestational Age Infants

Large for gestational age (LGA) fetuses, often defined as an EFW greater than 90th percentile, have an increased risk of intrapartum complications, including shoulder dystocia. A meta-analysis reported screening in the third trimester had a 54% sensitivity and a 94% specificity of predicting an LGA neonate at delivery.[24] However, despite the EFW being highly predictive of the neonate being LGA at delivery, EFW was only weakly predictive of shoulder dystocia.[24,26] A weak association between ultrasonic EFW greater than 90th percentile and the risk of shoulder dystocia is not surprising given that the actual weight of the infant is not strongly predictive of shoulder dystocia and most cases of shoulder dystocia occur in appropriately sized infants.[27] Interestingly, 2 blinded studies, the POP and Genesis studies, reported no association between diagnosis of an LGA fetus and shoulder dystocia.[26,28] Nonblinded studies may lead to ascertainment bias with an overreporting of shoulder dystocia as clinicians may have a lower threshold to initiate maneuvers for shoulder dystocia or to document that a delayed delivery is due to shoulder dystocia when the infant was suspected to be LGA. In the POP study, a combination of abdominal growth velocity and ultrasonic LGA was predictive of neonatal morbidity.[26] Those fetuses who had an EFW greater than the 90th percentile on their final ultrasound scan alongside a normal abdominal growth velocity were not at an increased risk of an adverse neonatal outcome, whereas those fetuses with an EFW greater than the 90th percentile and an accelerated abdominal growth velocity were at an increased risk of an adverse neonatal outcome. Therefore, the combination of the EFW and the abdominal growth velocity provides more promise as a third trimester screening test than EFW alone. The POP study demonstrated the equivalent finding for SGA, that is, that slow abdominal growth velocity discriminated SGA fetuses at increased risk of an adverse neonatal outcome, whereas fetal size alone did not.[21] In both cases (ie, SGA and LGA), the abdominal circumference percentile at the third trimester scan was compared with the abdominal circumference percentile at the mid-trimester anomaly scan. This approach (assessing trajectory) is important in interpreting third trimester estimates of fetal weight.

To improve pregnancy outcomes, an effective intervention is required for those women at higher risk of adverse outcomes. A randomized controlled trial indicated that routine induction of labor in the presence of suspected macrosomia may reduce the risk of shoulder dystocia.[29] The Big Baby Trial (Induction of labor for predicted macrosomia: the Big Baby trial"; ISRCTN1822989) is currently ongoing, which aims to further assess this finding. It is important to note that both of the preceding studies address the question of screening and intervention in a targeted population of women who meet criteria to have a third trimester scan. However, neither the published randomized controlled trial nor the Big Baby Trial address the question of induction of labor for an LGA fetus in the context of universal third trimester ultrasound in a low-risk population.

FOE
False Positives

When considering a screening test, some women will be incorrectly classified as high risk. Using routine ultrasonography to detect SGA fetuses improves the sensitivity of detection of SGA at the expense of reduced specificity.[21] In the POP study when selective ultrasound was used, 2% of women were incorrectly classified as SGA, but this increased to 10% when routine ultrasonography was used. This equates to 2 additional false positives for every 1 additional true positive result with the use of universal scanning. The women incorrectly classified as having an SGA fetus may be more likely to experience increased anxiety, inappropriate medicalization and resource allocation, and possible iatrogenic harm through unnecessary intervention. This was evident when routine ultrasonography was introduced in France where there were higher rates of adverse outcomes in the false positive women compared with those correctly identified as having an appropriately grown infant.[30] These adverse outcomes include a sixfold increased risk of neonatal resuscitation and a twofold increase in admission to the neonatal intensive care unit (NICU). This was likely secondary to a fourfold increase in delivery at preterm gestations in this group of women who were incorrectly classified as having an SGA baby.

Women incorrectly classified as carrying an LGA fetus are also at risk of iatrogenic harm. When routine third trimester ultrasound is completed, approximately 6% of women are given a false positive result, and the fetus is appropriately grown despite being categorized as LGA at the time of the ultrasound scan.[24] Despite the fetus being appropriately grown, these women have a higher risk of emergency cesarean delivery in labor.[31,32] It is probable that this risk is due to the clinician having a lower threshold to perform a cesarean delivery when the ultrasound scan has reported an LGA fetus.

Limited Options of Intervention

When considering routine ultrasonography as a method of preventing stillbirth, delivery is the single highly effective disease-modifying intervention that removes the subsequent risk of antepartum stillbirth.[15] However, medically indicated delivery involves earlier delivery of the neonate, potentially at early-term or preterm gestations. Preterm delivery to prevent stillbirth needs to be carefully balanced against the risk of prematurity, as prematurity is one of the major determinants of neonatal mortality and morbidity.[33,34] Early-term delivery should not be considered a completely safe option, as it is still associated with poorer short-term outcomes and an increased risk of special educational needs long-term.[35,36] The introduction of routine third trimester ultrasound scanning between 30 and 35 weeks' gestation in France highlights the potential risks.[30] Even the correct identification of an SGA fetus (true positive) was associated with increased adverse outcomes, such as resuscitation at delivery and need for admission to the NICU, compared with SGA infants who were not identified following an ultrasound scan (ie, false negatives). This indicates that the management of SGA fetuses may have resulted in further adverse outcomes compared with those who were not identified and therefore had no intervention. When considering intervention for an SGA cohort, there will be a proportion of these neonates who are healthy, constitutionally small infants. Furthermore, even among truly growth-restricted fetuses, the natural history for most remains benign with only a very small proportion having an adverse outcome such as stillbirth. Given the diverse pathways that lead to adverse outcomes, a truly pathologic population may be better identified by a combination of tests such as multiple ultrasound parameters or using ultrasound and blood biomarkers.[37–39] Identifying a truly pathologic cohort would then aid more targeted intervention.

One-third of stillbirths occur after 37 weeks of gestational age.[40] After this gestational age, intervention by delivery is relatively benign. However, the absolute risk of term stillbirth in the low-risk population remains small (approximately 1 in 1000 pregnancies), with most cases of stillbirth occurring in the antepartum period.[41] A meta-analysis of routine induction of labor at term in an unselected population of women compared with standard practice demonstrated a greater than 50% reduction in stillbirth together with a >85% reduction in perinatal death.[20] To prevent excessive levels of intervention, it is possible that a term ultrasound scan would help in risk-stratifying women in whom delivery of at-risk fetuses may reduce their risk of stillbirth. However, given the relative rarity of term stillbirth, it is still likely that with current methods, very large numbers of women would need to be induced to prevent each death.

Lack of Evidence

A critical element of the evidence base in screening is the quality of studies of diagnostic effectiveness. Ideally, the natural history of a positive test should be known. This requires that a research study had been performed where the result of the test was not revealed. However, there are few studies in which the clinicians have been blinded to the ultrasound scan findings. This can lead to multiple problems. For example, where the screening test was positive it may be more likely that the outcome was recorded as being present, that is, ascertainment bias, as discussed for LGA and shoulder dystocia, previously in this article. Without blinded studies, it is not possible to demonstrate a true association between the measured parameter and the adverse outcome. In studies in which there is no association between adverse ultrasound parameters and neonatal mortality or morbidity, this may be due to treatment paradox, in which interventions initiated by the clinician following the positive test may have prevented the given adverse outcome. However, it is also possible that the ultrasound parameters being measured were not predictive of adverse outcome in that population and are unlikely to be of benefit as a screening test. In such cases in which an association between a scan finding and an adverse outcome is demonstrated, this could be secondary to iatrogenic harm caused by the clinical intervention that was performed based on the positive test result. Before considering routine ultrasound as a screening test, the gold standard is to demonstrate an association between the ultrasound findings and adverse perinatal outcomes in a blinded study in a low-risk or unselected population. This would then allow the diagnostic effectiveness of the test to be clearly quantified. Unfortunately, blinded studies need to be prospective and involve significant cost and time, which makes it very challenging to power such studies for the outcomes of greatest interest, such as stillbirth.

When considering the use of an ultrasound scan in the third trimester to prevent stillbirth, current evidence is underpowered to detect the outcome of perinatal death.[42] It is unclear if the lack of evidence for the use of ultrasonography to prevent perinatal death is a true finding or because the current studies are underpowered. Previous studies have reported sample size calculations for a screening study to reduce perinatal mortality and demonstrated that current studies are profoundly underpowered even assuming an excellent screening test and a highly effective intervention. For example, assuming a background risk of perinatal death of 5 in 1000, a screening test with a 5% screen positive rate and a positive likelihood ratio of 10, coupled to an intervention that reduces the risk of stillbirth by 50%, the calculation indicated that a study would need to recruit about 130,000 women to be adequately powered, which is far in excess of the sample size achieved by the Cochrane review.[2,42]

Timing of Ultrasound

The timing of a routine third trimester ultrasound scan is critical and has varied from early to late in the third trimester in the current literature.[2] The timing of the scan influences how predictive the scan is of the infant's birthweight percentile. For example, ultrasound scans at 36 weeks are more predictive of an infant's weight percentile at delivery than those completed at 28 to 30 weeks.[43] As discussed previously, when an ultrasound scan is completed at preterm gestations it is possible that the risk of intervention and secondary complications of premature delivery is greater than the risk of stillbirth. In this setting, there is then a risk of the ultrasound doing more harm than good. One-third of stillbirths occur at term and there is a substantial increased risk of complications following preterm delivery. Thus, introduction of routine ultrasonography at approximately 36 weeks would identify those fetuses with evidence of FGR, and

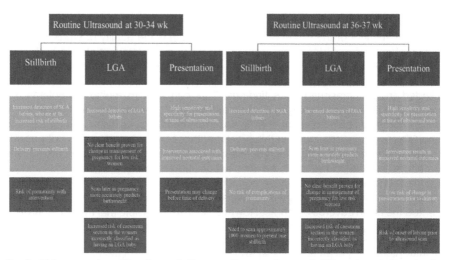

Fig. 2. Risks versus benefits of completing an ultrasound scan at different gestations in the third trimester. Green boxes demonstrate potential benefits, red boxes demonstrate potential risks.

intervention by early-term delivery would then be relatively benign (compared with iatrogenic delivery earlier in gestation). An ultrasound scan to determine the fetal presentation needs to be completed at the end of the third trimester to reduce the risk of a change in presentation before the onset of delivery. Further, an ultrasound at this gestation provides adequate time for the planning of the method of delivery for those infants who are breech or are LGA. **Fig. 2** summarizes the risks and benefits of a routine third trimester ultrasound completed at 30 to 34 weeks compared with 36 to 37 weeks.

SUMMARY

A routine third trimester ultrasound can be used to help identify high-risk fetuses who are breech, SGA, LGA, or those at higher risk of stillbirth. However, a cautious approach needs to be taken due to the lack of current evidence, first, for its ability to predict pathology in a low-risk population, and second, that intervention effectively improves outcomes for these infants. Current evidence strongly suggests preterm delivery is the strongest predictor of neonatal mortality and morbidity. Based on current evidence, no definitive conclusion can be drawn whether routine third trimester ultrasound to prevent antepartum stillbirth is a friend or foe. However, there is a case for considering routine late-preterm or early-term point-of-care ultrasound to detect breech presentation.

CLINICS CARE POINTS

- Routine third trimester ultrasound improves the sensitivity of detecting infants who are breech or LGA and is likely to help identify a higher proportion of infants at high risk of stillbirth.

- In a low-risk screening population, if an ultrasound is completed at preterm gestations with the aim to prevent stillbirth, intervention may result in poorer neonatal outcomes secondary to prematurity.

- We currently lack appropriately powered blinded trials to know if routine ultrasound could be used to improve pregnancy outcomes in low-risk women.

DISCLOSURE

GS: Received research support from Roche Diagnostics Ltd, GSK, Illumina, and Sera Prognostics (fetal growth restriction, preeclampsia, and preterm birth). Paid to attend advisory boards by GSK (preterm birth) and to speak at a meeting by Roche Diagnostics Ltd, Switzerland (fetal growth restriction). Paid consultant to GSK (preterm birth). Member of a GSK DMC (RSV vaccination in pregnancy). K. Stephens: None to declare.

REFERENCES

1. RCOG. RCOG green-top guideline No. 31: the investigation and management of the small-for-gestational-age-fetus. London, UK: RCOG; 2014.
2. Bricker L, Medley N, Pratt JJ. Routine ultrasound in late pregnancy (after 24 weeks' gestation). Cochrane Database Syst Rev 2015;(6):CD001451.
3. Al-Hafez L, Chauhan SP, Riegel M, et al. Routine third-trimester ultrasound in low-risk pregnancies and perinatal death: a systematic review and meta-analysis. Am J Obstet Gynaecol MFM 2020;2(4):100242.
4. Smith G. A critical review of the Cochrane meta-analysis of routine late-pregnancy ultrasound. BJOG 2020. https://doi.org/10.1111/1471-0528.16386.
5. Toijonen A, Heinonen S, Gissler M, et al. Risk factors for adverse outcomes in vaginal preterm breech labor. Arch Gynecol Obstet 2020. https://doi.org/10.1007/s00404-020-05731-y.
6. Hickok DE, Gordon DC, Milberg JA, et al. The frequency of breech presentation by gestational age at birth: a large population-based study. Am J Obstet Gynecol 1992;166(3):851–2.
7. Wastlund D, Moraitis AA, Dacey A, et al. Screening for breech presentation using universal late-pregnancy ultrasonography: a prospective cohort study and cost effectiveness analysis. PLoS Med 2019;16(4):e1002778.
8. Hannah ME, Hannah WJ, Hewson SA, et al. Planned caesarean section versus planned vaginal birth for breech presentation at term: a randomised multicentre trial. Term Breech Trial Collaborative Group. Lancet 2000;356(9239):1375–83.
9. Impey LWM, Murphy DJ, Griffiths M, et al. Management breech presentation. BJOG 2017;124(7).
10. Nassar N, Roberts CL, Cameron CA, et al. Diagnostic accuracy of clinical examination for detection of non-cephalic presentation in late pregnancy: cross sectional analytic study. BMJ 2006;333(7568):578–80.
11. Watson WJ, Welter S, Day D. Antepartum identification of breech presentation. J Reprod Med 2004;49(4):294–6.
12. Hofmeyr GJ, Hannah M, Lawrie TA. Planned caesarean section for term breech delivery. Cochrane Database Syst Rev 2015;(7):CD000166.
13. Hannah ME. Planned elective cesarean section: a reasonable choice for some women? CMAJ 2004;170(5):813–4.
14. Flenady V, Koopmans L, Middleton P, et al. Major risk factors for stillbirth in high-income countries: a systematic review and meta-analysis. Lancet 2011;377(9774):1331–40.
15. Alfirevic Z, Stampalija T, Dowswell T. Fetal and umbilical Doppler ultrasound in high-risk pregnancies. Cochrane Database Syst Rev 2017;6:CD007529.
16. Flood K, Unterscheider J, Daly S, et al. The role of brain sparing in the prediction of adverse outcomes in intrauterine growth restriction: results of the multicenter PORTO Study. Am J Obstet Gynecol 2014;211(3):288.e1–5.

17. Khalil A, Morales-Roselló J, Townsend R, et al. Value of third-trimester cerebropla-cental ratio and uterine artery Doppler indices as predictors of stillbirth and peri-natal loss. Ultrasound Obstet Gynecol 2016;47(1):74–80.
18. Figueroa L, McClure EM, Swanson J, et al. Oligohydramnios: a prospective study of fetal, neonatal and maternal outcomes in low-middle income countries. Reprod Health 2020;17(1):19.
19. Vollgraff Heidweiller-Schreurs CA, De Boer MA, Heymans MW, et al. Prognostic accuracy of cerebroplacental ratio and middle cerebral artery Doppler for adverse perinatal outcome: systematic review and meta-analysis. Ultrasound Ob-stet Gynecol 2018;51(3):313–22.
20. Middleton P, Shepherd E, Crowther CA. Induction of labour for improving birth outcomes for women at or beyond term. Cochrane Database Syst Rev 2018;5: CD004945.
21. Sovio U, White IR, Dacey A, et al. Screening for fetal growth restriction with uni-versal third trimester ultrasonography in nulliparous women in the Pregnancy Outcome Prediction (POP) study: a prospective cohort study. Lancet 2015; 386(10008):2089–97.
22. Gordijn SJ, Beune IM, Thilaganathan B, et al. Consensus definition of fetal growth restriction: a Delphi procedure. Ultrasound Obstet Gynecol 2016;48(3):333–9.
23. Alfirevic Z, Stampalija T, Medley N. Fetal and umbilical Doppler ultrasound in normal pregnancy. Cochrane Database Syst Rev 2015;(4):CD001450.
24. Smith G, Moraitis A, Wastlund D, et al. A systematic review and cost-effectiveness analysis of the case for screening nulliparous women in late preg-nancy using ultrasound. HTA J 2019. https://doi.org/10.17863/CAM.50647.
25. Baschat AA, Gembruch U, Weiner CP, et al. Qualitative venous Doppler wave-form analysis improves prediction of critical perinatal outcomes in premature growth-restricted fetuses. Ultrasound Obstet Gynecol 2003;22(3):240–5.
26. Sovio U, Moraitis AA, Wong HS, et al. Universal vs selective ultrasonography to screen for large-for-gestational-age infants and associated morbidity. Ultrasound Obstet Gynecol 2018;51(6):783–91.
27. Ouzounian JG. Shoulder dystocia: incidence and risk factors. Clin Obstet Gyne-col 2016;59(4):791–4.
28. Galvin DM, Burke N, Burke G, et al. 94: Accuracy of prenatal detection of macrosomia >4,000g and outcomes in the absence of intervention: results of the prospective multicenter genesis study. Am J Obstet Gynecol 2017;216:S68.
29. Boulvain M, Senat MV, Perrotin F, et al. Induction of labour versus expectant man-agement for large-for-date fetuses: a randomised controlled trial. Lancet 2015; 385(9987):2600–5.
30. Monier I, Blondel B, Ego A, et al. Poor effectiveness of antenatal detection of fetal growth restriction and consequences for obstetric management and neonatal outcomes: a French national study. BJOG 2015;122(4):518–27.
31. Little SE, Edlow AG, Thomas AM, et al. Estimated fetal weight by ultrasound: a modifiable risk factor for cesarean delivery? Am J Obstet Gynecol 2012;207(4): 309.e1–6.
32. Parry S, Severs CP, Sehdev HM, et al. Ultrasonographic prediction of fetal macro-somia. Association with cesarean delivery. J Reprod Med 2000;45(1):17–22.
33. Manuck TA, Rice MM, Bailit JL, et al. Preterm neonatal morbidity and mortality by gestational age: a contemporary cohort. Am J Obstet Gynecol 2016;215(1): 103.e1–14.
34. Saigal S, Doyle LW. An overview of mortality and sequelae of preterm birth from infancy to adulthood. Lancet 2008;371(9608):261–9.

35. MacKay DF, Smith GC, Dobbie R, et al. Gestational age at delivery and special educational need: retrospective cohort study of 407,503 schoolchildren. PLoS Med 2010;7(6):e1000289.
36. Spong CY. Defining "term" pregnancy: recommendations from the defining "Term" Pregnancy Workgroup. JAMA 2013;309(23):2445–6.
37. Heazell AE, Hayes DJ, Whitworth M, et al. Biochemical tests of placental function versus ultrasound assessment of fetal size for stillbirth and small-for-gestational-age infants. Cochrane Database Syst Rev 2019;5:CD012245.
38. Sovio U, Goulding N, McBride N, et al. A maternal serum metabolite ratio predicts fetal growth restriction at term. Nat Med 2020;26(3):348–53.
39. Gaccioli F, Aye ILMH, Sovio U, et al. Screening for fetal growth restriction using fetal biometry combined with maternal biomarkers. Am J Obstet Gynecol 2018; 218(2S):S725–37.
40. Draper ES, Kurinczuk JJ, Kenyon S. MBRRACE-UK Perinatal confidential enquiry: term, singleton, normally formed, antepartum stillbirth. Leicester, UK: the Infant Mortality and Morbidity Studies, Department of Health Sciences, University of Leicester; 2015.
41. Moraitis AA, Wood AM, Fleming M, et al. Birth weight percentile and the risk of term perinatal death. Obstet Gynecol 2014;124(2 Pt 1):274–83.
42. Flenady V, Wojcieszek AM, Middleton P, et al. Stillbirths: recall to action in high-income countries. Lancet 2016;387(10019):691–702.
43. Sovio U, Smith GCS. Comparison of estimated fetal weight percentiles near term for predicting extremes of birthweight percentile. Am J Obstet Gynecol 2020. https://doi.org/10.1016/j.ajog.2020.08.054.

Evaluation and Management of Suspected Fetal Growth Restriction

Claartje Bruin, MD[a],*, Stefanie Damhuis, MD[a,b],
Sanne Gordijn, MD, PhD[b], Wessel Ganzevoort, MD, PhD[a]

KEYWORDS

- Fetal growth restriction • Placental insufficiency • Small for gestational age
- Doppler ultrasound • Cardiotocography

KEY POINTS

- The diagnosis fetal growth restriction (FGR) is made when the fetus has clinical signs of malnourishment and/or hypoxia owing to placental insufficiency.
- There is no available effective "cure" for FGR, other than delivery.
- In early-onset FGR ("*easy diagnosis, difficult management*"), the obstetric challenge lies in timing of delivery, whereas in late-onset FGR ("*difficult diagnosis, easy management*"), the challenge is the detection of FGR.

INTRODUCTION

Prenatal care focuses on the early detection of several pregnancy-specific conditions. Impaired fetal growth due to placental insufficiency is among the most important of those conditions because it is a major contributor to adverse perinatal outcomes. In this article, the authors focus first on the evaluation by prenatal care providers that identifies fetal growth restriction (FGR) and potential causes. Second, the authors discuss management options, including potential therapeutic strategies, monitoring modalities, and how to inform the decision for iatrogenic delivery.

EVALUATION
Primary Assessment

The evaluation of suspected FGR typically commences when it is observed that the estimated fetal size is below a defined threshold of normality for gestational age, termed small for gestational age (SGA), or when a decline in growth percentile is

[a] Department of Obstetrics and Gynecology, Amsterdam University Medical Centers, University of Amsterdam, Room H4-205, PO Box 22660, Amsterdam 1105 AZ, The Netherlands;
[b] Department of Obstetrics and Gynecology, University Medical Center Groningen, University of Groningen, Huispostcode CB20, Hanzeplein 1, Groningen 9700 RB, The Netherlands
* Corresponding author.
E-mail address: c.m.bruin@amsterdamumc.nl

Obstet Gynecol Clin N Am 48 (2021) 371–385
https://doi.org/10.1016/j.ogc.2021.02.007   obgyn.theclinics.com

observed. In optimal conditions, the fetus grows according to its own intrinsic growth potential, determined by genetic and epigenetic factors. A fetus may be small in relation to a population reference or standard, yet be appropriate for its intrinsic growth potential. However, the more significant the deviation from the threshold of normality, the bigger the chance that a pathologic process underlies the observed smallness. This is described in Stefanie E. Damhuis and colleagues' article, "Abnormal Fetal Growth: SGA, FGR, LGA: Definitions and Epidemiology," in this issue. The core issue when confronted with a small fetus is determining if the fetal size is appropriate for this fetus. The aim of the clinical approach is primarily to discover if the fetus is compromised by placental insufficiency and at risk for morbidity or mortality.

For all diagnoses, it is important to first verify if the gestational age was calculated appropriately because this is key to the interpretation of fetal size. In high-income countries, a reliable due date will often be provided by routine first-trimester ultrasound, but this may not be the case in exceptional cases, for example, in (socially) deprived settings. If the gestational age has been reliably set, evaluation proceeds with an ultrasound to confirm the extent of abnormality of fetal size. It is important to understand that fetal size is the result of previous fetal growth. It is advisable to incorporate the results from all previous ultrasounds greater than 18 weeks of gestation in the evaluation to establish the growth pattern. Impaired placental function leads, if long-lasting or severe enough, to a decline in size centiles of biometric measurements plotted on a reference chart to "crossing centiles." As a screening tool, this is sometimes defined by a decline of 20 centiles or more, and for the diagnosis FGR, a decline of 50 centiles has been determined in consensus.[1,2]

Also, the medical, obstetric, and family history should be taken to understand if specific other factors contributing to impaired placental function can be identified. The most common are maternal or environmental smoke exposure and medical problems, such as hypertension.[3]

Placental insufficiency

The underlying pathologic mechanism of FGR is placental insufficiency, with or without maternal diseases, fetal chromosomal abnormalities, or infection. Pathologic smallness reflects malnourishment as well as hypoxia, as these processes go hand in hand.[4,5] Many causal placental lesions are known. However, the most common lesion is suboptimal remodeling of uterine spiral arteries (placentation) in early pregnancy; this is termed "maternal vascular malperfusion" (MVM). MVM occurs mostly when uterine artery remodeling is only shallow and the maternal vascular bed thereby retains smooth muscle cell vascular reactivity, which amounts to an incomplete physiologic transformation. High-resistance vessels persist, resulting in high-velocity blood flow into the intervillous space with shear stress and altered villous vascularization.[6,7]

Other well-described FGR-related placental lesions include fetal vascular malperfusion (FVM) and villitis of unknown etiology (VUE).[8] FVM is most often caused by obstructed fetal blood flow because of thrombosis or other lesions, such as those occurring in the cord (high- or low-coiling index) and hypercoagulability with and without thrombosis. VUE is only considered present when a nonspecific inflammatory process results in villitis.[8]

Antenatal detection of placental insufficiency

The increased vascular resistance in MVM can be detected by use of Doppler ultrasound to measure the blood flow patterns of both maternal and fetal arteries (**Fig. 1**). Many vessels, including the uterine artery, umbilical artery (UA), and middle cerebral artery (MCA), can be assessed throughout pregnancy and can provide an indication of actual placental function. Abnormal flow patterns can be used to identify the compromised fetus that is deprived of oxygen and nutrients. It is noteworthy that Doppler abnormalities are not necessarily seen in other placental lesions (**Table 1**).[9]

Uterine artery
In normal pregnancy, the uterine arteries, as an indirect measure of resistance in the spiral arteries, demonstrate a transition from a unit of high resistance to very low resistance in the first trimester.[6] The opening of the spiral arteries into low-resistance units causes the upstream resistance of the uterine artery to decrease to levels where the notching of the uterine artery disappears. If this does not occur sufficiently, the notching continues to be measurable, and/or the pulsatility index (PI) remains high. Retained high resistance of the uterine artery in the second trimester of pregnancy is associated with an increased risk for the development of especially early-onset preeclampsia and FGR.[10]

Umbilical artery
Many studies demonstrate the relationship between uteroplacental insufficiency and consequent increased impedance in the UA. Among the earliest phenomenon in early-onset FGR are abnormal UA flow velocity waveforms.[11,12] It is described quantitatively by increased PI and qualitatively by absent or reversed end-diastolic (ARED) flow. ARED-flow is specific for very-early-onset FGR and less so for term or late preterm FGR.[13] This phenomenon is merely the "tip of the iceberg" because ARED-flow is only observed when a larger proportion of the placental vascular bed is dysfunctional.[14] In later gestational ages, fetuses have little placental reserve, and UA waveforms do not typically become severely abnormal. Fetal distress in advanced pregnancy can become apparent through reduced fetal movements, abnormal

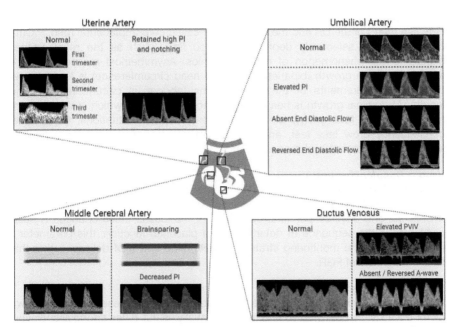

Fig. 1. Different Doppler flow patterns in maternal and fetal vessels relevant to placental function. PVIV, peak velocity index for the vein.

Table 1
Overview of relevant ultrasound parameters and their implications

Doppler Parameters	Indication	Abnormal Findings	Indicative for
Uterine artery	Screening high-risk FGR pregnancies	UtA-PI >95th centile[a]	Risk stratification for development of PE and FGR
Umbilical artery	(Suspected) FGR maternal hypertensive disorders	UA-PI >95th centile[a] AEDF REDF	Very early-onset FGR
Middle cerebral artery	(Suspected) FGR	MCA <5th centile[a] PSV	Fetal adaptation to hypoxemia Fetal anemia
Cerebroplacental ratio	(Suspected) FGR	CPR <5th centile[a]	Fetal redistribution
Ductus venosus	Severe early-onset FGR	PVIV >95th centile[a] Reversed A wave	Fetal cardiac compromise

Abbreviations: AEDF, absent end-diastolic flow; CPR, cerebroplacental ratio; PE, preeclampsia; PSV, peak systolic flow; REDF, reversed end-diastolic flow; UtA, uterine artery.
[a] Most often used cutoff for abnormal.

cardiotocogram (CTG), or death before deterioration of Doppler flows, partly because the indication to measure flow patterns is often only small size.[15]

Signs of redistribution in the fetal circulation
An early response to placental insufficiency is redistribution of blood flow in the fetal circulation. Blood flow is selectively redirected to the most important organs, including the heart, brain, and, in utero, the adrenal gland. This phenomenon has been dubbed the "brain-sparing effect" and can be expressed in an abnormal ratio between the PI of the UA and the MCA, the so-called cerebroplacental ratio.[16] Other organs may be selectively deprived of blood flow, such as the renal arteries, explaining the phenomenon of oligohydramnios. Asymmetrical measurements of size signify brain growth (biparietal diameter, head circumference) is less affected than the measurements of the other organs (abdominal circumference, femur length). Abdominal growth is heavily influenced by liver size, which is the predominant location of fetal energy storage. In energy-deprived situations, the liver will consequently grow less fast, and the abdominal circumference will be typically smaller relative to cerebral measurements.

Venous Doppler changes
Signs of FGR can also be observed in the fetal venous circulation. Both abnormal ductus venosus (DV) measurements and pulsations in the umbilical vein are related to fetal hypoxemia and adverse perinatal outcomes.[12,17] Because these changes typically occur late in the sequence of deterioration of placental function, this parameter is more useful for the monitoring strategy to determine timing of delivery rather than for the diagnosis of FGR.

Serum biomarkers
Placental dysfunction is also reflected in serum markers; of these, placental growth factor (PIGF) is the best studied and most potentially useful. It has strong associations with early-onset hypertensive disorders of pregnancy and its clinical manifestations, particularly if combined with soluble fms-like tyrosine kinase-1 (sFlt-1).[18] These

markers may be useful in identifying FGR fetuses,[19,20] although utility is diluted significantly if SGA is chosen as the endpoint rather than FGR.[21]

Decreased fetal movements

When placental insufficiency deteriorates to the extent whereby the fetus experiences hypoxemia, a decline in fetal activity can occur.[22] This phenomenon is one that can be recognized by the mother, and as such, can be considered an additional monitoring tool. Although efficacy is uncertain, most authorities recommend additional antenatal testing in cases of decreased fetal movement.

Differential diagnosis and maternal comorbidities

Clinicians, when confronted with a suspected small or growth-restricted fetus/newborn, must explore all possible pathophysiologic mechanisms besides and/or relating to placental insufficiency. These mechanisms are, among others, fetal infections, congenital anomalies, syndromes, genetic abnormalities, and maternal diseases. Each of these conditions requires different management and treatment strategies and should therefore be considered.

Fetal infections

An uncommon, but clinically important alternative diagnosis underlying SGA is congenital infection. The microorganisms that are the main contributors are toxoplasmosis, rubella, cytomegalovirus (CMV), herpes simplex virus, and malaria, as they have the potential to cause a placental and/or congenital infection.

Ultrasonographic abnormalities that are associated with these infections are fetal ventriculomegaly, intracranial calcifications, ascites, and hyperechogenic bowel. In severe fetal smallness, screening for CMV infection can be considered because this is the most common congenital viral infection, with a prevalence of 0.2% to 2% (average, 0.65%).[23]

Other infections should only be assessed if there is a specific pattern of ultrasound abnormalities or specific clinical risk factors, because the incidence of these infections in the absence of ultrasonographic abnormalities is very low.[24,25]

Syndromal abnormalities

In the case of early-onset FGR, an advanced obstetric sonogram can help to screen for chromosomal abnormalities, especially if other signs of placental insufficiency are absent. Structural anomalies can suggest an underlying syndrome and may justify invasive prenatal testing with amniocentesis or chorionic villus sampling. Noninvasive prenatal testing is currently only useful to screen for a small number of chromosomal abnormalities. Because placental insufficiency is more common in the context of chromosomal abnormalities, diagnostic testing (rather than screening) should be considered in early-onset FGR, especially when other ultrasound abnormalities are seen.[26]

Maternal comorbidities

The presence of maternal comorbidities may increase (or sometimes decrease) the likelihood that the observed fetal smallness is caused by placental insufficiency. Most noticeable are disorders that have impact on endothelial cell function, such as chronic hypertension, diabetes mellitus, renal disease, lupus, and cardiovascular disease, all of which can have an impact on early placental development.[27]

Maternal preeclampsia

Most of the pathophysiologic processes of hypertensive disorders of pregnancy are similar in FGR. Therefore, some of this knowledge can be extended into the field of

FGR. Preeclampsia is a serious complication of pregnancy, characterized by hypertension and proteinuria in the second half of pregnancy because of endovascular inflammation.[28] Poor placentation is particularly associated with the early-onset phenotype of both preeclampsia and FGR. Especially in earlier gestational ages, hypertensive disorders of pregnancy and FGR have a reciprocal association.[29]

MANAGEMENT

In this section, the authors discuss potential therapies influencing the root cause of the placental insufficiency. Next, they discuss how the main therapeutic approach remains determining the timing of delivery and how this is different in early-onset FGR and late-onset FGR. In early-onset FGR ("*easy diagnosis, difficult management*"), obstetric management focuses on timing of delivery, whereas in late-onset FGR ("*difficult diagnosis, easy management*"), the focus lies on the detection of FGR.

Therapeutic strategies

Particularly in early-onset FGR, MVM with retained smooth muscle cell function of the spiral arteries appears to be the predominant pathophysiologic pathway. This suboptimal remodeling of uterine spiral arteries has led to pharmacologic strategies that influence uteroplacental vascular function through the endothelial nitric oxide pathway and vasodilatation, depicted in **Fig. 2**.[30] No strategy with established efficacy is currently available. Such an intervention is particularly wanted for the severe phenotype of early-onset FGR, because any option that can prolong pregnancy and decrease the consequences of prematurity after iatrogenic delivery can have a tremendous impact on perinatal outcomes.

Sildenafil

Early evaluations of phosphodiesterase-5 inhibitors (sildenafil) as therapeutic treatment for early-onset severe FGR with high risk of fetal demise appeared promising.[31,32] However, in an international collaboration (acronym STRIDER), randomized controlled trials (RCTs) of antenatal sildenafil citrate for FGR showed no benefit and possible harm.[33–35]

Antioxidants: arginine

An increasing number of studies on the therapeutic use of antioxidants, such as L-arginine, have become available.[36] This option is appealing, as it is a nutritional supplement, unlikely to have unexpected unwanted side effects, such as seen with sildenafil exposure in the Dutch STRIDER RCT.[35] A recent cross-species meta-analysis combining all available data from human and nonhuman studies suggests that arginine family supplementation, in particular, arginine and nitrogen carbamoyl glutamate, improves fetal growth in complicated pregnancies.[37] Rigorous research in complicated human pregnancies is needed before determining efficacy in the treatment of FGR.

Gene therapy

A promising and more radical approach is vascular endothelial growth factor (VEGF) gene therapy, in which adenoviral vectors encoding for proteins, such as VEGF, are introduced to the maternal uterine artery.[38] In preclinical studies, it has been shown to increase uterine blood flow and reduce vascular contractility. These functional findings correspond with the anatomic findings of vascular remodeling with increased endothelial cell proliferation in the perivascular adventitia of treated uterine arteries. This method is anticipated to be safe, because no vector seems to spread to the fetus, and no adverse effects on either the mother or fetus have been observed. However,

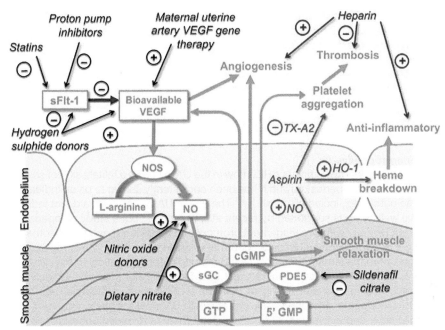

Fig. 2. Possible interventions to treat FGR by site of action influencing the vascular smooth muscle and endothelium metabolism. 5′ GMP, guanosine monophosphate; cGMP, cyclic guanosine monophosphate; GTP, guanosine-5′-triphosphate; HO-1, heme oxygenase-1; NO, nitric oxide; NOS, nitric oxide synthase; PDE5, phosphodiesterase type 5 inhibitor; sGC, soluble guanylate cyclase; TX-A2, thromboxane A2. (*From* Groom KM, David AL. The role of aspirin, heparin, and other interventions in the prevention and treatment of fetal growth restriction. Am J Obstet Gynecol. 2018;218(2S):S829-S840.)

this bold strategy still requires many steps, including extensive clinical trials, before it can be implemented into clinical practice. Furthermore, the high cost associated with gene therapy may restrict this option to high-income health care settings.

Monitoring for delivery in early-onset fetal growth restriction

Although the term "fetal growth restriction" implies that the fetus suffers most from poor nutritional exchange, sustained starvation is rarely the cause of fetal demise. It is the lack of oxygen supply to the fetus, resulting in chronic or acute hypoxia that leads to perinatal death. Obstetric management aims to minimize the risk of fetal demise. The only management that "treats" placental insufficiency is delivery, which prevents stillbirth but predisposes to postnatal death from prematurity. Despite the fact that early-onset FGR is rare (0.3% of all pregnancies), this extreme phenotype has significant societal and individual impact owing to the aggravated effects of prematurity: death or survival with severe impairment.[39] All severe morbidities are essentially expressions of underdeveloped organ function, including lungs (bronchopulmonary dysplasia, respiratory distress syndrome), bowels (necrotizing enterocolitis), immune system (sepsis and meningitis), and cerebral blood vessels (intracerebral hemorrhage, periventricular leukomalacia).

Timing of delivery is therefore based on the estimated balance of the risks of ongoing intrauterine hypoxia versus the consequences of iatrogenic premature delivery. In the previable/periviable period, consideration of expectant management is warranted even when fetal death is expected because delivery often confers near certainty of postnatal death.[40] In scenarios whereby severe fetal compromise is present before viability, pregnancy termination should be made available, especially when continued expectant management is associated with maternal risk. Of note is that viability may occur at later gestational ages for fetuses with FGR, and the determination of the moment of esteemed viability depends on the expertise of the obstetric and neonatal staff along with local resources. Once a viable gestation is reached, the main clinical dilemma is which surveillance test should guide the decision on timing of birth: CTG, fetal Doppler ultrasound, and/or serum biomarkers.[12,41,42] At the moment, published national guidelines on the matter vary considerably.[43]

Indication for delivery
Umbilical Artery. The finding of ARED flow in the UA in FGR is a telltale sign of severely impaired placental perfusion, and it has been consistently shown to be an indicator of adverse outcomes, including death.[17,44] The use of UA Dopplers as a direct indicator for fetal well-being is supported by recent study results,[45] but a study comparing the use of UA Doppler with a management protocol that remains expectant until other parameters of fetal condition become abnormal is lacking. Currently, UA Doppler is variably part of management protocols as a direct indicator for delivery in the extremely preterm period. The most recent Society for Maternal-Fetal Medicine Guideline for FGR recommends general timing of delivery at 37 weeks' gestational age in the case of UA Doppler PI > p95, delivery at 33 to 34 weeks if there is absent end-diastolic flow, and delivery at 30 to 32 weeks if there is reversed end-diastolic flow. However, in the case of repetitive late decelerations on CTG tracing, delivery is advised after the fetal viability.[25]

Cardiotocography. Fetal heart rate (FHR) is a function of the autonomic nervous system. At the onset of hypoxia, FHR variability decreases, whereas progressive hypoxia and acidemia result in spontaneous decelerations. When repeated decelerations occur, unprovoked by uterine contractions, there is strong consensus that imminent delivery is warranted because hypoxia is likely present, and the risk of stillbirth is high.[43]

The importance of low FHR variability is less clear. Short-term variation (STV) is a measurement of FHR variability that is calculated by computer analysis, which avoids the high interobserver and intraobserver variability of visual CTG observation.[46] It has recently been made available as freeware.[47] STV has been established as a reflection of fetal acid-base status.[48] However, no studies exist with sufficient power to detect an association of STV at any threshold with the most important outcomes, stillbirth, and long-term infant health.[49]

In an indirect comparison of visual CTG versus STV assessment with computerized CTG (cCTG) using data from the GRIT and TRUFFLE trials, it was suggestive that monitoring with cCTG improved outcomes.[41] Notwithstanding the lack of conclusive comparative evidence, some advocate that cCTG should be the gold standard.[50] However, clinical practice shows variable implementation: although STV has been adopted as a standard of care in many European centers (but far from all), it has not been adopted in the United States. Because of these firm beliefs and practice variation, cCTG needs to be tested rigorously to determine whether its use improves outcomes compared with visual CTG interpretation.

Ductus Venosus. Use of the DV Doppler waveform in addition to CTG to determine timing of delivery appears to improve neurocognitive outcome at the age of 2 among surviving infants, although this finding is nonsignificant when stillbirths and perinatal deaths are included in comparison groups.[42] It is likely that intrauterine malnutrition and hypoxia affect some fetal organs before others. In fetuses with early-onset FGR, cardiac dysfunction (as reflected in abnormal DV assessment) can precede cerebral dysfunction (as reflected in low STV).[51] The combination of CTG and Doppler evaluation of the DV as monitoring modalities to time delivery is likely to be synergistic in achieving optimal results. The findings of the TRUFFLE trial are difficult to generalize to practice settings in the United States, where cCTG has not been widely adopted and Doppler evaluation of the DV waveform has not been endorsed by professional societies.[25]

Biophysical Profile. The biophysical profile score (BPS) is a crude composite score of a combined assessment of fetal movements, reactivity of the CTG, and assessment of amniotic fluid. The association of an abnormal BPS with the adverse outcomes of interest is not as good as other available parameters.[52] Nevertheless, in the difficult decision of iatrogenic preterm delivery in the context of borderline abnormal findings of cCTG, the presence or absence of fetal movements may sometimes sway decisions in practice.

Late-Onset Fetal Growth Restriction: From Diagnosis to Delivery

In late-onset FGR when placental reserve is already challenged, the interval between the onset of nutritional deprivation and life-threatening hypoxia is typically shorter than in early-onset FGR. In this gestational age period, the concept is "easy to manage, difficult to diagnose." This concept is reflected in the fact that a significant number of fetuses suffer from the consequences of hypoxia without apparently being challenged in growth, as they are not small.[53,54]

The Small for Gestational Age Approach

Because the aforementioned signs of placental insufficiency are unlikely to be observed in late-onset FGR, differentiation between FGR (failure to meet growth potential) and SGA (constitutionally small but healthy) is difficult. Despite the low absolute risk, adverse outcomes are devastating and include stillbirth and short- and long-term effects of hypoxia (neonatal intensive care unit admission, hypoxic-ischemic encephalopathy). On the other hand, unnecessary iatrogenic (relatively) preterm birth in women with small but healthy infants also confers low absolute risk of postnatal morbidity but translates into significant societal impact.

Because serious perinatal morbidity from delivery in the late preterm pregnancy is unlikely,[55] clinicians may have a low threshold for delivering small fetuses relatively later in gestation. Imperfections with approaches that depend exclusively on assessments of fetal size lead to "undertreatment" of fetuses of normal size but who are affected by FGR and "overtreatment" of fetuses who are small but healthy. The DIGITAT study randomized women with fetuses suspected to have FGR at 37 weeks' gestation to delivery or expectant management and showed no difference in the primary outcome of short-term perinatal morbidity.[56] However, more fetuses in the expectant management were in the lowest birth weight percentile group, and these were the fetuses at risk of later developmental delay.[57] This study shows that selection of "the fetus at risk" is still imperfect, and the ideal approach is still not known.

The individual risk approach

Further risk stratification is necessary to identify the fetus that should be delivered early.[58] The same variables that are identified in early-onset FGR can be used for an individualized risk approach. The most commonly used marker is the brain-sparing phenomenon.[59] Cohort studies have consistently shown that abnormal MCA Dopplers (low PI) are associated with adverse outcomes.[13,60] However, in a recent individual patient data meta-analysis, it was found that, if continuous data of UA and MCA Doppler indices were used, the diagnostic performance of both UA and MCA variables and their ratio (cerebroplacental ratio) was similar.[61] Ongoing studies are further evaluating these discrepancies and whether UA Doppler velocities that were previously considered normal may actually represent evidence of compromised placental function.

Management: other aspects

Prevention of Fetal Growth Restriction/Acetyl Salicylic Acid

Low-dose aspirin (acetyl salicylic acid 80–150 mg) has long been recognized as effective for reducing the risk of developing preeclampsia, provided it is started in early pregnancy.[62] Considering the fact that preeclampsia and FGR share risk factors with MVM as the most common pathologic underlying lesion, these data have been extrapolated to FGR by some. Its use in decreasing the risk of FGR is studied with mixed results[63] and will be reviewed in more detail in Nathan Blue and colleagues' article, "Recurrence Risk of Fetal Growth Restriction: Management of Subsequent Pregnancies," in this issue. Also, the risk of SGA infants is reduced with low-dose aspirin, although this was assessed as a secondary outcome in most studies. One approach is to offer it to women with the highest risk of developing the disorder, using algorithms provided by the Fetal Medicine Foundation algorithm, or US Preventive Services Task Force.[64,65]

Mode of Delivery

Severe fetal compromise often affects mode of delivery planning. In situations where it is unlikely that the fetus will be able to withstand the challenges of uterine contractions, a cesarean section without a trial of labor should be considered. If it is estimated that the placental reserve will allow vaginal delivery, continuous fetal CTG is warranted. Because it can be difficult to accurately predict whether a fetus will tolerate labor, shared decision making is critical.

Corticosteroids and Magnesium Sulfate

Once it is estimated that the antenatal risks surpass the neonatal risk and intensive monitoring is underway with the intent to deliver a fetus, it is also important to optimally anticipate imminent delivery. The benefit of a single course of antenatal corticosteroids to accelerate fetal lung maturation for spontaneous premature delivery has been unequivocally established remote from term.[66] Whether this is also valid in the context of severe early-onset FGR is uncertain, as these high-risk pregnancies were often excluded from trials included in meta-analyses. Nonetheless, it is appropriate to offer this potentially potent preventive therapy, as it is endorsed by professional societies.[25]

A serendipitous finding from studies assessing magnesium sulfate for prevention of eclamptic seizures was a reduction in the risk of cerebral palsy, and several studies have since confirmed that magnesium sulfate has a neuroprotective effect and can reduce the incidence of cerebral palsy when given to women at risk of early preterm (<32 weeks) birth.[67–69]

Postnatal Pediatric Care

The need for specialized pediatric care is self-evident if birth is very preterm. Given the potential for the need of specialized postnatal pediatric care, clinicians should be prompted to consider referral to a center where such specialized care is available. Specific attention should be given to the problems associated with long-standing metabolic challenges, such as an increased risk of necrotizing enterocolitis and difficulties in achieving full enteral feeding. However, if growth restriction is suspected in a neonate born at term, transitional problems above and beyond those associated with preterm birth should be anticipated. These problems include neonatal hypoglycemia and jaundice.

Summary and future perspectives

Currently, there is no proven therapeutic option in FGR other than timed delivery. In early-onset FGR, Doppler assessment of UA, MCA, and DV, along with visual or computerized CTG assessment can be used to guide delivery timing. However, the optimal combination of how to use these modalities remains unclear. Some may be indicative in themselves (recurrent FHR decelerations) but most seem to be interdependent. In the future, the integration of these variables in decision support tools is likely to be of great value. The development of such tools would require a collaborative effort to analyze prospectively collected data that include all known prognostic factors: cCTG, fetal sex, gestational age, Doppler measurements of fetal (UA, MCA, DV) and maternal (uterine artery) blood vessels, and maternal characteristics (age, body mass index, blood pressure) as well as serum biomarkers (PIGF, sFLT). In the development of such a model, several sources of bias, including intervention bias and competing risks, need to be accounted for. Moreover, before implementation of decision support, the approach needs to be prospectively evaluated with a randomization element with outcomes that include long-term neonatal follow-up.

In late-onset FGR, identifying the fetus that is at risk for immediate hypoxia and benefits from expedited delivery is the challenge. In most cases, available parameters have imperfect correlation with important outcomes, particularly when considered dichotomously and as stand-alone prognosticators. It is likely that studies in the next decades will provide evidence on how to use estimated fetal size in combination with other identifiers of placental insufficiency in risk models that include these identifiers as continuous variables.

CLINICS CARE POINTS

- The most common mechanism in fetal growth restriction is suboptimal remodeling of uterine spiral arteries, leading to smooth muscle cell vascular reactivity of the maternal vascular bed, resulting in high-resistance placental circulation without a constant large amount of low-velocity maternal blood flow into the intervillous space.

- Doppler ultrasound of the uterine artery, umbilical artery, and middle cerebral artery can be measured throughout pregnancy and provides an indication of placental function.

- The main obstetric decision for fetal growth restriction remains timing of delivery. In early-onset fetal growth restriction, management hinges on weighing the risk of prematurity versus the risk of fetal hypoxia; in late-onset fetal growth restriction, the clinical challenge is the correct diagnosis of the fetus at risk for hypoxia.

DISCLOSURE

The authors S. Gordijn and W. Ganzevoort report the in-kind contribution of study materials from Roche Diagnostics for investigator-initiated studies. The authors C. Bruin and S. Damhuis have nothing to disclose.

REFERENCES

1. Verfaille V, de Jonge A, Mokkink L, et al. Multidisciplinary consensus on screening for, diagnosis and management of fetal growth restriction in the Netherlands. BMC Pregnancy Childbirth 2017;17(1):353.

2. Gordijn SJ, Beune IM, Thilaganathan B, et al. Consensus definition of fetal growth restriction: a Delphi procedure. Ultrasound Obstet Gynecol 2016;48(3):333–9.
3. Ko TJ, Tsai LY, Chu LC, et al. Parental smoking during pregnancy and its association with low birth weight, small for gestational age, and preterm birth offspring: a birth cohort study. Pediatr Neonatol 2014;55(1):20–7.
4. Dunsworth HM, Warrener AG, Deacon T, et al. Metabolic hypothesis for human altriciality. Proc Natl Acad Sci U S A 2012;109(38):15212–6.
5. Thilaganathan B. Ultrasound fetal weight estimation at term may do more harm than good. Ultrasound Obstet Gynecol 2018;52(1):5–8.
6. Bell E. A bad combination. Nat Rev Immunol 2004;4:1.
7. Burton GJ, Jauniaux E. Placental oxidative stress: from miscarriage to preeclampsia. J Soc Gynecol Investig 2004;11(6):342–52.
8. Khong TY, Mooney EE, Ariel I, et al. Sampling and definitions of placental lesions: Amsterdam Placental Workshop Group Consensus Statement. Arch Pathol Lab Med 2016;140(7):698–713.
9. Kingdom JC, Audette MC, Hobson SR, et al. A placenta clinic approach to the diagnosis and management of fetal growth restriction. Am J Obstet Gynecol 2018;218(2S):S803–17.
10. Leslie K, Whitley GS, Herse F, et al. Increased apoptosis, altered oxygen signaling, and antioxidant defenses in first-trimester pregnancies with high-resistance uterine artery blood flow. Am J Pathol 2015;185(10):2731–41.
11. Baschat AA, Gembruch U, Harman CR. The sequence of changes in Doppler and biophysical parameters as severe fetal growth restriction worsens. Ultrasound Obstet Gynecol 2001;18(6):571–7.
12. Hecher K, Bilardo CM, Stigter RH, et al. Monitoring of fetuses with intrauterine growth restriction: a longitudinal study. Ultrasound Obstet Gynecol 2001;18(6):564–70.
13. Schreurs CA, de Boer MA, Heymans MW, et al. Prognostic accuracy of cerebro-placental ratio and middle cerebral artery Doppler for adverse perinatal outcomes: a systematic review and meta-analysis. Ultrasound Obstet Gynecol 2018;51(3):313–22.
14. Thompson RS, Stevens RJ. Mathematical model for interpretation of Doppler velocity waveform indices. Med Biol Eng Comput 1989;27(3):269–76.
15. Efkarpidis S, Alexopoulos E, Kean L, et al. Case-control study of factors associated with intrauterine fetal deaths. MedGenMed 2004;6(2):53.
16. Flood K, Unterscheider J, Daly S, et al. The role of brain sparing in the prediction of adverse outcomes in intrauterine growth restriction: results of the multicenter PORTO Study. Am J Obstet Gynecol 2014;211(3):288.e1-5.
17. Baschat AA, Cosmi E, Bilardo CM, et al. Predictors of neonatal outcome in early-onset placental dysfunction. Obstet Gynecol 2007;109(2 Pt 1):253–61.
18. Chappell LC, Duckworth S, Seed PT, et al. Diagnostic accuracy of placental growth factor in women with suspected preeclampsia: a prospective multicenter study. Circulation 2013;128(19):2121–31.
19. Benton SJ, Hu Y, Xie F, et al. Can placental growth factor in maternal circulation identify fetuses with placental intrauterine growth restriction? Am J Obstet Gynecol 2012;206(2):163.e1-7.
20. Calabrese S, Cardellicchio M, Mazzocco M, et al. Placental growth factor (PLGF) maternal circulating levels in normal pregnancies and in pregnancies at risk of developing placental insufficiency complications. Reprod Sci 2012;19(3):211A–2A.

21. Griffin M, Seed P, Webster L, et al. Placental growth factor (PLGF) and ultrasound parameters for predicting the small for gestational age infant (SGA) in suspected small for gestational age: Pelican FGR study. J Matern Fetal Neonatal Med 2014; 27:121–2.

22. Arduini D, Rizzo G, Caforio L, et al. Behavioural state transitions in healthy and growth retarded fetuses. Early Hum Dev 1989;19(3):155–65.

23. Kenneson A, Cannon MJ. Review and meta-analysis of the epidemiology of congenital cytomegalovirus (CMV) infection. Rev Med Virol 2007;17(4):253–76.

24. Yamamoto R, Ishii K, Shimada M, et al. Significance of maternal screening for toxoplasmosis, rubella, cytomegalovirus and herpes simplex virus infection in cases of fetal growth restriction. J Obstet Gynaecol Res 2013;39(3):653–7.

25. Society for Maternal-Fetal Medicine, Electronic address pso, Martins JG, et al. Society for Maternal-Fetal Medicine Consult Series #52: diagnosis and management of fetal growth restriction: (replaces clinical guideline number 3, April 2012). Am J Obstet Gynecol 2020;223(4):B2–17.

26. Guseh SH, Little SE, Bennett K, et al. Antepartum management and obstetric outcomes among pregnancies with Down syndrome from diagnosis to delivery. Prenat Diagn 2017;37(7):640–6.

27. Redman CW, Sargent IL, Staff AC. IFPA senior award lecture: making sense of pre-eclampsia - two placental causes of preeclampsia? Placenta 2014; 35(Suppl):S20–5.

28. Tranquilli AL, Dekker G, Magee L, et al. The classification, diagnosis and management of the hypertensive disorders of pregnancy: a revised statement from the ISSHP. Pregnancy Hypertens 2014;4(2):97–104.

29. Groom KM, North RA, Poppe KK, et al. The association between customised small for gestational age infants and pre-eclampsia or gestational hypertension varies with gestation at delivery. BJOG 2007;114(4):478–84.

30. Groom KM, David AL. The role of aspirin, heparin, and other interventions in the prevention and treatment of fetal growth restriction. Am J Obstet Gynecol 2018; 218(2S):S829–40.

31. von Dadelszen P, Dwinnell S, Magee LA, et al. Sildenafil citrate therapy for severe early-onset intrauterine growth restriction. BJOG 2011;118(5):624–8.

32. Paauw ND, Terstappen F, Ganzevoort W, et al. Sildenafil during pregnancy: a preclinical meta-analysis on fetal growth and maternal blood pressure. Hypertension 2017;70(5):998–1006.

33. Sharp A, Cornforth C, Jackson R, et al. Maternal sildenafil for severe fetal growth restriction (STRIDER): a multicentre, randomised, placebo-controlled, double-blind trial. Lancet Child Adolesc Health 2018;2(2):93–102.

34. Groom KM, McCowan LM, Mackay LK, et al. STRIDER NZAus: a multicentre randomised controlled trial of sildenafil therapy in early-onset fetal growth restriction. BJOG 2019;126(8):997–1006.

35. Pels A, Derks J, Elvan-Taspinar A, et al. Maternal sildenafil vs placebo in pregnant women with severe early-onset fetal growth restriction: a randomized clinical trial. JAMA Netw Open 2020;3(6):e205323.

36. Chen J, Gong X, Chen P, et al. Effect of L-arginine and sildenafil citrate on intrauterine growth restriction fetuses: a meta-analysis. BMC Pregnancy Childbirth 2016;16:225.

37. Terstappen F, Tol AJC, Gremmels H, et al. Prenatal amino acid supplementation to improve fetal growth: a systematic review and meta-analysis. Nutrients 2020; 12(9):2535.

38. David AL. Maternal uterine artery VEGF gene therapy for treatment of intrauterine growth restriction. Placenta 2017;59(Suppl 1):S44–50.

39. Spencer R, Rossi C, Lees M, et al. Achieving orphan designation for placental insufficiency: annual incidence estimations in Europe. BJOG 2019;126(9): 1157–67.

40. Gaugler-Senden IP, Huijssoon AG, Visser W, et al. Maternal and perinatal outcome of preeclampsia with an onset before 24 weeks' gestation. Audit in a tertiary referral center. Eur J Obstet Gynecol Reprod Biol 2006;128(1–2):216–21.

41. Ganzevoort W, Thornton JG, Marlow N, et al. Comparative analysis of 2-year outcomes in GRIT and TRUFFLE trials. Ultrasound Obstet Gynecol 2020;55(1): 68–74.

42. Lees CC, Marlow N, van Wassenaer-Leemhuis A, et al. 2 year neurodevelopmental and intermediate perinatal outcomes in infants with very preterm fetal growth restriction (TRUFFLE): a randomised trial. Lancet 2015;385(9983):2162–72.

43. McCowan LM, Figueras F, Anderson NH. Evidence-based national guidelines for the management of suspected fetal growth restriction: comparison, consensus, and controversy. Am J Obstet Gynecol 2018;218(2S):S855–68.

44. Karsdorp VH, Van Vugt JM, Van Geijn HP, et al. Clinical significance of absent or reversed end diastolic velocity waveforms in umbilical artery. Lancet 1994; 344(8938):1664–8.

45. Morsing E, Brodszki J, Thuring A, et al. Infant outcome after active management of early-onset fetal growth restriction with absent or reverse umbilical artery blood flow. Ultrasound Obstet Gynecol 2020.

46. Dawes GS, Redman CW, Smith JH. Improvements in the registration and analysis of fetal heart rate records at the bedside. Br J Obstet Gynaecol 1985;92(4): 317–25.

47. Wolf H, Bruin C, Dobbe JGG, et al. Computerized fetal cardiotocography analysis in early preterm fetal growth restriction - a quantitative comparison of two applications. J Perinat Med 2019;47(4):439–47.

48. Street P, Dawes GS, Moulden M, et al. Short-term variation in abnormal antenatal fetal heart rate records. Am J Obstet Gynecol 1991;165(3):515–23.

49. Pels A, Mensing van Charante NA, Vollgraff Heidweiller-Schreurs CA, et al. The prognostic accuracy of short term variation of fetal heart rate in early-onset fetal growth restriction: a systematic review. Eur J Obstet Gynecol Reprod Biol 2019; 234:179–84.

50. Bilardo CM, Hecher K, Visser GH, et al. Severe fetal growth restriction at 26–32 weeks: key messages from the TRUFFLE study. Ultrasound Obstet Gynecol 2017;50(September):285–90.

51. Ganzevoort W, Mensing Van Charante N, Thilaganathan B, et al. How to monitor pregnancies complicated by fetal growth restriction and delivery before 32 weeks: post-hoc analysis of TRUFFLE study. Ultrasound Obstet Gynecol 2017;49(6):769–77.

52. Turan S, Turan OM, Berg C, et al. Computerized fetal heart rate analysis, Doppler ultrasound and biophysical profile score in the prediction of acid-base status of growth-restricted fetuses. Ultrasound Obstet Gynecol 2007;30(5):750–6.

53. Vasak B, Koenen SV, Koster MP, et al. Human fetal growth is constrained below optimal for perinatal survival. Ultrasound Obstet Gynecol 2015;45(2):162–7.

54. Moraitis AA, Wood AM, Fleming M, et al. Birth weight percentile and the risk of term perinatal death. Obstet Gynecol 2014;124(2 Pt 1):274–83.

55. Delnord M, Zeitlin J. Epidemiology of late preterm and early term births - an international perspective. Semin Fetal Neonatal Med 2019;24(1):3–10.

56. Boers KE, Vijgen SM, Bijlenga D, et al. Induction versus expectant monitoring for intrauterine growth restriction at term: randomised equivalence trial (DIGITAT). BMJ 2010;341:c7087.
57. van Wyk L, Boers KE, van der Post JA, et al. Effects on (neuro)developmental and behavioral outcome at 2 years of age of induced labor compared with expectant management in intrauterine growth-restricted infants: long-term outcomes of the DIGITAT trial. Am J Obstet Gynecol 2012;206(5):406.e1-7.
58. Ganzevoort W, Thilaganathan B, Baschat A, et al. Point: fetal growth and risk assessment: is there an impasse? Am J Obstet Gynecol 2019;220(1):9.
59. Figueras F, Gratacos E. An integrated approach to fetal growth restriction. Best Pract Res Clin Obstet Gynaecol 2017;38:48–58.
60. Morris RK, Selman TJ, Verma M, et al. Systematic review and meta-analysis of the test accuracy of ductus venosus Doppler to predict compromise of fetal/neonatal wellbeing in high risk pregnancies with placental insufficiency. Eur J Obstet Gynecol Reprod Biol 2010;152(1):3–12.
61. Vollgraff Heidweiller-Schreurs CA, van Osch IR, Heymans MW, et al. Cerebroplacental ratio in predicting adverse perinatal outcome: a meta-analysis of individual participant data. BJOG 2020.
62. Bujold E, Roberge S, Nicolaides KH. Low-dose aspirin for prevention of adverse outcomes related to abnormal placentation. Prenat Diagn 2014;34(7):642–8.
63. Bettiol A, Lombardi N, Crescioli G, et al. Pharmacological interventions for the prevention of fetal growth restriction: protocol for a systematic review and network meta-analysis. BMJ Open 2019;9(7):e029467.
64. LeFevre ML, Force USPST. Low-dose aspirin use for the prevention of morbidity and mortality from preeclampsia: U.S. Preventive Services Task Force recommendation statement. Ann Intern Med 2014;161(11):819–26.
65. Rolnik DL, Wright D, Poon LC, et al. Aspirin versus placebo in pregnancies at high risk for preterm preeclampsia. N Engl J Med 2017;377(7):613–22.
66. Roberts D, Brown J, Medley N, et al. Antenatal corticosteroids for accelerating fetal lung maturation for women at risk of preterm birth. Cochrane Database Syst Rev 2017;(3):CD004454.
67. Altman D, Carroli G, Duley L, et al. Do women with pre-eclampsia, and their babies, benefit from magnesium sulphate? The Magpie Trial: a randomised placebo-controlled trial. Lancet 2002;359(9321):1877–90.
68. Doyle LW, Crowther CA, Middleton P, et al. Magnesium sulphate for women at risk of preterm birth for neuroprotection of the fetus. Cochrane Database Syst Rev 2009;(1):CD004661.
69. Crowther CA, Middleton PF, Voysey M, et al. Assessing the neuroprotective benefits for babies of antenatal magnesium sulphate: an individual participant data meta-analysis. PLoS Med 2017;14(10):e1002398.

Evaluation and Management of Fetal Macrosomia

Michelle T. Nguyen, MD, Joseph G. Ouzounian, MD, MBA*

KEYWORDS

- Macrosomia • Ultrasound • Shoulder dystocia

KEY POINTS

- Macrosomia is most commonly defined as a birthweight exceeding 4000 g. Large for gestational age (LGA) is defined as birthweight greater than the 90th percentile at a given gestational age.
- Risk factors for macrosomia include maternal prepregnancy characteristics, maternal co-morbidities, maternal obstetric history, fetal characteristics, and (rarely) genetic syndromes.
- Macrosomia can be diagnosed using clinical techniques, ultrasound, and maternal estimation. MRI is also being investigated. All techniques have limited accuracy in predicting macrosomia.
- Fetal macrosomia can result in shoulder dystocia, neonatal brachial plexus injury, and clavicle fracture.

INTRODUCTION

Suspected fetal macrosomia is common in modern obstetrics. The delivery of large fetuses is clinically important because of the risk for maternal and neonatal complications. Data from the National Center for Health Statistics shows that in 2018, 7.8% of liveborn infants in the United States weighed more than 4000 g at birth, and 1% weighed more than 4500 g. About 0.1% weighed more than 5000 g.[1] Potential maternal risks of macrosomia include an increased risk for Cesarean birth, protracted labor, uterine rupture, postpartum hemorrhage, third- and fourth-degree perineal lacerations, and infection. Potential neonatal risks include shoulder dystocia, bone fracture, brachial plexus injuries, low 5-minute Apgar scores, neonatal intensive care unit admission, hypoglycemia, polycythemia, meconium aspiration, respiratory problems, and in rare cases, asphyxial injury.[2–4] Some studies suggest that fetal macrosomia can lead to childhood obesity, glucose intolerance, and development of metabolic syndrome later in life.[5,6]

Department of Obstetrics and Gynecology, USC/Keck School of Medicine, 2020 Zonal Avenue, IRD 236, Los Angeles, CA 90033, USA
* Corresponding author.
E-mail address: joseph.ouzounian@med.usc.edu

Obstet Gynecol Clin N Am 48 (2021) 387–399
https://doi.org/10.1016/j.ogc.2021.02.008
0889-8545/21/© 2021 Elsevier Inc. All rights reserved.

DEFINITION OF MACROSOMIA

The terms macrosomia and large for gestational age (LGA) both refer to excessive fetal growth. Even though there is no universal agreement regarding the absolute threshold for macrosomia, historically it has been defined as a birthweight exceeding 4000 g independent of gestational age. The term large for gestational age refers to infants whose birthweight exceeds the 90th percentile for growth at a specific gestational age. The American College of Obstetricians and Gynecologists (ACOG) acknowledges that there is increased morbidity in infants with a birthweight greater than 4000 g, and the risks of adverse outcomes increase on a continuum as the birthweight increases. Thus, infants with a birthweight over 5000 g have higher morbidity than infants weighing 4500 to 4999 g, who in turn have higher morbidity than infants weighing 4000 to 4499 g.[2,7] These increments of increased risk serve as the basis for a macrosomia grading system used by some clinicians in the decision-making process for mode of delivery: grade 1 for weight of 4000 to 4499 g, grade 2 for weight of 4500 to 4999 g, and grade 3 for weight over 5000 g.[2]

RISK FACTORS FOR MACROSOMIA

There are several historic risk factors described in association with macrosomia. These risk factors, listed in **Table 1**, include maternal prepregnancy characteristics, maternal comorbidities, maternal obstetric history, fetal characteristics, and (rarely) genetic syndromes.[8–15] One study found that macrosomia in a prior pregnancy was the single strongest individual risk factor for recurrent macrosomia.[8] Many of the risk factors for macrosomia (male sex, parity, prior history of macrosomia, and maternal prepregnancy weight) are predetermined at conception and are not modifiable. Overall, less than 40% of macrosomic infants are born to women with identifiable risk factors.[16]

In normal-weight women with gestational diabetes, 13.6% give birth to an LGA infant, while 22.3% of obese women with gestational diabetes give birth to LGA infants.[17] Conversely, in diabetic women with good glycemic control, the rate of macrosomia approaches that of the general population (10%–13%). Even though the risk of accelerated fetal growth in infants of diabetic mothers increases with worsening hyperglycemia, there is no known universal threshold value of hyperglycemia that predisposes the fetus to macrosomia.

Poorly understood factors that relate to increased fetal growth include genetic predisposition, fetal intrauterine metabolism, and placental nutrient transport. Some or all of these factors likely contribute to the intrauterine environment and influence fetal growth. Fetal hyperinsulinism is an example of altered fetal metabolism that can lead to excessive intrauterine growth and an increased risk for type 2 diabetes in later life. However, fetal hyperinsulinism appears to affect only a minority of pregnancies complicated by diabetes and does not correlate well with maternal glycemic control. This lack of association between fetal hyperinsulinism and maternal glucose levels may explain why good glycemic control does not eliminate the risk of macrosomia in some diabetic pregnancies.[18]

DIAGNOSIS OF MACROSOMIA

Available methods for diagnosis of macrosomia are ultrasound measurements, MRI measurements, clinical assessment via Leopold maneuvers or fundal height measurements, and maternal estimation. A comparison of these diagnostic techniques, including sensitivities and specificities, is provided in **Table 2**.[19–26] Unfortunately,

Table 1
Risk factors associated with macrosomia

Category	Examples	Odds Ratio (OR)	Studies
Maternal prepregnancy characteristics	Ethnicity Height ≥80th percentile Own birth weight >4000g	0.54–1.15 1.71 1.378	Bowers et al,[8] 2013 Marshall et al,[9] 2019 Su et al,[10] 2016
Maternal comorbidities	Diabetes (pregestational) Diabetes (gestational) Hypertriglyceridemia Obesity (body mass index [BMI] ≥30 kg/m²) Excessive gestational weight gain	6.97 1.48–2.77 1.19 2.08–5.64 1.55–5.45	Jolly et al,[11] 2003 Jolly et al,[11] 2003 Bowers et al,[8] 2013 Jin et al,[12] 2016 Jolly et al,[11] 2003 Usta et al,[13] 2017 Bowers et al,[8] 2013 Usta et al,[13] 2017
Maternal obstetric history	History of macrosomia Multiparity Advanced maternal age	3.62 1.31–2.20 1.22–1.86	Bowers et al, 2013 Jolly et al,[11] 2003 Bowers et al,[8] 2013 Usta et al,[13] 2017 Bowers et al,[8] 2013 Jolly et al,[11] 2003 Usta et al,[13] 2017
Fetal characteristics	Male fetus Post-term (gestational age ≥42 weeks)	1.89–2.0 2.62	Usta et al,[13] 2017 Sheiner et al,[14] 2004 Maoz et al,[15] 2019
Genetic syndromes	Beckwith Wiedemann Weaver Sotos Perlman Costello Pallister-Killian	N/A	N/A

accurate detection of macrosomia prior to birth remains a clinical conundrum. Although accelerated fundal height growth may provide an early clinical clue for suspected macrosomia, fundal height measurements themselves are not reliable with birthweight greater than 4000 g.[23] With birthweights between 2500 and 4000 g, good evidence demonstrates the superiority of ultrasound-derived fetal weight estimates over clinical estimation. However, all techniques lose accuracy as birthweight increases over 4000 g.[27]

There are over 30 different formulas for ultrasound estimates of fetal weight, but most use the fetal biparietal diameter, head circumference, abdominal circumference, and femur length alone or in combination to estimate fetal weight. In studies comparing the most common formulas, Hadlock's formula (which incorporates biparietal diameter, femur length, and abdominal circumference) produced the most accurate estimates of fetal weight, whereas Shepard's formula (which incorporates only biparietal diameter and abdominal circumference) produced the least accurate estimates.[28,29] Other formulas have been derived specifically for diabetic patients and specifically for patients with clinically suspected macrosomia. However, these formulas have not been shown to be useful in distinguishing macrosomic fetuses from normal-weight fetuses.[30–32] Overall, ultrasound estimates of fetal weight have a low

Table 2
Methods for diagnosing macrosomia

Diagnostic Method	Sensitivity	Specificity	Studies
Fundal height measurement	20%–70%	>90%	Persson et al,[24] 1986 Goetzinger et al,[23] 2013
Abdominal palpation or Leopold's maneuvers	16%–68%	90%–99%	Chauhan et al. 1998 Weiner et al,[25] 2002 Noumi et al,[22] 2005 Peregrine et al,[26] 2007
Ultrasound (for infants weighing >4000 g)	10%–45%	57%–99%	Malin et al,[19] 2016
Ultrasound (for infants weighing >4500 g)	56%	92%	Malin et al,[19] 2016
MRI	85%–93%	95%–97%	Malin et al,[19] 2016 Kadji et al,[21] 2019

sensitivity (10%–45%), but a high specificity (57%–99%) and high negative predictive value (92%–99%) for detecting macrosomia.[20,25,33,34] However, the American Institute of Ultrasound in Medicine reports that even the best fetal weight detection methods yield error rates of approximately 15%.[35] Other reports show error rates as high as 38% in infants weighing over 4500 g.[36]

When studied individually, abdominal circumference may be the most clinically useful biometric parameter in the sonographic evaluation for macrosomia, particularly in diabetic patients. Even when the overall estimated fetal weight is less than the 90th percentile, an abdominal circumference measuring greater than the 90th percentile or 2 to 3 weeks ahead of gestational age may be a sign of impending macrosomia. Some data suggest that if the abdominal circumference measures less than the 90th percentile on 2 consecutive ultrasounds, the likelihood of developing macrosomia is low.[37] In 1 study, using large fetal abdominal circumference as a criterion for starting insulin in patients with gestational diabetes resulted in a reduction in birthweight.[38]

Another ultrasound measurement that has been studied in the context of macrosomia is fetal soft tissue thickness. Measurements of the subcutaneous fat can be performed in multiple areas including the shoulder, midhumerus, abdominal wall, thigh, and buccal area.[39–43] Initial studies show that soft tissue thickness may predict macrosomia and correlates well with skin fold measurements at birth.[44–46] Increased soft tissue thickness and increased skin fold thickness are most commonly seen in pregnancies with poorly controlled diabetes. Although this technique has not been adopted widely in clinical practice, these initial studies are promising and warrant further investigation.

Other studies show that the ratio of head circumference (HC) to abdominal circumference (AC) in diabetic pregnancies may indicate disproportionate fetal growth. In fact, these earlier studies demonstrated that an HC/AC ratio of less than 0.80 suggested disproportionate central body growth and was associated with an increased risk for shoulder dystocia and birth trauma. However, more recent data show that the ultrasound-derived fetal abdominal diameter-biparietal diameter difference is not a reliable predictor of shoulder dystocia or brachial plexus injury.[47–49]

In addition to ultrasonography, MRI is another imaging modality that may be used to estimate fetal weight. Recent studies found that MRI has a higher sensitivity and specificity than ultrasonography for detecting macrosomia.[19,21] However, the clinical utility of MRI may be limited by cost, availability, and the inability to image some patients adequately because of maternal obesity or claustrophobia. In addition, ultrafast MRI protocols are needed to image a live mobile fetus floating in amniotic fluid. As technology and techniques are refined, fetal MRI may be used more regularly in clinical practice. Although promising, at this time, fetal MRI to detect macrosomia is considered investigational.

As noted previously, clinical estimates of fetal weight can also be achieved by abdominal palpation (Leopold maneuvers) and fundal height measurements. Some studies indicate that in experienced hands, clinical estimates approach the accuracy of ultrasound estimates for fetal weight.[20,22,50–53] Other studies show that a mother's estimate of her own baby's weight can be as accurate as clinical or ultrasound estimates.[26,54] In clinical practice, it is reasonable to use maternal and clinical estimates to estimate fetal weight, but in cases where macrosomia is suspected, ultrasound examination should be considered. Despite the inherent limitations of all available methods for fetal weight estimation, a combination of clinical estimates, ultrasound assessment, and clinical history can help craft an appropriate management plan when macrosomia is suspected.

PREVENTION OF MACROSOMIA

Overall, our ability to prevent macrosomia is limited, because many of the risk factors discussed are not modifiable. However, there are some strategies that can, at a minimum, mitigate the degree of macrosomia encountered. These include exercise, bariatric surgery for patients with class 2 or class 3 obesity, and appropriate glycemic control for diabetic patients.

There are multiple benefits of exercise during pregnancy including less weight gain, which is associated with lower risk of macrosomia or LGA infants, and lower risk of cesarean delivery.[55–57] These benefits have been observed with both resistance training and aerobic exercise. Exercise has not been associated with an increased risk of preterm birth or small for gestational age (SGA) infants. In contrast, patients who undergo bariatric surgery are at increased risk of delivering SGA infants and possibly preterm birth. The degree of pregnancy risks and long-term weight-loss benefits of bariatric surgery vary depending on the type of procedure. When compared with adjustable gastric banding (AGB), Roux-en-Y gastric bypass (RYGB) and sleeve gastrectomy (SG) are associated with more rapid weight loss in the immediate postoperative period,[58] in addition to higher rates of excess weight loss at 10-year follow-up.[59] Patients with RYGB or SG typically achieve optimal weight loss and weight stabilization by 1 year after surgery, as opposed to patients with AGB, who typically do not achieve these goals until 2 years after surgery; therefore, the recommended delay in conception after surgery is shorter for RYGB and SG than for AGB. However, RYGB and SG are associated with less gestational weight gain than AGB, and insufficient gestational weight gain in turn is strongly associated with adverse neonatal outcomes including low birth weight.[58] Furthermore, patients with RYGB are at increased risk of developing internal herniation during pregnancy, while patients with AGB are at increased risk of gastric band slippage during pregnancy.[58] For patients with class 2 or class 3 obesity, the aforementioned risks of bariatric surgical intervention must be weighed against the benefits of a lower likelihood of developing gestational diabetes and LGA infants.[60,61]

In women with diabetes, diet therapy to control maternal hyperglycemia can decrease macrosomia by as much as 73%.[62] In nondiabetic women, a low-glycemic diet may reduce excessive gestational weight gain; however, it is unclear whether diet alone reduces the risk of macrosomia in these patients.[63] Thus, women who are at risk for developing macrosomia should be advised to exercise and (if they are diabetic) to maintain euglycemia with an appropriate low glycemic diet. Furthermore, preconception counseling for patients with class 2 or class 3 obesity should include a discussion of the risks and benefits of bariatric surgery. If the patient elects to have bariatric surgery, it should be performed at least 6 months before a pregnancy is achieved.

MANAGEMENT OF SUSPECTED MACROSOMIA

Even though macrosomia is technically a statistical definition and not a true disease, the risk for potentially serious maternal, fetal, and neonatal morbidity mandates thoughtful management plans in patients with suspected macrosomia.

The clinical dilemma encountered most often by clinicians managing a patient with suspected macrosomia at term is whether or not to allow labor or to proceed with cesarean section. Here again, the effectiveness of prophylactic cesarean delivery in reducing fetal and neonatal morbidity in these cases has not been evaluated in randomized clinical trials. In addition, as outlined earlier, available techniques to estimate fetal weight in and of themselves are inaccurate. Finally, cesarean section reduces, but does not completely eliminate the risk for birth trauma and brachial plexus injury associated with vaginal birth.[64–66] Thus, while clinically it may be tempting to select a route of delivery based solely on estimated fetal weight, such a decision should take into account all pertinent risk factors and the patient's personal preferences and future reproductive plans as part of detailed informed consent. Patient counseling and shared decision making is warranted in these cases, and such counseling at a minimum should address several points:

> Accurate prediction of actual birthweight and/or shoulder dystocia antenatally is limited
> The incidence of shoulder dystocia and brachial plexus injuries is low even when macrosomia is present, and most macrosomic fetuses do not experience shoulder dystocia during vaginal delivery
> Brachial plexus injuries can occur even with cesarean delivery

Thus, vaginal delivery can be a reasonable plan in patients with suspected macrosomia but only after appropriate informed consent. Although a trial of labor after cesarean (TOLAC) is not contraindicated for patients with suspected macrosomia, these patients should be counseled on the increased risk of uterine rupture and the decreased likelihood of a successful vaginal birth after cesarean (VBAC).[67–70]

Current guidelines from ACOG do not support a planned cesarean delivery unless estimated fetal weight exceeds 4500 g in diabetic women or 5000 g in nondiabetic women.[7] These are broad guidelines, however, and care must be individualized and based on informed consent and clinical judgment. The benefits of induction of labor as opposed to expectant management for suspected macrosomia are uncertain, especially prior to 39 weeks gestation. Some studies have shown that induction of labor for suspected macrosomia at any gestational age increases the risk of cesarean delivery but does not reduce shoulder dystocia or neonatal morbidity.[71–73] Other studies, some of which included patients induced prior to 39 weeks gestation,[74–76] have shown that induction of labor was not associated with a lower risk of shoulder dystocia and was possibly associated with a slightly lower risk of cesarean delivery.[77,78] Further studies are needed to clarify the optimal timing for delivery of infants with suspected macrosomia and whether induction of labor improves outcomes in such cases. At present, induction at 39 weeks for suspected macrosomia (or electively) is reasonable in cases with appropriate informed consent and shared decision making. Induction prior to 39 weeks is not as well supported by the current literature but may still be considered carefully in select cases, especially if there are other maternal comorbidities such as poorly controlled diabetes.

If a patient with macrosomia has been appropriately counseled and desires to attempt a trial of labor, careful intrapartum monitoring of the labor curve and fetal heart tracing are required. The obstetrician should anticipate and be prepared for the possibility of postpartum hemorrhage and shoulder dystocia at the time of delivery. Uterotonic medications (eg, oxytocin, methylergonovine, 15-methyl prostaglandin $F_{2\alpha}$, and misoprostol), tranexamic acid, and an intrauterine balloon tamponade should be available at bedside in case the patient experiences heavy bleeding because of uterine atony. The obstetrician should also consider obtaining a type and crossmatch at the time of admission to have appropriate blood products available for a possible transfusion, especially if the patient is anemic. Furthermore, the obstetrician should ensure that other staff members are available and qualified to assist in case of shoulder dystocia. Shoulder dystocia simulations and team-based drills effectively improve communication and utilization of obstetric maneuvers while potentially reducing the risk of transient brachial plexus injuries.[79,80]

Operative vaginal delivery, especially midpelvic procedures, increase the risk of shoulder dystocia and brachial plexus injury and should be used with extreme caution in patients with suspected macrosomia. The risk is even higher in patients with suspected macrosomia and a prolonged second stage of labor or arrest of descent.[81] In these circumstances, cesarean delivery is preferable. At a minimum, extensive informed consent is required prior to attempting operative vaginal delivery in patients with suspected macrosomia. Such counseling should address not only the increased risk of shoulder dystocia and brachial plexus injury, but also the increased risk of third- or fourth-degree perineal lacerations (which themselves lead to hemorrhage, pain, dyspareunia, and fecal incontinence).

MANAGEMENT OF SHOULDER DYSTOCIA

Shoulder dystocia occurs in 0.15% to 2.0% of all vaginal deliveries, but the incidence is as high as 14% when the birthweight exceeds 4500 g.[7] Once a shoulder dystocia is encountered, standardized maneuvers usually relieve the impaction and accomplish delivery. These include, but are not limited to, McRobert maneuver, suprapubic pressure, delivery of the posterior arm, and rotational maneuvers (Rubin and Wood). Although no randomized controlled trials have demonstrated the superior efficacy of one maneuver over another, it is reasonable to begin with McRobert maneuver, because it is relatively simple and will resolve the shoulder dystocia in about 40% of cases.[82] Addition of suprapubic pressure will resolve about 60% of shoulder dystocia cases, and three maneuvers will resolve 95% of cases.[82] If all these maneuvers are unsuccessful, Gaskin all-fours maneuver (positioning the patient on her hands and knees and applying downward traction on the posterior shoulder) and episiotomy may be employed. Then, if still unsuccessful, the maneuvers can be repeated. In extreme cases where the shoulder dystocia is not alleviated after the aforementioned techniques have been exhausted, heroic measures such as intentional clavicular fracture (which involves pulling the anterior clavicle outward to decrease the bisacromial diameter) and Zavanelli maneuver (which involves pushing the fetal head back into the vagina in preparation for cesarean delivery) can be performed as a last resort. Intentional clavicular fracture is technically challenging and may cause injury to underlying vascular and pulmonary structures, but it is less morbid than the Zavanelli maneuver.[83]

Although shoulder dystocia can result in neonatal brachial plexus palsy and clavicle fracture, these outcomes are uncommon, and most cases resolve without permanent sequalae. Brachial plexus palsies (both transient and permanent) affect 1.5 per 1000 total births, while clavicle fractures affect 0.4% to 0.6% of all births and can occur in women with and without shoulder dystocia.[84–86] However, fetal macrosomia increases the risk for brachial plexus palsy. In women with a history of shoulder dystocia in a prior pregnancy, cesarean section should be recommended, as the risk of recurrent shoulder dystocia can be as high as 17%.[87–91]

SUMMARY

Macrosomia results from abnormal fetal growth and can lead to serious consequences for both the mother and fetus. From a practical perspective, most known risk factors are not easily modifiable. Techniques to diagnose macrosomia include ultrasound examination, clinical estimation, maternal estimation, and MRI. The ability to accurately predict birthweight remains limited, and all techniques have an error rate of 15% to 20% or higher, especially as birthweight increases. In cases of suspected macrosomia, patients must be counseled carefully regarding a delivery plan, and cesarean section should be considered when indicated. Although induction for suspected macrosomia typically is not advisable before 39 weeks gestation, it may be considered in select cases after shared decision-making and with careful informed consent. In all deliveries with suspected macrosomia, extreme caution is advised with regard to operative vaginal delivery. Although shoulder dystocia can occur in any vaginal delivery, increasing birthweight is associated with a higher incidence of shoulder dystocia and concomitant brachial plexus injury, and these factors must be weighed carefully in devising an appropriate delivery plan.

CLINICS CARE POINTS

- Ultrasound assessment may be the most clinically useful method to assess for macrosomia, particularly in diabetic patients.
- Some strategies that can mitigate the degree of macrosomia include exercise, bariatric surgery for patients with class 2 or class 3 obesity, and appropriate glycemic control for diabetic patients.
- Cesarean delivery is recommended when the estimated fetal weight is 4500 g in diabetic patients or 5000 g in nondiabetic patients.
- For patients with macrosomia, induction of labor may be considered on an individualized basis and only with appropriate informed consent.
- Women with suspected macrosomia are at increased risk for postpartum hemorrhage and shoulder dystocia at the time of delivery.

DISCLOSURE

The authors have nothing to disclose.

REFERENCES

1. Martin JA, Hamilton BE, Osterman MJK, et al. Births: final data for 2018. Natl Vital Stat Rep 2019;68:1–47.
2. Boulet SL, Alexander GR, Salihu HM, et al. Macrosomic births in the united states: determinants, outcomes, and proposed grades of risk. Am J Obstet Gynecol 2003;188(5):1372–8.

3. King JR, Korst LM, Miller DA, et al. Increased composite maternal and neonatal morbidity associated with ultrasonographically suspected fetal macrosomia. J Matern Fetal Neonatal Med 2012;25(10):1953–9.
4. Gillean JR, Coonrod DV, Russ R, et al. Big infants in the neonatal intensive care unit. Am J Obstet Gynecol 2005;192(6):1948–53 [discussion: 1953–5].
5. Cnattingius S, Villamor E, Lagerros YT, et al. High birthweight and obesity–a vicious circle across generations. Int J Obes (Lond) 2012;36(10):1320–4.
6. Sparano S, Ahrens W, De Henauw S, et al. Being macrosomic at birth is an independent predictor of overweight in children: results from the IDEFICS study. Matern Child Health J 2013;17:1373–81.
7. American College of Obstetricians and Gynecologists. Macrosomia. Practice Bulletin no. 216. Washington, DC: ACOG; 2019.
8. Bowers K, Laughon SK, Kiely M, et al. Gestational diabetes, pre-pregnancy obesity and pregnancy weight gain in relation to excess fetal growth: variations by race/ethnicity. Diabetologia 2013;56:1263–71.
9. Marshall NE, Biel FM, Boone-Heinonen J, et al. The association between maternal height, body mass index, and perinatal outcomes. Am J Perinatol 2019;36(6):632–40.
10. Su R, Zhu W, Wei Y, et al. Relationship of maternal birth weight on maternal and neonatal outcomes: a multicenter study in Beijing. J Perinatol 2016;36(12):1061–6.
11. Jolly MC, Sebire NJ, Harris JP, et al. Risk factors for macrosomia and its clinical consequences: a study of 350,311 pregnancies. Eur J Obstet Gynecol Reprod Biol 2003;111(1):9–14.
12. Jin WY, Lin SL, Hou RL, et al. Associations between maternal lipid profile and pregnancy complications and perinatal outcomes: a population-based study from China. BMC Pregnancy Childbirth 2016;16:60.
13. Usta A, Usta CS, Yildiz A, et al. Frequency of fetal macrosomia and the associated risk factors in pregnancies without gestational diabetes mellitus. Pan Afr Med J 2017;26:62.
14. Sheiner E, Levy A, Katz M, et al. Gender does matter in perinatal medicine. Fetal Diagn Ther 2004;19:366–9.
15. Maoz O, Wainstock T, Sheiner E, et al. Immediate perinatal outcomes of post-term deliveries. J Matern Fetal Neonatal Med 2019;32(11):1847–52.
16. Little SE, Edlow AG, Thomas AM, et al. Estimated fetal weight by ultrasound: a modifiable risk factor for cesrean delivery? Am J Obstet Gynecol 2012;207:309.e1-6.
17. Black MH, Sacks DA, Xiang AH, et al. The relative contribution of prepregnancy overweight and obesity, gestational weight gain, and IADPSG-defined gestational diabetes mellitus to fetal overgrowth. Diabetes Care 2013;36:56–62.
18. Metzger BE, Lowe LP, Dyer AR, et al. HAPO study collaborative research group. N Engl J Med 2008;258:1991–2002.
19. Malin GL, Bugg GJ, Takwoingi Y, et al. Antenatal magnetic resonance imaging versus ultrasound for predicting neonatal macrosomia: a systematic review and meta-analysis. BJOG 2016;123:77–88.
20. Chauhan SP, Hendrix NW, Magann EF, et al. Limitations of clinical and sonographic estimates of birthweight: experience with 1034 parturients. Obstet Gynecol 1998;91:72–7.
21. Kadji C, Cannie MM, Resta S, et al. Magnetic resonance imaging for prenatal estimation of birthweight in pregnancy: review of available data, techniques, and future perspectives. Am J Obstet Gynecol 2019;220:428–39.

22. Noumi G, Collado-Khoury F, Bombard A, et al. Clinical and sonographic estimation of fetal weight performed during labor by residents. Am J Obstet Gynecol 2005;192:1407–9.
23. Goetzinger KR, Tuuli MG, Odibo AO, et al. Screening for fetal growth disorders by clinical exam in the era of obesity. J Perinatol 2013;33:352–7.
24. Persson B, Stangenberg M, Lunell NO, et al. Prediction of size of infants at birth by measurement of symphysis fundus height. Br J Obstet Gynaecol 1986;93:206–11.
25. Weiner Z, Ben-Shlomo I, Beck-Fruchter R, et al. Clinical and ultrasonographic weight estimation in large for gestational age fetus. Eur J Obstet Gynecol Reprod Biol 2002;105:20–4.
26. Peregrine E, O'Brien P, Jauniaux E. Clinical and ultrasound estimation of birthweight prior to induction of labor at term. Ultrasound Obstet Gynecol 2007;29:304–9.
27. Scioscia M, Vimercati A, Ceci O, et al. Estimation of birthweights by two-dimensional ultrasonography: a critical appraisal of its accuracy. Obstet Gynecol 2008;111:57–65.
28. Faschingbauer F, Voigt F, Goecke TW, et al. Fetal weight estimation in extreme macrosomia ($\geq$ 4,500 g): comparison of 10 formulas. Ultraschall Med 2012; 33:E62.
29. Rosati P, Arduini M, Giri C, et al. Ultrasonographic weight estimation in large for gestational age fetuses: a comparison of 17 sonographic formulas and four models algorithms. J Matern Fetal Neonatal Med 2010;23:675.
30. Cesnaite G, Domza G, Ramasauskaite D, et al. The Accuracy of 22 Fetal Weight Estimation Formulas in Diabetic Pregnancies. Fetal Diagn Ther 2020;47(1):54–9.
31. Porter B, Neely C, Szychowski J, et al. Ultrasonographic fetal weight estimation: should macrosomia-specific formulas be utilized? Am J Perinatol 2015;32(10):968–72.
32. Weiss C, Enengl S, Enzelsberger SH, et al. Does the Porter formula hold its promise? A weight estimation formula for macrosomic fetuses put to the test. Arch Gynecol Obstet 2020;301(1):129–35.
33. Aviram A, Yogev Y, Ashwal E, et al. Different formulas, different thresholds and different performance-the prediction of macrosomia by ultrasound. J Perinatol 2017;37:1285–91.
34. O'Reilly-Green CP, Divon MY. Receiver operating characteristic curves of sonographic estimated fetal weight for prediction of macrosomia in prolonged pregnancies. Ultrasound Obstet Gynecol 1997;9:403–8.
35. AIUM-ACR-ACOG-SMFM-SRU. Practice parameter for the performance of standard diagnostic obstetric ultrasound examinations. J Ultrasound Med 2018; 37(11):E13–24.
36. Lindell G, Källén K, Maršál K. Ultrasound weight estimation of large fetuses. Acta Obstet Gynecol Scand 2012;91(10):1218–25.
37. Schaefer-Graf UM, Wendt L, Sacks DA, et al. How many sonograms are needed to reliably predict the absence of fetal overgrowth in gestational diabetes mellitus pregnancies? Diabetes Care 2011;34:39.
38. Kjos SL, Schaefer-Graf U, Sardesi S, et al. A randomized controlled trial using glycemic plus fetal ultrasound parameters versus glycemic parameters to determine insulin therapy in gestational diabetes with fasting hyperglycemia. Diabetes Care 2001;24:1904.
39. Mintz MC, Landon MB, Gabbe SG, et al. Shoulder soft tissue width as a predictor of macrosomia in diabetic pregnancies. Am J Perinatol 1989;6:240.

40. Sood AK, Yancey M, Richards D. Prediction of fetal macrosomia using humeral soft tissue thickness. Obstet Gynecol 1995;85:937.
41. Petrikovsky BM, Oleschuk C, Lesser M, et al. Prediction of fetal macrosomia using sonographically measured abdominal subcutaneous tissue thickness. J Clin Ultrasound 1997;25:378.
42. Santolaya-Forgas J, Meyer WJ, Gauthier DW, et al. Intrapartum fetal subcutaneous tissue/femur length ratio: an ultrasonographic clue to fetal macrosomia. Am J Obstet Gynecol 1994;171:1072.
43. Abramowicz JS, Sherer DM, Woods JR Jr. Ultrasonographic measurement of cheek-to-cheek diameter in fetal growth disturbances. Am J Obstet Gynecol 1993;169:405.
44. Chauhan SP, West DJ, Scardo JA, et al. Antepartum detection of macrosomic fetus: clinical versus sonographic, including soft-tissue measurements. Obstet Gynecol 2000;95:639.
45. Rossi AC, Vimercati A, Greco P, et al. [Echographic measurement of subcutaneous adipose tissue as fetal growth index]. Acta Biomed Ateneo Parmense 2000; 71(Suppl 1):379.
46. Maruotti GM, Saccone G, Martinelli P. Third trimester ultrasound soft-tissue measurements accurately predicts macrosomia. J Matern Fetal Neonatal Med 2017; 30:972.
47. Cohen B, Penning S, Major C, et al. Sonographic prediction of shoulder dystocia in infants of diabetic mothers. Obstet Gynecol 1996;88:10–3.
48. Miller RS, Devine PC, Johnson EB. Sonographic fetal asymmetry predicts shoulder dystocia. J Ultrasound Med 2007;26:1523–8.
49. Rajan PV, Chung JH, Porto M, et al. Correlation of increased fetal asymmetry with shoulder dystocia in the nondiabetic woman with suspected macrosomia. J Reprod Med 2009;54:478–82.
50. Chauhan SP, Cowan BD, Magann EF, et al. Intrapartum detection of a macrosomic fetus: clinical versus 8 sonographic models. Aust N Z J Obstet Gynaecol 1995;35:266–70.
51. Sherman DJ, Arieli S, Tovbin J, et al. A comparison of clinical and ultrasonic estimation of fetal weight. Obstet Gynecol 1998;91:212–7.
52. Hendrix NW, Grady CS, Chauhan SP. Clinical vs. sonographic estimate of birthweight in term parturients. A randomized clinical trial. J Reprod Med 2000;45: 317–22.
53. Weiner E, Mizrachi Y, Fainstein N, et al. Comparison between three methods of fetal weight estimation during the active stage of labor performed by residents: a prospective cohort study. Fetal Diagn Ther 2017;42:117–23.
54. Harlev A, Walfisch A, Bar-David J, et al. Maternal estimation of fetal weight as a complementary method of fetal weight assessment: a prospective clinical trial. J Reprod Med 2006;51:515–20.
55. Wiebe HW, Boule NG, Chari R, et al. The effect of supervised prenatal exercise on fetal growth: a meta-analysis. Obstet Gynecol 2015;125:1185–94.
56. Davenport MH, Meah VL, Ruchat SM, et al. Impact of prenatal exercise on neonatal and childhood outcomes: a systematic review and meta-analysis. Br J Sports Med 2018;52:1386–96.
57. Physical activity and exercise during pregnancy and the postpartum period. Committee Opinion No. 650. American College of Obstetricians and Gynecologists. Obstet Gynecol 2015;126:e135–42.

58. Shawe J, Ceulemans D, Akhter Z, et al. Pregnancy after bariatric surgery: consensus recommendations for periconception, antenatal and postnatal care. Obes Rev 2019;20(11):1507–22.

59. O'Brien PE, Hindle A, Brennan L, et al. Long-term outcomes after bariatric surgery: a systematic review and meta-analysis of weight loss at 10 or more years for all bariatric procedures and a single-centre review of 20-year outcomes after adjustable gastric banding. Obes Surg 2019;29(1):3–14.

60. Yi XY, Li QF, Zhang J, et al. A meta-analysis of maternal and fetal outcomes of pregnancy after bariatric surgery. Int J Gynaecol Obstet 2015;130:3–9.

61. Galazis N, Docheva N, Simillis C, et al. Maternal and neonatal outcomes in women undergoing bariatric surgery: a systematic review and meta-analysis. Eur J Obstet Gynecol Reprod Biol 2014;181:45–53.

62. Wei J, Heng W, Gao J. Effects of low glycemic index diets on gestational diabetes mellitus: a meta-analysis of randomized controlled clinical trials. Medicine (Baltimore) 2016;95:e3792.

63. Muktabhant B, Lawrie TA, Lumbiganon P, et al. Diet or exercise, or both, for preventing excessive weight gain in pregnancy. Cochrane Database Syst Rev 2015;(6):CD007145.

64. Ecker JL, Greenberg JA, Norwitz ER, et al. Birthweight as a predictor of brachial plexus injury. Obstet Gynecol 1997;89:643–7.

65. Gherman RB, Goodwin TM, Ouzounian JG, et al. Brachial plexus palsy associated with cesarean section: an in utero injury? Am J Obstet Gynecol 1997;177:1162–4.

66. Gregory KD, Henry OA, Ramicone E, et al. Maternal and infant complications in high and normal weight infants by method of delivery. Obstet Gynecol 1998;92:507–13.

67. Barger MK, Weiss J, Nannini A, et al. Risk factors for uterine rupture among women who attempt a vaginal birth after a previous cesarean: a case-control study. J Reprod Med 2011;56(7–8):313–20.

68. Jastrow N, Roberge S, Gauthier RJ, et al. Effect of birth weight on adverse obstetric outcomes in vaginal birth after cesarean delivery. Obstet Gynecol 2010;115(2 Pt 1):338–43.

69. Elkousy MA, Sammel M, Stevens E, et al. The effect of birth weight on vaginal birth after cesarean delivery success rates. Am J Obstet Gynecol 2003;188:824–30.

70. Zelop CM, Shipp TD, Repke JT, et al. Outcomes of trial of labor following previous cesarean delivery among women with fetuses weighing >4000 g. Am J Obstet Gynecol 2001;185:903–5.

71. Combs CA, Singh NB, Khoury JC. Elective induction versus spontaneous labor after sonographic diagnosis of fetal macrosomia. Obstet Gynecol 1993;81:492–6.

72. Friesen CD, Miller AM, Rayburn WF. Influence of spontaneous or induced labor on delivering the macrosomic fetus. Am J Perinatol 1995;12:63–6.

73. Leaphart WL, Meyer MC, Capeless EL. Labor induction with a prenatal diagnosis of fetal macrosomia. J Matern Fetal Med 1997;6:99–102.

74. Boulvain M, Senat MV, Perrotin F, et al. Induction of labour versus expectant management for large-for-date fetuses: a randomised controlled trial. Groupe de Recherche en Obstetrique et Gynecologie, (GROG). Lancet 2015;385:2600–5.

75. Walker K, Thornton J. Induction of labour at 37 weeks for suspected fetal macrosomia may reduce birth trauma. Evid Based Med 2017;22(4):148.

76. Rozenberg P. En cas de macrosomie fœtale, la meilleure stratégie est le déclenchement artificiel du travail à 38 semaines d'aménorrhée [In case of fetal

macrosomia, the best strategy is the induction of labor at 38 weeks of gestation]. J Gynecol Obstet Biol Reprod (Paris) 2016;45(9):1037–44.

77. Cheng YW, Sparks TN, Laros RKJr, et al. Impending macrosomia: will induction of labour modify the risk of caesarean delivery? BJOG 2012;119:402–9.

78. Vendittelli F, Riviere O, Neveu B, et al, Audipog Sentinel Network. Does induction of labor for constitutionally large-for-gestational-age fetuses identified in utero reduce maternal morbidity? BMC Pregnancy Childbirth 2014;14:15–156.

79. Grobman WA, Miller D, Burke C, et al. Outcomes associated with introduction of a shoulder dystocia protocol. Am J Obstet Gynecol 2011;205:513–7.

80. Inglis SR, Feier N, Chetiyaar JB, et al. Effects of shoulder dystocia training on the incidence of brachial plexus injury. Am J Obstet Gynecol 2011;204:322.e1-6.

81. Benedetti TJ, Gabbe SG. Shoulder dystocia. A complication of fetal macrosomia and prolonged second stage of labor with midpelvic delivery. Obstet Gynecol 1978;52:526–9.

82. Gherman R, Ouzounian JG. American College of Obstetricians and Gynecologists. Shoulder dystocia. Practice Bulletin no. 178. Washington, DC: ACOG; 2017.

83. Davis DD, Roshan A, Canela CD, et al. Shoulder dystocia. In: StatPearls. Treasure Island (FL): StatPearls Publishing; 2020. p. 1–8. Available at: https://www.ncbi.nlm.nih.gov/books/NBK470427/. Accessed January 24, 2021.

84. Gherman R, Ouzounian JG, Grobman W, et al. Neonatal brachial plexus palsy. Washington, DC: American College of Obstetricians and Gynecologists; 2014.

85. Ahn ES, Jung MS, Lee YK, et al. Neonatal clavicular fracture: recent 10 year study. Pediatr Int 2015;57:60–3 (Level II-3).

86. Perlow JH, Wigton T, Hart J, et al. Birth trauma. A five-year review of incidence and associated perinatal factors. J Reprod Med 1996;41:754–60.

87. Baskett TF, Allen AC. Perinatal implications of shoulder dystocia. Obstet Gynecol 1995;86:14–7.

88. Ouzounian JG, Gherman RB, Chauhan S, et al. Recurrent shoulder dystocia: analysis of incidence and risk factors. Am J Perinatol 2012;29:515–8.

89. Smith RB, Lane C, Pearson JF. Shoulder dystocia: what happens at the next delivery? Br J Obstet Gynaecol 1994;101:713–5.

90. Ginsberg NA, Moisidis C. How to predict recurrent shoulder dystocia. Am J Obstet Gynecol 2001;184:1427–9 [discussion: 1429–30].

91. Lewis DF, Raymond RC, Perkins MB, et al. Recurrence rate of shoulder dystocia. Am J Obstet Gynecol 1995;172:1369–71.

Fetal Growth in Multiple Gestations
Evaluation and Management

Nicholas Behrendt, MD*, Henry L. Galan, MD

KEYWORDS

- Multifetal gestation • Twins • Growth evaluation
- Selective intrauterine growth restriction • Twin-twin transfusion syndrome
- Multifetal pregnancy reduction

KEY POINTS

- Multifetal pregnancies have different growth trajectories than their singleton counterparts.
- Evaluation of growth in twins is unique and management of selective intrauterine growth restriction is complex.
- Doppler studies assist in the management of selective intrauterine growth restriction.
- Multifetal pregnancy reduction and selective reduction are options in the management of multifetal gestation pregnancies.

INTRODUCTION

The rate of twin births has declined in the United States over the past several years (32.6 twins per 1000 births in 2018 as compared with a rate of 33.9 per 1000 births in 2014). However, they remain common: 123,536 infants were born in twin deliveries in 2018 in the United States alone.[1] Practice guidelines implemented by the American Society for Reproductive Medicine over the past 2 decades has significantly reduced the triplet and higher-order multiple gestation rates from a peak in 2003 of approximately 250 per 100,000 births to fewer than 120 per 100,000 births in 2018.[1] Despite this improvement in decreasing numbers of higher-order multiple gestations, the rate of twins with current reproductive medicine practices remains steady.[2]

Twin births continue to be a significant source of perinatal morbidity mainly due to complications of preterm birth, with approximately 20% delivering before 34 weeks' gestation and up to 80% delivering before 37 weeks' gestation.[1] In addition to preterm birth, twin pregnancies have higher rates of hypertensive disorders of pregnancy, gestational diabetes, cesarean delivery, congenital anomalies, genetic abnormalities, and stillbirth.[3]

Division of Maternal-Fetal Medicine, University of Colorado, Children's Hospital Colorado, Colorado Fetal Care Center, 12631 East 17th Avenue, Box B198-5, Aurora, CO 80045, USA
* Corresponding author.
E-mail address: Nicholas.behrendt@cuanschutz.edu

Obstet Gynecol Clin N Am 48 (2021) 401–417
https://doi.org/10.1016/j.ogc.2021.02.009
0889-8545/21/© 2021 Elsevier Inc. All rights reserved.

Another common occurrence at the time of delivery in twins is low birthweight. In 2018, 56% of twins had a birthweight less than 2500 g with 9% having a birthweight less than 1500 g.[1] This leads to a further increase in morbidity and mortality, above and beyond that noted with preterm birth alone.[4] These issues have led to an increased focus on fetal evaluation in twin pregnancies. With the continued improvement in fetal evaluation technology, we can now better evaluate fetal growth disorders before birth and potentially improve outcomes.

The purpose of this article was to review data on twin growth abnormalities across gestational ages, focusing on evaluation, prediction, and management, including potential interventions.

CHORIONICITY AND AMNIONICITY

Twins have been traditionally referred to as monozygotic (arising from one fertilized ovum) versus dizygotic (arising from 2 fertilized ova). Why this occurs is not completely understood, but recent data have called into question the exact mechanisms that lead to twinning.[5] Although this is academically intriguing, the more important distinction is the chorion and amnion number for the twins. The chorion is the embryonic structure that eventually matures into the placenta. There can be 1 or 2 chorions in twins that are referred to as monochorionic or dichorionic, depending on the number of placentas visualized. The amnion refers to the amniotic sac membrane and is similarly described as monoamniotic or diamniotic. Therefore, twins are commonly referred to as dichorionic-diamniotic, monochorionic-diamniotic, or monochorionic-monoamniotic, depending on ultrasound evaluation of the numbers of placentas and amniotic sacs. Ideally this is determined in the first trimester, which is the most accurate time to determine the number of chorions and amnions.[6] This distinction is important, as each version of twins comes with a unique set of potential complications.

Monochorionic twins have the highest complication rates due to disease processes specific to sharing a placenta. These include twin-to-twin transfusion syndrome (TTTS), twin anemia-polycythemia sequence (TAPS), and selective intrauterine growth restriction (sIUGR). These unique complications are due to the almost inevitable placental vascular anastomoses occurring between the halves of monochorionic placentas.[7] These vascular connections cause TTTS in 10% to 20% of monochorionic twins, which accounts for at least 15% of perinatal mortality in twins.[8,9] Monochorionic-monoamniotic twins also have a high incidence of morbidity and mortality occurring as a result of more frequent fetal anomalies, TTTS, TAPS, and cord entanglement. The perinatal mortality in these pregnancies has traditionally approached 50% with more recent estimates approximating 10% to 20%.[6]

Dichorionic-diamniotic twin complications are primarily attributable to preterm birth. However, they are also more predisposed to a full range of obstetric complications such as congenital anomalies, hypertensive disorders of pregnancy, gestational diabetes, and others.[10] Although there are rare reports of TTTS in dichorionic twins, TTTS and TAPS do not occur commonly.[11] Although these complications in dichorionic twins and complications in other twin pregnancies such as monoamniotic and conjoined twins are not the focus of this review, they are important to mention as they often occur concomitantly with abnormal fetal growth and can therefore complicate its clinical management.[12,13] As such, the obstetric complications, surveillance, and general management specific for dichorionic, monochorionic, and conjoined twins are summarized in **Table 1**. As fetal anomalies are increased in all twin gestations, a detailed anatomy survey is recommended. In addition, as fetal cardiac abnormalities are more common in monochorionic twins of all types, fetal echocardiography

Table 1
Summary of obstetric complications and management recommendations by type of twin gestation

Twin Gestation Type	Obstetric Complications	Management Recommendations

Dichorionic Diamniotic	• Fetal anomalies
	• Twin growth abnormality
	• Preterm Labor
		• Detailed anatomy surveys
		• Serial growth ultrasound every 4 wk
		• Preterm labor surveillance
		• Timing of delivery:
		  ○ Uncomplicated: 38° wk
		  ○ sIUGR present: individualized

Monochorionic Diamniotic	• Fetal anomalies
	• Twin growth abnormality
	• TTTS
	• TAPS
	• sIUGR
		• Fetal anatomy survey
		• Fetal echocardiogram
		• Serial growth ultrasound every 4 wk
		• TTTS, TAPS, sIUGR assessment at least every 2 wk starting at 16 wk for the duration of the pregnancy. If present, consider referral to fetal treatment center
		• Timing of delivery:
		  ○ Uncomplicated - 37° wk
		  ○ sIUGR present: individualized
		  ○ TTTS/TAPS: individualized

Monochorionic Monoamniotic	• Fetal anomalies
	• Twin growth abnormality
	• TTTS
	• TAPS
	• sIUGR
	• Cord entanglement
	• Spontaneous fetal demise
		• Fetal anatomy surveys
		• Fetal echocardiograms
		• Serial growth ultrasound every 4 wk
		• TTTS, TAPS, sIUGR assessment at least every 2 wk starting at 16 wk for the duration of the pregnancy. If present, consider referral to fetal treatment center
		• Inpatient admission to AP service for TID hour long external FHR monitoring at viability
		• Timing of delivery:
		  ○ Uncomplicated: 32°–34° wk
		  ○ sIUGR present: individualized
		  ○ TTTS/TAPS: individualized

Conjoined twins	Fetal anomalies SAB Spontaneous fetal demise	• Fetal anatomy survey • Fetal echocardiogram/s • Growth ultrasound every 4 wk • Viability checks every 1–2 wk • Consider referral to fetal/neonatal treatment center • Timing of delivery: Individualized

Abbreviations: AP, antepartum; FHR, fetal heart rate; SAB, spontaneous abortion; sIUGR, selective intrauterine growth restriction; TAPS, twin anemia-polycythemia sequence; TID, twice a day; TTTS, twin-to-twin transfusion syndrome.

is recommended.[14] Specific considerations for twin growth are described further in the following sections. The timing of delivery of multiple gestations is commonly influenced by coexisting maternal or fetal concurrent conditions. Timing of delivery for the different twin pregnancies in **Table 1** is consistent with the recommendations previously published by the American College of Obstetricians and Gynecologists and Society for Maternal-Fetal Medicine.[15]

TWIN GROWTH: FIRST TRIMESTER EVALUATION

Very early size discrepancies between twin embryonic/fetal poles are not considered disorders of growth because small differences are likely not important, and larger differences are likely to lead to demise of one fetus, or a "vanishing twin." Therefore, we focus on discrepancies measured at ≥7 weeks, which is the stage in gestation when a crown rump length (CRL) can be measured.

CRL measurements are expected to be concordant among all twin pairs. Significant discrepancies in CRL measurements (calculated as the percent difference between them) are associated with fetal loss at 11 to 14 weeks. D'Antonio and colleagues[16] evaluated 1356 twin pairs with CRLs performed between 7 weeks 0 days and 9 weeks 6 days. CRLs with less than 20% discordance had a very low rate (0.8%–4.5%) of at least a single fetal loss at 11 to 14 weeks. A CRL discrepancy greater than 30% conferred a single fetal loss rate greater than 45%. Further analysis showed that a CRL discrepancy ≥19% was associated with a relative risk of at least one fetal loss of 52.9 compared with lesser degrees of discordance. This analysis is consistent with data from prior studies with smaller sample sizes in finding a correlation between discrepant CRLs and initial adverse outcomes.[17]

Later CRL discordance (at 11–14 weeks) is less correlated with adverse outcomes according to the STORK analysis performed by D'Antonio and colleagues.[18] However, smaller studies have shown some association between CRL discordance of at least 10% and adverse outcomes including preterm delivery, low birth weight, birth weight discordance, and adverse pregnancy outcomes.[19,20] Another study found that twins with CRL discordance of greater than 10% had significantly increased risk of fetal structural anomalies (22.2% vs 2.8%; $P = .01$) as well as increased genetic abnormalities.[21] Therefore, counseling and evaluation for genetic abnormalities as well as structural anomalies may be warranted. No additional modifications in clinical care are necessary for CRL differences at 11 to 14 weeks.

Although the focus of this review is twin growth, we would be remiss to not mention nuchal translucency (NT). Performing an NT measurement between 11 and 14 weeks in twins is common for genetic screening, just as it is in singleton pregnancies. Discordant NT measurements in dichorionic twins have not been associated with adverse outcomes above and beyond those described in singletons, such as genetic anomalies and anatomic abnormalities.[22] However, in monochorionic twins, there are data to suggest that a discrepancy in NT measurements is associated with an increased risk for other pathologic processes. Kagan and colleagues[23] showed that NT discordance of greater than 20% was associated with a risk of 34% for serious complications including TTTS or fetal death, whereas NT discrepancy less than this was only associated with a 9.5% risk of these complications. Similarly, another study showed that an NT discrepancy greater than 20% had positive predictive value of 50% to predict TTTS development, versus a discrepancy less than 20%, which had a negative predictive value for TTTS development of 86%.[24] Another study by Mackie and colleagues[25] showed only a moderate association between discrepant NTs (≥10%) and TTTS (odds ratio, 2.29). Because of the possibility that discrepant NTs may identify those at increased risk for adverse outcomes such as TTTS, it is reasonable to consider increased surveillance in these patients. At our institution, we consider weekly TTTS surveillance rather than every other week surveillance in these patients, although efficacy is uncertain.

TWIN GROWTH: SECOND TRIMESTER EVALUATION

Evaluating fetal size during the second trimester is common in all pregnancies because most fetuses receive an anatomy ultrasound at approximately the 20th week of gestation. Traditionally, the expectation for fetal size and growth in the second (and into the third trimester) is that the fetuses show "concordant" growth, with "discordant" growth betraying potential pathology. The American College of Obstetricians and Gynecologists defines twin discordance as at least a 20% difference in estimated fetal weights.[26] Whether this level of discrepancy is clinically relevant is debatable, as studies have not been able to show a strong correlation between intertwin weight discordance and adverse neonatal outcomes. There have been weak and inconsistent associations with adverse outcomes such as hyperbilirubinemia, birth weight discrepancy, and need for neonatal intensive care unit admission.[27,28]

Fox and colleagues[29] performed an analysis assessing second trimester estimated fetal weight discordance and adverse outcomes. Using a cutoff of 15% discordance in the second trimester, they found a significant association with birth weight discordance, low birth weights, and birth weight below the 10th percentile and 5th percentile for gestational age. Subgroup analysis in this study showed that in dichorionic twins, the size discordance was associated with low birth weights and low birth weight percentiles. This was not seen when analyzing monochorionic twins; however, the study was underpowered for this analysis so an association cannot be ruled out. In another STORK analysis, 2399 twin pregnancies were evaluated for estimated fetal weight discordance in the second trimester and its relation to adverse outcomes during the pregnancy.[30] Similar to prior studies, this large cohort analysis failed to show associations between discordant birth weights and adverse outcomes when structural anomalies, chromosome abnormalities, and TTTS were excluded. These same results were seen even when separately analyzing dichorionic and monochorionic twin pairs. It is relatively common to find a condition referred to as sIUGR starting in the mid-second trimester. This unique condition for twins is discussed separately in this article.

TWIN GROWTH: THIRD TRIMESTER EVALUATION

The American College of Obstetricians and Gynecologists states that in twins "it seems reasonable that serial ultrasonographic surveillance be performed every 4 to 6 weeks in the absence of evidence of fetal growth restriction or other pregnancy complications."[26] Given this statement, along with routine surveillance that is advised in monochorionic twins occurring at least every 4 weeks to exclude TTTS, most twin pregnancies have growth studies performed through the second and third trimesters (see **Table 1**).

It is well accepted that fetal growth in twins mirrors that of singletons until approximately 30 weeks' gestation, when growth trajectory of twins begins to slow relative to singletons at the same gestational ages (**Fig. 1**).[31,32]

Therefore, after 30 to 32 weeks, a perceived slowing in fetal weight in twins is not necessarily a sign of pathology. In fact, a slower trajectory of fetal growth later in pregnancy may represent a helpful physiologic adaptation for twins as it is likely a sign of nutritional management and attempting to not over distend the growing uterus. Blickstein[32] breaks twin growth phases into A, B, and C. Phase A is from early pregnancy until 28 weeks for twins in whom size trajectory is similar to singletons. Phase B starts at approximately 30 weeks, at which time there is a decrease in birth weights in twins compared with singletons. He suggests that at this point the uterus cannot maintain the trajectory of singleton growth, so twin birth weights become progressively smaller than singletons and are approximately 15% to 20% lower by the beginning of phase C. Blickstein[32] suggests this is not pathologic but potentially adaptive. During phase C (from 32 weeks until birth) this 15% to 20% difference is maintained and therefore the weight difference between twins and singletons plateaus. Further supporting these

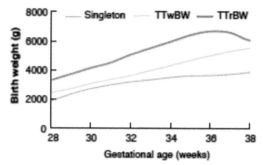

Fig. 1. Total twin and triplet birth weight versus 90th percentile for singletons. TTrBW, total triplet birth weight; TTwBW, total twin birth weight. (*From* Blickstein I. Is it normal for. multiples to be smaller than singletons? *Best Pract Res Clin Obstet Gynaecol.* Aug 2004;18(4):613-23. https://doi.org/10.1016/j.bpobgyn.2004.04.008.)

observations, the National Institute of Child Health and Human Development (NICHD) Fetal Growth Studies showed that in dichorionic twins, estimated fetal weights are similar to singletons up until 32 weeks, but after that up to 40% of twins would be considered small for gestational age when using singleton growth charts.[33] Based on his prior research, Blickstein[32] theorized that pregnancy has physiologically adapted to prioritize gestational age over size at birth in multiples. This theory is consistent with the observed initial decrease and then plateau in fetal size in late twin gestations. This is also supported by studies that have shown that twins, even with significant discordance between each other or when compared with singletons, have similar outcomes when controlled for gestational age.[34]

Similar to estimated fetal weight discordance in the second trimester, third trimester fetal weight discordance does not necessarily predict adverse outcomes but may actually represent physiologic adaptation to multiple gestations. Therefore, no changes in obstetric surveillance are recommended even with large estimated weight discordances. However, if one fetus qualifies as having fetal growth restriction (FGR) then modification in surveillance may be necessary. The NICHD twin growth study contains excellent nomogram data for fetal biometry and estimated weights in graphical and tabular formats.[33] When one fetus in a dichorionic twin set is considered to have FGR, monitoring usually mirrors that of singleton fetuses with growth restriction. This is discussed in the next section.

Twin Growth Surveillance Recommendations: We advocate for early ultrasound for any pregnancy, and especially in twins. Determining the amnionicity and chorionicity early is critical to guide counseling and management. In dichorionic twin pregnancies, we recommend growth ultrasounds every 4 weeks after anatomy ultrasound (approximately 20 weeks). If FGR is found then Doppler velocimetry monitoring at least every 2 weeks is warranted. For monochorionic twins, we recommend growth ultrasounds every 4 weeks from 16 weeks until the end of pregnancy. See later in this article for discussion on FGR in monochorionic twins. These recommendations are also summarized in **Table 1**.

SELECTIVE INTRAUTERINE GROWTH RESTRICTION

sIUGR refers to a twin pair in which one fetus qualifies as having FGR compared with its co-twin. A standardized definition has not been established. However, traditionally one fetus having an estimated fetal weight less than the 10th percentile compared with a singleton growth chart has been used to define sIUGR. Other definitions include a small abdominal circumference in one twin or even estimated fetal weight discordance beyond a certain threshold.

sIUGR in dichorionic twins is usually cared for similarly to singleton gestations with growth restriction, including the use of Doppler velocimetry and increased antepartum surveillance for the growth restricted fetus. However, because these fetuses are not integrally connected through the placenta, evaluation can be separate and even when severe growth restriction is present it does not necessarily pose a risk for the normally grown fetus. In a metanalysis, Ong and colleagues[35] showed that when demise of one fetus occurred, the risk of co-twin demise was 4% in dichorionic twins and 12% in monochorionic twins. Of note, the risk of co-twin demise was sixfold higher when a single-twin death occurred after 20 weeks' gestation. Furthermore, after single-twin demise, the risk of co-twin neurologic injury was 1% in dichorionic twins versus 18% in monochorionic twins. Therefore, we advocate for treating surveillance with sIUGR in dichorionic twins similar to singleton growth restriction. Delivery timing should be based on the severity of growth restriction, gestational age, and other factors. If demise of a fetus is imminent and the pregnancy is either previable or very preterm, then expectant care may be appropriate to optimize the outcome for the non–growth restricted fetus.[36] In contrast, at later gestational ages, medically indicated delivery may be appropriate to optimize outcome for the sIUGR twin, despite causing preterm birth of the healthy twin.

sIUGR in monochorionic twins is more problematic in that the placental connections between the fetuses cause compromise or stillbirth of one fetus to pose a risk for the other fetus. Indeed, death of one fetus in a monochorionic set presents a significant risk of death or potential neurologic injury in the co-twin. This was illustrated in a recent meta-analysis by Mackie and colleagues[37] showing a co-twin death rate of 41% and a fetal MRI brain abnormality rate of 20%. The rate of brain abnormalities increased to a 43% after birth if the co-twin survived. This confirms prior smaller studies that indicated an increased rate of neurodevelopmental impairment in surviving co-twins of approximately 20%.[38,39]

sIUGR in a monochorionic twin conveys a significant risk of fetal loss in the growth restricted fetus. Evaluation in these complicated pregnancies is similar to singleton pregnancies affected by FGR with respect to the use of Doppler evaluation of the umbilical arteries, middle cerebral arteries, and ductus venosus. However, the natural history of the evolution in these Dopplers for monochorionic twins is not always the same as in singleton pregnancies. For instance, Vanderheyden and colleagues[40] showed that in monochorionic twins, the average latency between the diagnosis of absent end diastolic velocity in the umbilical arteries and progression to reversed end diastolic velocity was significantly longer (54 days) than dichorionic twins (30 days) or comparable singletons (11 days). This is likely because of several factors including earlier age of onset and placental vascular connections that complicate the traditional pathophysiology of FGR which is usually due to placental microvascular disease.[41] This makes the prediction of disease severity and disease progression challenging in sIUGR.

Gratacos and colleagues[42] published a staging system for describing sIUGR in monochorionic-diamniotic twins. Type I is defined by the presence of forward end diastolic velocity in the umbilical arteries. Type II is characterized by the consistent absence or reversal of end diastolic velocity in the umbilical arteries. Type III is defined as absent and reversed end diastolic flow seen alternating over a short period with forward diastolic velocity. They showed that Type I usually does not deteriorate over the course of pregnancy and rarely results in stillbirth. This pattern appears to mimic singleton FGR with an overall positive outlook with close surveillance. Fetuses with type II sIUGR showed in utero deterioration in a large proportion of pregnancies (90%) but none died unexpectedly. This pattern of consistently abnormal umbilical artery Doppler studies also seemed to mimic singleton FGR in that the consistent abnormality heralds deterioration. Fortunately, this pattern appears to be relatively predictable and therefore timely intervention (eg, delivery before stillbirth) may be possible. In utero deterioration was uncommon in the sIUGR fetus with type III abnormalities. However, fetuses with type III patterns had high rates of unexpected fetal demise in both the larger fetus (6.2%) and the sIUGR fetus (15.4%). This is problematic because the variability of the abnormal umbilical artery Doppler pattern makes in utero deterioration and death nearly impossible to predict. **Table 2** shows the unanticipated loss rate, average age at delivery and risk of central nervous system injury by Gratacos category of sIUGR.

Management options for sIUGR include expectant management, delivery, and selective reduction. At our institution, we manage each stage and clinical scenario differently. Type I and type II sIUGR are managed similarly to singleton pregnancies with similar Doppler patterns. Type I disease is routinely managed on an outpatient basis, with Doppler evaluations every 1 to 2 weeks and weekly antenatal testing with delivery timing depending on gestational age and testing results. Type II is also managed with frequent use of Doppler studies to identify deterioration and progression to worse disease. When a gestational age is reached in which the fetuses could potentially survive outside the womb, we will often increase the frequency of testing. If a pattern of obvious decline in Doppler studies is seen, including progression from absent end diastolic flow to reversed end diastolic flow in the umbilical arteries or abnormalities in the ductus venosus, then delivery is considered.[43] This management option obviously necessitates delivery of both fetuses at whatever gestational age is achieved, potentially putting both at risk for prematurity complications.

In monochorionic twins in whom the sIUGR fetus is at significant risk for spontaneous death and the pregnancy is too preterm for survival after delivery or the pregnancy is at a gestational age in which the morbidity and mortality is high due to early gestational age, selective feticide may be an option with the goal of maximizing the outcome for the larger fetus and minimizing the morbidity and mortality from the loss of the sIUGR fetus. Deciding when selective feticide is indicated is extremely challenging. If the procedure is performed too early it may result in unnecessary loss of the

Table 2
Outcomes in monochorionic-diamniotic twin pregnancies by Gratacos stage

Gratacos Stage of sIUGR	Unanticipated Loss Rate of sIUGR Fetus (%)	Average GA at Delivery (wk)	Rate of CNS Injury
I	0.0%	35	<5%
II	2.5%	31	<5%
III	15.8%	31	18.9%

Abbreviations: CNS, central nervous system; GA, gestational age; sIUGR, selective intrauterine growth restriction.

Data from Gratacos E, Lewi L, Munoz B, et al. A classification system for selective intrauterine growth restriction in monochorionic pregnancies according to umbilical artery Doppler flow in the smaller twin. *Ultrasound Obstet Gynecol.* Jul 2007;30(1):28-34. https://doi.org/10.1002/uog. 4046.

sIUGR fetus, whereas performing it too late mate lead to loss of both infants. Decision making is further complicated by the often early onset of sIUGR and the varied and unpredictable time course and evolution of Doppler abnormalities.[37] In the study by Vanderheyden and colleagues,[40] sIUGR was diagnosed on average at 20 weeks in monochorionic twins, whereas (s)IUGR in singleton and dichorionic twins was diagnosed approximately 27 weeks. Selective feticide can be safely performed in the affected sIUGR fetus in monochorionic twins using radiofrequency ablation or cord coagulation. This avoids complications such as death or neurologic injury to the co-twin by potentially avoiding a "watershed" decrease in blood flow. Outcomes for the surviving twin appear to be improved after selective feticide when compared with when the growth restricted fetus passes spontaneously.[44,45] Selective feticide may not be selected by a patient on initial evaluation but remains an option should the smaller fetus show deterioration based on Doppler studies or a lack of growth. Further discussion on selective feticide is beyond the scope of this review.

Type III sIUGR presents a challenging scenario because of the relatively high rate of unexpected fetal death that occurs.[42] At our institution, we consider selective feticide if the type III pattern is seen before viability with the goal of avoiding spontaneous fetal demise and the accompanying morbidity and mortality in the co-twin. We counsel the patient on the up to 15% risk of spontaneous death of the fetus with this abnormal pattern and the subsequent risk to the other fetus. If the ductus venosus shows an absent or reversed a-wave we are more concerned about imminent death and counsel more toward intervention. If sIUGR is diagnosed after a viable gestational age is reached or if the plan is for initial expectant management, we routinely admit the patient to the hospital to perform more intensive monitoring, similar to monoamniotic twin gestations. This usually involves non–stress tests 3 times a day and Doppler studies twice a week to identify deterioration before demise so that delivery can occur. We routinely deliver these patients at 32 to 34 weeks. Although not formally studied, we have not seen the high rate of spontaneous fetal demise that Gratacos and colleagues[42] found with this intensive monitoring schedule and plan for delivery. Of course, efficacy remains uncertain.

sIUGR Recommendations: In dichorionic twins, we recommend growth ultrasounds every 4 weeks after anatomy ultrasound. If sIUGR is found, then Doppler velocimetry studies are warranted. Management depends on gestational age and severity of Doppler changes; however, if demise of one fetus occurs, the risk of co-twin demise is unlikely and therefore selective feticide is not routinely recommended. In monochorionic twins, we recommend growth ultrasounds every 4 weeks starting at 16 weeks (in addition to more frequent TTTS surveillance, see **Table 1**). If sIUGR is found, we routinely recommend Doppler velocimetry studies at least every week given the significant risk to the larger fetus. If type II or type III sIUGR is found before viability, then a surgical procedure focused on reducing risk to the larger fetus should be considered. If this is found after viability, then we will often recommend hospital admission for more intense monitoring or delivery, depending on the patient's desires.

SELECTIVE INTRAUTERINE GROWTH RESTRICTION AND TWIN-TO-TWIN TRANSFUSION SYNDROME

Although TTTS is discussed elsewhere in this issue, it is important to note that sIUGR is commonly found in TTTS and its presence has a substantial impact on outcome. In an unpublished series (Ehrig J and colleagues, 2018) of patients with TTTS undergoing fetoscopic laser photocoagulation from our center, the presence of sIUGR significantly reduces the dual survival rates. **Table 3** shows survival outcomes at our center

Table 3
Preoperative risk factors and TTTS outcome following fetoscopic laser photocoagulation at the Colorado Fetal Care Center

Risk Factor				Probability		Odds Ratio	
				1 or More Survival, %	Both Survival, %	1 or More Survival	Both Survival
Anterior Placenta	Selective IU6R	Short Cervix	GA <18 wk				
n = 52	n = 67	n = 12	n = 19				
				96.50	82.80	11.12	4.87
X				92.30	71.00	9.1	4.63
	X			91.80	65.00	8.48	2.7
		X		85.40	58.90	4.44	3.51
			X	84.10	58.20	4.01	2.63
X	X			90.10	63.80	6.94	2.57
X		X		82.70	57.60	3.64	1.33
X			X	81.20	57.00	3.28	2.5
	X	X		81.70	50.70	3.39	1.95
	X		X	80.10	50.10	3.06	1.46
		X	X	67.90	43.60	1.6	1.9
X	X	X		78.50	49.40	2.77	1.85
X	X		X	76.70	48.80	2.5	1.39
X		X	X	63.30	42.40	1.31	1.8
	X	X	X	61.70	35.80	1.22	1.05
X	X	X	X	a			

n, represents the number of pregnancies and not the number of fetuses. X, represents risk factor.
Abbreviations: GA, gestational age; TTTS, twin-to-twin transfusion syndrome.
[a] Only 1 case with all 4 complications.

for 108 twin pregnancies following fetoscopic laser photocoagulation for severe stage TTTS (Quintero 3 or greater) in whom a variety of previously published risk factors were evaluated.[46–50] In our population of patients, the presence of sIUGR reduced the chance of dual twin survival, and any combination of preoperative risk factors also reduced survival of one or both twins (see **Table 3**).

These decreased survival numbers, especially with sIUGR present, are consistent with previous studies evaluating this as a risk factor for decreased survival. **Fig. 2** is an adaptation of a previous study showing fetal survival outcomes when TTTS and sIUGR are present in 571 cases.[51]

Performing a fetoscopic laser photocoagulation for sIUGR in the absence of TTTS appears to be associated with a similar outcome for the sIUGR twin as in the presence of TTTS. However, survival of the larger twin appears to be reduced when using fetoscopic laser photocoagulation for sIUGR versus when used in TTTS. Further, selective feticide by radiofrequency ablation (RFA) performed in the setting of sIUGR is associated with significantly greater survival of the larger twin than has been reported when fetoscopic laser photocoagulation is used for sIUGR in the absence of TTTS. Peeva and colleagues[51] showed a survival rate of 89.1% in the larger twin when selective feticide was used. Thus, selective feticide for severe sIUGR in the absence of TTTS should be a consideration, if not preferred.

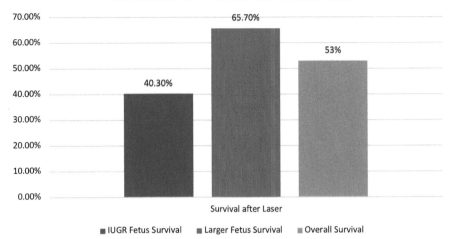

Fig. 2. Twin survival after laser procedure with sIUGR present. (*Data from* Peeva G, Bower S, Orosz L, Chaveeva P, Akolekar R, Nicolaides KH. Endoscopic Placental Laser Coagulation in Monochorionic Diamniotic Twins with Type II Selective Fetal Growth Restriction. *Fetal Diagn Ther.* 2015;38(2):86-93. https://doi.org/10.1159/000374109.)

In conclusion, sIUGR in monochorionic twins presents a challenging clinical scenario given the multifactorial etiology of growth restriction and abnormal Doppler studies. Additional research is needed so our understanding of the disease process can progress and our clinical management can improve.

HIGHER-ORDER MULTIPLE GESTATIONS

One of the greater challenges encountered in obstetrics is the management and complications seen in triplets and higher-order multiple gestations. Compared with singleton and twin gestations, they confer significantly greater risk for preterm birth and low birth weight deliveries, as depicted in **Fig. 3**, which is adapted from the National Vital Statistics Reports.[1]

In addition, the impact on maternal health in higher-order pregnancies is considerable, resulting in higher rates of anemia, postpartum hemorrhage, hospitalization, and time lost from work. These triplet and higher-order multiple gestations are at risk for the previously reviewed complications of monochorionic gestations. In addition, the additional fetuses make potential therapeutic interventions more complicated, in part because of difficulty achieving access to allow for completion of the procedure. For these reasons, together with the improved outcomes for survival of 1 or 2 fetuses in a given pregnancy, multifetal pregnancy reduction is a reasonable option that is an important part of patient counseling in early pregnancy.

The terms multifetal pregnancy reduction and selective reduction or feticide are often used interchangeably but represent different procedures with different goals. The purpose of multifetal pregnancy reduction is to reduce the number of fetuses early in gestation to optimize outcomes and decrease morbidity/mortality in survivors of higher-order pregnancies by reducing the number of fetuses in the gestation. These fetuses are usually selected at random or based on location, as ease of access is important to minimize complications from this procedure. Multifetal pregnancy reduction is typically used when there are 3 or more fetuses in a gestation, as reduction of a

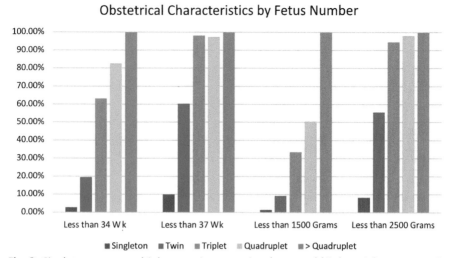

Fig. 3. Singleton versus multiple gestation gestational age and birth weight outcomes in 2018 per the National Vital Statistics Report. (*Data from* Martin JA, Hamilton BE, Osterman MJK, Driscoll AK. Births: Final Data for 2018. *Natl Vital Stat Rep.* Nov 2019;68(13):1-47.)

twin pregnancy to singleton is more controversial because improved outcomes are less certain. However, the American College of Obstetrics and Gynecology has stated in a committee opinion that reduction from twins to singletons is medically justified and is more commonly used with a comorbid condition or obstetric indication in the mother.[52] Preprocedural considerations include relationship of gestational sacs to one another, chorionicity, fetal anatomy and aneuploidy markers, and determining which fetuses are most accessible to chorionic villus sampling (CVS) and reduction procedures. CVS is performed in 44% of patients before multifetal pregnancy reduction and is performed at 10 to 13 weeks in 1 or more of the fetuses.[53] CVS does not increase loss rate with multifetal pregnancy reduction and actually reduces it, as fetuses with aneuploidy can be identified.[54–57] Traditionally, potassium chloride (KCL) is used for multifetal pregnancy reduction, but cannot be used in monochorionic placentation because fetal vascular connections within the placenta.

Pregnancy outcomes after multifetal pregnancy reduction are broadly improved. In a meta-analysis of triplet pregnancies reduced to twins (vs conservatively managed), outcomes including pregnancy loss <24 weeks, preterm delivery and perinatal mortality were improved in the twins group as reported by Wimalasundera and colleagues[58] (**Table 4**). Of course, the option of multifetal pregnancy reduction requires a clear discussion of the potential risks and benefits with a focus on shared decision making and an effort to center on the patient's goals and values.

Selective reduction is commonly seen as a reduction in the number of fetuses so as to interrupt a pathologic disease process (TTTS, sIUGR, TAPS, fetal anomalies) in the cases of monochorionic placentation in which KCL injection would put each fetus at risk due to placental vascular connections. This is usually performed in diamniotic pregnancies with RFA in which the RFA device is placed into the cord insertion for the abnormal fetus and radiofrequency is used to interrupt blood flow. This causes fetal cardiac activity to cease and importantly decreases the complications in the co-twin seen in spontaneous fetal demise. In monoamniotic pregnancies RFA is an option, but most experts advocate for cord coagulation and release. This involves

Table 4
Pregnancy outcomes after reduction from triplets to twins versus triplet pregnancies

Pregnancy Outcome	MPR Triplet to Twin	Triplet	OR; 95% CI
SAB <24 wk, %	5.10	11.50	0.45; 0.3–0.6
Delivery <28 wk, %	2.90	8.60	0.35; 0.2–0.6
Delivery <32 wk, %	10.10	20.30	0.5; 0.37–0.66
PMR/pregnancy	26.6/1000	92/1000	0.3:0.2–0.5
Take Home Baby Rate per pregnancy, %	93	79	0.3; 0.2–0.7

Abbreviations: CI, confidence interval; MPR, multipregnancy reduction; OR, odds ratio; PMR, perinatal mortality rate, SAB, spontaneous abortion.

Data from Wimalasundera RC, Trew G, Fisk NM. Reducing the incidence of twins and triplets. *Best Pract Res Clin Obstet Gynaecol.* Apr 2003;17(2):309-29. https://doi.org/10.1016/ s1521-6934(02) 00135-9.

using a bipolar device to stop blood flow in the cord of 1 fetus. Then, either fetoscopic scissors or laser is used to cut this cord to decrease the chance of cord entanglement complications. SR is used to improve the survival of one or more fetuses when monochorionicity and some pathologic process is found.

Higher-order multiple gestations recommendations: We recommend increased surveillance, including growth ultrasounds every 4 weeks starting at 16 weeks until delivery along with additional monitoring (such as for TTTS), depending on chorionicity. Shared decision making should be instituted when discussing the option of multifetal pregnancy reduction. If a pathologic disease process is found, then selective reduction should be considered depending on gestational age, chorionicity, amnionicity, and the patient's wishes.

SUMMARY

Disorders of fetal growth in multifetal pregnancies present unique clinical management challenges. Discrepancies in fetal size may be a predictor of eventual complications, especially in monochorionic twins. Monochorionic twins present unique challenges because of the inevitable placental vascular anastomoses between them, which makes a unique set of diseases possible. These connections also complicate matters because the loss of one fetus presents a risk to the other. Fortunately, most growth abnormalities can be detected through serial sonograms and surveillance and in many cases, effective therapy is available.

CLINICAL PEARLS AND PITFALLS

More than 120,000 infants born in the United States each year are from twin deliveries.

One in 5 twin births occur before 34 weeks' gestation.

Monochorionic twins have a unique set of potential complications that must be monitored for, including TTTS, TAPS, and sIUGR.

Discordant CRL measurements in early gestation have are associated with an increased chance of fetal loss.

Traditional literature uses a 20% discordance in estimated fetal weight as a marker of potential complications; however, there are no studies showing significant risk in these patients.

After 30 weeks' gestation, twin growth curve trajectory flattens compared with singleton pregnancies, likely as a mechanism to prolong gestation.

sIUGR in monochorionic twins comes with risks including stillbirth and neurologic injury.

The management of sIUGR depends on umbilical artery Doppler patterns, as described in categories I, II, and III by Gratacos and colleagues.[42] Category III, in which forward, absent, and reversed end diastolic flow is seen, has at least a 15% risk of spontaneous fetal loss.

The combination of TTTS and selective intrauterine growth restriction significantly lowers the chance of survival post laser procedure for the donor fetus.

DISCLOSURE

The authors have nothing to disclose.

REFERENCES

1. Martin JA, Hamilton BE, Osterman MJK, et al. Births: final data for 2018. Natl Vital Stat Rep 2019;68(13):1–47.
2. Practice Committee of American Society for Reproductive Medicine. Multiple gestation associated with infertility therapy: an American Society for Reproductive Medicine Practice Committee opinion. Fertil Steril 2012;97(4):825–34.
3. Norwitz ER, Edusa V, Park JS. Maternal physiology and complications of multiple pregnancy. Semin Perinatol 2005;29(5):338–48.
4. Townsend R, Khalil A. Fetal growth restriction in twins. Best Pract Res Clin Obstet Gynaecol 2018;49:79–88.
5. McNamara HC, Kane SC, Craig JM, et al. A review of the mechanisms and evidence for typical and atypical twinning. Am J Obstet Gynecol 2016;214(2): 172–91.
6. Simpson LL. Ultrasound in twins: dichorionic and monochorionic. Semin Perinatol 2013;37(5):348–58.
7. Zhao D, Lipa M, Wielgos M, et al. Comparison between monochorionic and dichorionic placentas with special attention to vascular anastomoses and placental share. Twin Res Hum Genet 2016;19(3):191–6.
8. Blickstein I. Monochorionicity in perspective. Ultrasound Obstet Gynecol 2006; 27(3):235–8.
9. Society for Maternal-Fetal M, Simpson LL. Twin-twin transfusion syndrome. Am J Obstet Gynecol 2013;208(1):3–18.
10. Boyle B, McConkey R, Garne E, et al. Trends in the prevalence, risk and pregnancy outcome of multiple births with congenital anomaly: a registry-based study in 14 European countries 1984-2007. BJOG 2013;120(6):707–16.
11. Cavazza MC, Lai AC, Sousa S, et al. Dichorionic pregnancy complicated by a twin-to-twin transfusion syndrome. BMJ Case Rep 2019;12(10):e231614.
12. Grubbs BH, Benirschke K, Korst LM, et al. Role of low placental share in twin-twin transfusion syndrome complicated by intrauterine growth restriction. Placenta 2011;32(8):616–8.
13. Groene SG, Tollenaar LSA, van Klink JMM, et al. Twin-twin transfusion syndrome with and without selective fetal growth restriction prior to fetoscopic laser surgery: short and long-term outcome. J Clin Med 2019;8(7):969.
14. Hoskins IA, Combs CA. Society for Maternal-Fetal Medicine Special Statement: Updated checklists for management of monochorionic twin pregnancy. Am J Obstet Gynecol 2020;223(5):B16–20.

15. ACOG committee opinion no. 560: Medically indicated late-preterm and early-term deliveries. Obstet Gynecol 2013;121(4):908–10.
16. D'Antonio F, Khalil A, Mantovani E, et al. Embryonic growth discordance and early fetal loss: the STORK multiple pregnancy cohort and systematic review. Hum Reprod 2013;28(10):2621–7.
17. Papaioannou GI, Syngelaki A, Maiz N, et al. Prediction of outcome in dichorionic twin pregnancies at 6-10 weeks' gestation. Am J Obstet Gynecol 2011;205(4):348.e1-5.
18. D'Antonio F, Khalil A, Pagani G, et al. Crown-rump length discordance and adverse perinatal outcome in twin pregnancies: systematic review and meta-analysis. Ultrasound Obstet Gynecol 2014;44(2):138–46.
19. Johansen ML, Oldenburg A, Rosthoj S, et al. Crown-rump length discordance in the first trimester: a predictor of adverse outcome in twin pregnancies? Ultrasound Obstet Gynecol 2014;43(3):277–83.
20. Grande M, Gonce A, Stergiotou I, et al. Intertwin crown-rump length discordance in the prediction of fetal anomalies, fetal loss and adverse perinatal outcome. J Matern Fetal Neonatal Med 2016;29(17):2883–8.
21. Kalish RB, Gupta M, Perni SC, et al. Clinical significance of first trimester crown-rump length disparity in dichorionic twin gestations. Am J Obstet Gynecol 2004;191(4):1437–40.
22. Cimpoca B, Syngelaki A, Litwinska E, et al. Increased nuchal translucency at 11-13 weeks' gestation and outcome in twin pregnancy. Ultrasound Obstet Gynecol 2020;55(3):318–25.
23. Kagan KO, Gazzoni A, Sepulveda-Gonzalez G, et al. Discordance in nuchal translucency thickness in the prediction of severe twin-to-twin transfusion syndrome. Ultrasound Obstet Gynecol 2007;29(5):527–32.
24. Linskens IH, de Mooij YM, Twisk JW, et al. Discordance in nuchal translucency measurements in monochorionic diamniotic twins as predictor of twin-to-twin transfusion syndrome. Twin Res Hum Genet 2009;12(6):605–10.
25. Mackie FL, Hall MJ, Morris RK, et al. Early prognostic factors of outcomes in monochorionic twin pregnancy: systematic review and meta-analysis. Am J Obstet Gynecol 2018;219(5):436–46.
26. American College of O, Gynecologists, Society for Maternal-Fetal M. ACOG Practice Bulletin No. 144: Multifetal gestations: twin, triplet, and higher-order multifetal pregnancies. Obstet Gynecol 2014;123(5):1118–32.
27. Cohen SB, Elizur SE, Goldenberg M, et al. Outcome of twin pregnancies with extreme weight discordancy. Am J Perinatol 2001;18(8):427–32.
28. Chen X, Zhou Q, Xiao X, et al. The value of ultrasound in predicting isolated inter-twin discordance and adverse perinatal outcomes. Arch Gynecol Obstet 2019;299(2):459–68.
29. Fox NS, Saltzman DH, Schwartz R, et al. Second-trimester estimated fetal weight and discordance in twin pregnancies: association with fetal growth restriction. J Ultrasound Med 2011;30(8):1095–101.
30. D'Antonio F, Khalil A, Thilaganathan B. Southwest Thames Obstetric Research C. Second-trimester discordance and adverse perinatal outcome in twins: the STORK multiple pregnancy cohort. BJOG 2014;121(4):422–9.
31. Alexander GR, Kogan M, Martin J, et al. What are the fetal growth patterns of singletons, twins, and triplets in the United States? Clin Obstet Gynecol 1998;41(1):114–25.
32. Blickstein I. Is it normal for multiples to be smaller than singletons? Best Pract Res Clin Obstet Gynaecol 2004;18(4):613–23.

33. Grantz KL, Grewal J, Albert PS, et al. Dichorionic twin trajectories: the NICHD Fetal Growth Studies. Am J Obstet Gynecol 2016;215(2):221.e1-6.

34. Garite TJ, Clark RH, Elliott JP, et al. Twins and triplets: the effect of plurality and growth on neonatal outcome compared with singleton infants. Am J Obstet Gynecol 2004;191(3):700–7.

35. Ong SS, Zamora J, Khan KS, et al. Prognosis for the co-twin following single-twin death: a systematic review. BJOG 2006;113(9):992–8.

36. Hillman SC, Morris RK, Kilby MD. Single twin demise: consequence for survivors. Semin Fetal Neonatal Med 2010;15(6):319–26.

37. Mackie FL, Rigby A, Morris RK, et al. Prognosis of the co-twin following spontaneous single intrauterine fetal death in twin pregnancies: a systematic review and meta-analysis. BJOG 2019;126(5):569–78.

38. Pharoah PO, Adi Y. Consequences of in-utero death in a twin pregnancy. Lancet 2000;355(9215):1597–602.

39. Hillman SC, Morris RK, Kilby MD. Co-twin prognosis after single fetal death: a systematic review and meta-analysis. Obstet Gynecol 2011;118(4):928–40.

40. Vanderheyden TM, Fichera A, Pasquini L, et al. Increased latency of absent end-diastolic flow in the umbilical artery of monochorionic twin fetuses. Ultrasound Obstet Gynecol 2005;26(1):44–9.

41. Gratacos E, Lewi L, Carreras E, et al. Incidence and characteristics of umbilical artery intermittent absent and/or reversed end-diastolic flow in complicated and uncomplicated monochorionic twin pregnancies. Ultrasound Obstet Gynecol 2004;23(5):456–60.

42. Gratacos E, Lewi L, Munoz B, et al. A classification system for selective intrauterine growth restriction in monochorionic pregnancies according to umbilical artery Doppler flow in the smaller twin. Ultrasound Obstet Gynecol 2007;30(1):28–34.

43. Galan HL, Ferrazzi E, Hobbins JC. Intrauterine growth restriction (IUGR): biometric and Doppler assessment. Prenat Diagn 2002;22(4):331–7.

44. Bebbington MW, Danzer E, Moldenhauer J, et al. Radiofrequency ablation vs bipolar umbilical cord coagulation in the management of complicated monochorionic pregnancies. Ultrasound Obstet Gynecol 2012;40(3):319–24.

45. van Klink J, Koopman HM, Middeldorp JM, et al. Long-term neurodevelopmental outcome after selective feticide in monochorionic pregnancies. BJOG 2015;122(11):1517–24.

46. Snowise S, Moise KJ, Johnson A, et al. Donor death after selective fetoscopic laser surgery for twin-twin transfusion syndrome. Obstet Gynecol 2015;126(1):74–80.

47. Van Winden KR, Quintero RA, Kontopoulos EV, et al. Perinatal survival in cases of twin-twin transfusion syndrome complicated by selective intrauterine growth restriction. J Matern Fetal Neonatal Med 2015;28(13):1549–53.

48. Stirnemann JJ, Nasr B, Essaoui M, et al. A nomogram for perioperative prognostic risk-assessment in twin-twin transfusion syndrome. Prenat Diagn 2013;33(2):103–8.

49. Diehl W, Diemert A, Grasso D, et al. Fetoscopic laser coagulation in 1020 pregnancies with twin-twin transfusion syndrome demonstrates improvement in double-twin survival rate. Ultrasound Obstet Gynecol 2017;50(6):728–35.

50. Chavira ER, Khan A, Korst LM, et al. Are patients with twin-twin transfusion syndrome and a very short cervix candidates for laser surgery? J Ultrasound Med 2009;28(5):633–9.

51. Peeva G, Bower S, Orosz L, et al. Endoscopic placental laser coagulation in monochorionic diamniotic twins with type II selective fetal growth restriction. Fetal Diagn Ther 2015;38(2):86–93.
52. Committee Opinion No. 719 Summary: Multifetal Pregnancy Reduction. Obstet Gynecol 2017;130(3):670–1.
53. Stone J, Belogolovkin V, Matho A, et al. Evolving trends in 2000 cases of multifetal pregnancy reduction: a single-center experience. Am J Obstet Gynecol 2007; 197(4):394.e1-4.
54. Brambati B, Tului L, Baldi M, et al. Genetic analysis prior to selective fetal reduction in multiple pregnancy: technical aspects and clinical outcome. Hum Reprod 1995;10(4):818–25.
55. Jenkins TM, Wapner RJ. The challenge of prenatal diagnosis in twin pregnancies. Curr Opin Obstet Gynecol 2000;12(2):87–92.
56. Eddleman KA, Stone JL, Lynch L, et al. Chorionic villus sampling before multifetal pregnancy reduction. Am J Obstet Gynecol 2000;183(5):1078–81.
57. Ferrara L, Gandhi M, Litton C, et al. Chorionic villus sampling and the risk of adverse outcome in patients undergoing multifetal pregnancy reduction. Am J Obstet Gynecol 2008;199(4):408.e1-4.
58. Wimalasundera RC, Trew G, Fisk NM. Reducing the incidence of twins and triplets. Best Pract Res Clin Obstet Gynaecol 2003;17(2):309–29.

Recurrence Risk of Fetal Growth Restriction
Management of Subsequent Pregnancies

Nathan R. Blue, MD[a],*, Jessica M. Page, MD, MSCI[b],
Robert M. Silver, MD[c]

KEYWORDS

- Fetal growth restriction • Small for gestational age • Stillbirth • Perinatal morbidity
- Recurrence • Prevention • Low-dose aspirin • Low-molecular-weight heparin

KEY POINTS

- Women with a history of a small for gestational age (SGA) newborn have a 20% to 30% risk of SGA recurrence in a subsequent pregnancy; this may reflect genetic programming and/or recurrence of pathology.
- Smoking is the most impactful modifiable risk factor for fetal growth restriction (FGR), and earlier cessation during pregnancy reduces the risk of SGA.
- FGR surveillance in subsequent pregnancies should consist of fetal growth assessment, with the number and frequency of ultrasounds determined by the severity of the index presentation of FGR.
- Low-dose aspirin reduces the risk of birth weight less than 10th percentile by 14% in women at risk of preeclampsia, whereas unfractionated and low-molecular-weight heparins are not effective.
- No pharmacologic interventions are effective for treatment of FGR once it develops, so none are recommended in the absence of another indication outside of research protocols.

INTRODUCTION

Fetal growth restriction (FGR) occurs when fetuses do not meet their genetic growth potential, leading to stillbirth in the most severe cases. In addition to a substantial increase in stillbirth risk, FGR is also associated with increased risks for neonatal intensive care unit admission, respiratory distress, and neonatal death.[1] Beyond perinatal

[a] Maternal-Fetal Medicine, University of Utah Health, Intermountain Healthcare, 30 North 1900 East, 2A200, Salt Lake City, UT 84132, USA; [b] Maternal-Fetal Medicine, Intermountain Healthcare, University of Utah Health, 5121 South Cottonwood Street, Suite 100, Murray, UT 84107, USA; [c] Maternal-Fetal Medicine, University of Utah Health, 30 North 1900 East, 2A200, Salt Lake City, UT 84132, USA
* Corresponding author.
E-mail address: nblue1297@gmail.com
Twitter: @Nateyblue (N.R.B.); @jess_m_page (J.M.P.)

Obstet Gynecol Clin N Am 48 (2021) 419–436
https://doi.org/10.1016/j.ogc.2021.03.002
0889-8545/21/© 2021 Elsevier Inc. All rights reserved.

morbidity and mortality, growth-restricted fetuses are at increased risk for cerebral palsy, early markers of metabolic syndrome, and childhood mortality.[2–4] They also undergo adaptive metabolic programming and cardiovascular remodeling that persists into adulthood, predisposing the child to a host of enduring morbidities, including metabolic syndrome, hypertension, and early vascular disease.[5] As many as 7% to 10% of pregnancies are affected by suboptimal fetal growth, such that the global burden of lifelong morbidity and mortality from FGR is considerable.[6]

Clinicians who offer pregnancy care are commonly asked for recommendations on how to avoid pregnancy complications that occurred in a prior pregnancy. Indeed, prior experiences of a pregnancy complication can cause feelings of foreboding in a newly pregnant person, and when complications were experienced as traumatic, their recurrence may feel inevitable.[7] In such cases, clinicians have an important role characterized by reassurance, carefully timed surveillance, and measured recommendations for evidence-based dietary and lifestyle interventions. In this article, we summarize the risk of and risk factors for FGR recurrence, recommendations for antenatal surveillance in subsequent pregnancies, and available evidence on pharmacologic and lifestyle preventive strategies.

TERMINOLOGY

Small for gestational age (SGA) is a term denoting size for gestational age less than 10th percentile and can be applied to both a fetus based on ultrasonographic estimated fetal weight (EFW) and a neonate based on birth weight. Used this way, SGA does not denote any abnormality but rather a statistical deviation from the expected weight. Conversely, FGR refers to a condition of pathologic smallness that indicates a degree of compromise, which predisposes to morbidity and mortality. Antenatally, FGR can be applied to more precisely denote a clinical concern for poor growth based on evidence of fetal compromise obtained using tools such as Doppler velocimetry or nonstress tests. FGR can also be applied both antenatally to a fetus and postnatally to a newborn to distinguish between pathologic and constitutional smallness. In clinical guidelines and research, SGA is often used only to refer to birth weight and not EFW and FGR to refer to antenatal fetal size less than 10th percentile. In this article, the authors use FGR to refer to both the prenatal diagnosis of small fetal size and as an umbrella term for the global condition of poor fetal growth. SGA is used as a designation of birth weight less than 10th percentile.

RECURRENCE RISK OF FETAL GROWTH RESTRICTION

A major concern of patients with a history of pregnancies complicated by FGR is the likelihood of recurrence in a subsequent pregnancy. In an analysis of 259,481 births in the Netherlands, SGA in the first pregnancy was independently associated with recurrent SGA after controlling for maternal age, ethnicity, socioeconomic status, and year of birth (adjusted odds ratio [OR] 8.1, 95% confidence interval [CI] 7.8–8.5).[8] In an analysis of 305,654 women who delivered their first 2 live births in Missouri from 1987 to 1997, 24% of women whose firstborn infant was less than 10th percentile at birth had a subsequent SGA birth, which conferred an OR of 3.9 (95% CI 3.7–4.0).[9] Recurrence risks between 20% and 30% have been confirmed in multiple analyses.[10,11]

The generalizability of these population-scale analyses may be limited for clinical application, however, as FGR has a variety of causes, each of which has unique considerations for a subsequent pregnancy. When FGR occurs as a feature of a congenital infection or genetic syndrome such as aneuploidy, the recurrence risk is related to the recurrence risk of the specific underlying condition and is expected to be low if the underlying condition has a low recurrence risk. It is also possible that SGA is less likely to recur when it first occurred in the context of a hypertensive disorder of pregnancy than when it occurs without concomitant hypertension. In an individual patient data meta-analysis of more than 99,000 pregnancies, van Oostward and colleagues found that when SGA occurs in the context of a hypertensive disorder of pregnancy, it recurs in just 6.6% of subsequent pregnancies.[12] This recurrence rate seems to be a low outlier given other reports, but some other investigators note similar results. The previously cited analysis of 259,481 births in the Netherlands performed a stratified analysis by the presence of a hypertensive disorder of pregnancy.[8] They noted that SGA recurrence rates are only slightly higher when the index pregnancy did not have a hypertensive disorder (23.7 vs 21.0%, P<.003).[8] These estimates must be interpreted cautiously, however, as they do not account for the fact that SGA recurrence may simply reflect familial programming for smaller neonatal size rather than a recurrence of placental insufficiency. Therefore, it is possible that the recurrence risk for FGR characterized by fetal compromise is lower than these estimates suggest.

When the index case is most likely attributable to placental insufficiency or has an unclear cause, the recurrence risk may depend on placental histologic findings. In a case-control study comparing placental histopathology in cases of recurrent FGR with that of placentas from normally grown fetuses, recurrent cases of FGR were strongly associated with lesions of fetal vascular malperfusion and maternal vascular malperfusion.[13] These lesions are common and are present to some degree in approximately 30% of uncomplicated pregnancies, suggesting that although associated with recurrence, they are unlikely to be highly accurate in predicting recurrent FGR.[14,15] Conversely, high-grade villitis of unknown cause, chronic histiocytic intervillositis, and massive perivillous fibrin deposition are uncommon, denote more severe placental dysfunction, and have recurrence rates ranging from 15% to 70%.[16] Although information is lacking for guidance based on specific findings, the presence of these placental histologic findings in a prior pregnancy affected by FGR of uncertain cause suggests placental insufficiency as an underlying cause, and women may be considered at increased risk of subsequent placenta-mediated complications.

Risk Factors for Recurrence

Among those with a history of FGR-affected pregnancy, several factors can be considered risk factors for recurrence. Advanced maternal age (AMA, age ≥35 at delivery) is an independent risk factor for SGA birth weight (OR 1.4, 95% CI 1.1–1.8).[17] However, this association has not been consistent. In a systematic review and meta-analysis, Lean and colleagues assessed the relationship of AMA with various adverse pregnancy outcomes.[18] Although AMA had an overall association with SGA (OR 1.2, 95% CI 1.01–1.52), subanalysis by maternal age categories (age 35–39, 40–44, and 45–50 years) showed the association only was significant at or older than 40 years. In 2 analyses specifically assessing risk factors for recurrent FGR (combined N = 13,828), AMA was not independently associated with recurrence of SGA[11,19]; this suggests that AMA women with a history of FGR likely do not warrant additional surveillance beyond what is recommended for prior FGR alone, especially when younger than 40 years.

Interpregnancy interval has been identified as a modifiable risk factor for various adverse outcomes, but it does not seem to be an important driver of fetal growth or FGR. Reports consistently show either a modest effect[20] or no effect after accounting for familial confounding or other measures of pregnancy intention and socioeconomic status.[21–23] In the 2 studies assessing risk factors for SGA recurrence, interpregnancy interval was not independently associated with recurrence.[11,19]

Maternal smoking and passive smoke exposure during pregnancy is perhaps the most important modifiable risk factor for adverse outcomes, including FGR. Prenatal tobacco use decreases birth weight in a dose-responsive fashion,[24] and the risk diminishes earlier in pregnancy that cessation can be achieved.[25] Smoking has not been extensively studied as a risk factor for FGR recurrence, and studies are mixed on whether it is independently associated with recurrence.[11,19] However, given the many health and obstetric harms associated with smoking, tobacco use should be actively screened for and cessation pursued. The associations between selected factors and SGA birth weight are summarized in **Table 1**.

In recent well-designed studies, inherited thrombophilias have consistently not been associated with FGR and so inherited thrombophilia testing in women with a history of FGR is not recommended.[26–29] Studies evaluating obstetric outcomes in obstetric antiphospholipid syndrome (APS) report an association with SGA at birth.[30] However, this is somewhat circular and may overestimate the association because FGR requiring delivery before 34 weeks is considered a diagnostic criterion for APS. Indeed, studies evaluating antiphospholipid antibodies rather than the diagnosis of APS find they are not consistently associated with FGR. A meta-analysis of 28 studies found that lupus anticoagulant was associated with FGR in case-control studies but not cohort studies, and anticardiolipin antibodies were not associated with FGR in either case-control or cohort studies.[31] Only one study (N = 1108) assessed anti-β2 glycoprotein antibodies and found a strong association with FGR (OR 20.03, 95% CI 4.59–87.4).[31] However, a subsequently published case-control study of 1000 women reported that anti-β2 glycoprotein antibodies were not associated with a composite outcome of placenta-mediated complications that included SGA.[32]

Table 1	
Associations of selected prenatal factors with small for gestational age	
Prenatal Factor	**OR (95% CI)**
Advanced maternal age (≥35 y)[18]	1.2 (1.01–1.52)
Age <35 y	Referent
35–39 y	1.06 (0.86–1.31)
≥40 y	1.20 (1.07–1.33)
Smoking and cessation timing[25]	1.12 (0.98–1.28)
Preconception cessation	1.26 (1.05–1.52)
First trimester cessation	2.0 (1.6–2.5)
Second trimester cessation	2.46 (2.28–2.67)
No cessation	
Preconception bariatric surgery any type[37]	1.87 (1.61–2.17)
Roux-en-Y or biliopancreatic diversion	2.72 (2.32–3.2)
Laparoscopic adjustable gastric banding and/or sleeve gastrectomy	1.25 (0.62–2.51)
Iron deficiency[47]	2.2 (1.1–4.1)
Serum ferritin <15 mg/dL at 12 wk	3.0 (1.0–9.0)
Maternal hemoglobin <11.0 g/dL	
Iron supplementation[a]	0.82 (0.55–1.22)
Daily[49]	1.07 (0.31–3.74)
Intermittent[48]	

Abbreviations: CI, confidence interval; OR, odds ratio.
References with supporting data are denoted by superscript numbers.
[a] For the outcome of birth weight less than 2500 g.

It is important to distinguish between women meeting clinical and laboratory criteria for APS and those with isolated FGR or normal pregnancies but positive tests for antiphospholipid antibodies. There are data indicating that the former group benefits from APS testing and treatment and the latter does not. For example, FGR requiring delivery before 34 weeks is considered an indication for APS testing. However, data do not support testing or treatment of APS in most of the FGR cases.[26]

Fetal Growth Surveillance in Subsequent Pregnancies

In women with a history of FGR from a cause such as unexplained placental insufficiency, which may recur, additional surveillance in later pregnancies is reasonable. Although the ideal surveillance regimen in the setting of a prior FGR-affected pregnancy has not yet been determined, American College of Obstetricians and Gynecologists (ACOG) and Society for Maternal Fetal Medicine (SMFM) specifically state that prenatal fetal heart rate testing, biophysical profile testing, and umbilical artery Doppler velocimetry are not recommended in the absence of another indication.[26] For fetal growth surveillance, local resource constraints, severity of the index clinical presentation, and estimated recurrence risk are all factors to consider. A reasonable approach is to perform one additional third trimester fetal growth scan at 28 to 32 weeks in women with a history of FGR. In severe cases, when multiple risk factors are present, or when a diagnosis of FGR would require prenatal referral to a regional medical center for a higher level of postnatal support, the number of fetal growth scans can be increased based on clinical judgment, with the first planned at or before the approximate gestational age at which the diagnosis was previously made. Although other investigators may advocate for fetal growth ultrasounds every 3 or 4 weeks starting at 24 weeks until delivery in all women with a history of FGR, high-quality evidence does not exist to justify the cost and resource utilization required by such an approach. Therefore, the authors' practice is to recommend such intensive serial growth surveillance only in women at the very highest risk of morbidity from FGR, such as those with active autoimmune disease, preexisting renal disease, or a history of FGR leading to stillbirth. Additional research is needed to identify the optimal fetal growth surveillance regimen in pregnancies at risk of FGR, including in those whose primary risk factor is their obstetric history.

Preventive Strategies

Although development of novel pharmacologic options is an area of intense focus, modifiable risk factors remain an important opportunity to reduce the risk of FGR recurrence. Maternal diabetes, hypertension, and obesity are 3 examples of well-characterized risk factors for complications of placental insufficiency that are modifiable either because they are potentially reversible through lifestyle interventions or because they can be optimized before attempting pregnancy. Diabetes and obesity are typically associated with fetal overgrowth, but they can also predispose to FGR insofar, as they cause maternal vascular disease that limits the maternal vascular adaptations required for normal placental and fetal development. Pregestational diabetes mellitus (DM) deserves consideration because it can often be improved or reversed through intensive lifestyle intervention. In cases when it cannot be reversed, such as in type 1 diabetes, preconception optimization of maternal glucose control seems to have benefits. In a case-control analysis of 154 women with pregnancy complicated by pregestational diabetes, FGR was closely linked to the development of hypertensive disorders of pregnancy (HDP).[33] Women with type 2 diabetes who developed HDP had nearly 9-fold higher odds of developing FGR (OR 8.88, 95% CI 2.04–38.7). In another cohort of 1505 women with pregestational DM, Glinianaia and colleagues reported that modifiable risk factors associated with decreased birth weight included a lack of prepregnancy care, smoking during pregnancy, and increased preconception hemoglobin A1c, although none of these were independently associated with SGA at birth.[34] Despite the fact that data are lacking to specifically recommend pregestational DM optimization as an FGR prevention strategy, optimization confers other concrete benefits for pregnancy, including reduction in congenital malformations, hypertensive disorders of pregnancy, and stillbirth.[33]

Uncontrolled hypertension clearly predisposes to adverse pregnancy outcomes, but there is controversy about the ideal blood pressure (BP) range when considering antihypertensive therapy during pregnancy.[35] Although tight control may reduce the development of severe hypertension or other severe features of preeclampsia, it has also been associated with SGA birth weight.[36] The chronic hypertension and pregnancy study is an ongoing randomized controlled trial (RCT) in the United States testing the effect of different target BP ranges in women with chronic hypertension on incidence of SGA birth weight (Clinicaltrials.gov NCT02299414). The ideal preconception approach to obesity is also unclear. A meta-analysis compared outcomes in 14,880 pregnancies after bariatric surgery with those of 3,979,978 controls.[37] The investigators found that preconception bariatric surgery is associated with less fetal overgrowth but also higher risk of perinatal mortality, congenital anomalies, preterm birth, and neonatal intensive care unit admission, as well as SGA birth weight. The fact that this analysis did not account for stabilization of weight loss or the time interval between surgery and pregnancy makes preconception counseling on the optimal approach difficult because outcomes are generally reported to be good if pregnancy occurs after weight loss stabilizes and at least 12 months elapses after surgery.[38] Furthermore, this meta-analysis did not assess the effect of bariatric surgery on maternal morbidity and mortality, an important consideration given the well-established associations between maternal obesity and adverse outcomes.[39]

Diet and Fetal Growth

Patients often ask whether specific diets are recommended to optimize fetal growth and prevent FGR. Multiple supplements have been tested for potential favorable effects on fetal growth, but none have demonstrated effectiveness, including zinc,[40] calcium,[41] magnesium,[42] vitamins C,[43] D,[44] E,[45] and omega-3 fatty acids.[46] Although iron deficiency during pregnancy has been associated with SGA, iron supplementation does not seem to improve fetal growth.[47] Cochrane reviews evaluating iron supplementation conclude that intermittent oral iron supplementation did not alter birth weight or prevent low birth weight,[48] although daily iron supplementation led to slightly higher birth weights of limited clinical significance (24g mean difference, 95% CI 3–51g).[49] Another Cochrane review found that use of lipid-based nutritional supplements in low- and middle-income countries reduced the risk of SGA (3 trials, N = 4823; RR 0.94, 95% CI 0.89–0.99) when compared with iron folic acid supplements but not when compared with multiple micronutrient supplementation (3 studies, N = 2393; RR 0.93, 95% CI 0.84–1.07).[50] Similarly, a multiple-micronutrient supplementation confers a slightly decreased risk of SGA in low- and middle-income countries but no effect was seen in high-income countries.[51]

L-arginine has been tested as an intervention for fetal growth and other placenta-mediated complications based on its ability to augment nitric oxide availability, possibly leading to increased placental blood flow.[52] A meta-analysis of prenatal amino acid supplementation to treat FGR in animal and human studies found that branched chain amino acids and methyl donors had no effect on fetal growth.[53] However, the investigators found that prenatal supplementation with arginine decreased the risk of SGA in at-risk human populations (8 studies, N = 629; pooled OR 0.45, 95% CI 0.27–0.75). Although intriguing, there was significant heterogeneity, and most trials did not report enough information for full risk of bias assessment. Taken in the context of as-yet unproved benefit of sildenafil, the validity of these results remains uncertain, and further study is required before arginine supplementation can be considered for use in clinical practice.

In terms of more general dietary recommendations, many associations have been reported but few have been tested in interventional trials. Periconceptional and prenatal fruit and vegetable intake have been associated with higher birth weight and lower risk of SGA,[54–56] along with antiinflammatory and dietary approaches to stop hypertension diet,[57] shellfish,[58] and fish.[59] Conversely, 2 prospective cohort studies (N = 2635 and N = 7346) assessing caffeine use during pregnancy reported modest dose-responsive increases in the risk of SGA.[60,61] One of these studies prospectively assessed caffeine intake using a validated caffeine assessment instrument and reported increased risks of FGR with the highest risk conferred by use in the third trimester (OR range 1.4–1.8 for doses >100 mg/d compared with <100 mg daily).[60] Whether and how to integrate these findings into clinical practice is complex, as diet is difficult to accurately characterize, and associations reported in observational studies are likely to be driven by other economic and lifestyle factors that often are not replicated in interventional trials. Several approaches have been tested in RCTs and were meta-analyzed in a Cochrane review.[62] High-protein supplementation was associated with an increased risk of SGA (relative risk [RR] 1.58, 95% CI 1.03–2.41), whereas balanced energy and protein supplementation was associated with an increase in birth weight (mean difference 41g, 95% CI 5–77g) and decreased risk of SGA (RR 0.79, 95% CI 0.69–0.90). Finally, prenatal nutritional education increased birth weight in 2 trials of undernourished women (N = 320, mean difference 490g, 95% CI 428–552g) but not for adequately nourished women (1 trial, N = 406).

For women inquiring about dietary approaches to optimize fetal growth, the authors recommend a well-rounded diet with daily fruit and vegetable intake, preference of lean meat over fatty and red meat, and avoidance of excessive caffeine intake. They also recommend proactive correction of iron deficiency. Although the benefit to prevent FGR may be limited or uncertain, these represent modifiable behaviors with other health benefits and little risk and therefore are reasonable to consider.

Pharmacologic Prevention

Pharmacologic approaches to prevention and treatment of FGR can be grouped as follows: antiplatelet agents, unfractionated heparin (UFH) and low-molecular-weight heparins (LMWH), phosphodiesterase inhibitors, and other investigational agents.

Aspirin has multiple effects on vascular processes and function that are relevant for placental development and could plausibly prevent FGR. In addition to the long-known inhibition of platelet formation of thromboxane A2 and aggregation, aspirin also increases endothelial nitric oxide release and heme catabolism, which suppresses inflammation, oxidative stress, and improves endothelial function.[63,64] Although most level 1 evidence assessing aspirin use targets preeclampsia prevention, enough trials report SGA as a secondary outcome to allow for preliminary conclusions to be reached. Two meta-analyses published in 2018 (one using individual patient data[65] and one using study-level data[66]) both showed that aspirin initiation before 17 weeks conferred a significant reduction in the risk of SGA (RR 0.56, 95% CI 0.44–0.70; 0.76, 0.61–0.94), whereas initiation after 17 weeks did not. However, these findings were not replicated in the Aspirin for Evidence-Based Preeclampsia Prevention (ASPRE) trial, which was not included in either meta-analysis.[67] A subsequent Cochrane Review analyzing the effect of low-dose aspirin on preeclampsia and related complications (including SGA) was published in 2019 and analyzed data from 35,761 participants from 50 trials, including the ASPRE trial.[68] The Cochrane review found that low-dose aspirin conferred a modest reduction in the risk of birth weight less than 10th percentile (RR 0.86, 95% CI 0.75–0.99) with a number needed to treat of 142. There was no difference in birth weight less than fifth or third percentiles. However because of conflicting evidence and the fact that most trials evaluating low-dose aspirin were designed for prevention of preeclampsia and not FGR, aspirin is not recommended by SMFM or ACOG for the sole indication of FGR prevention.[26,69] However, professional societies in Canada, Australia and New Zealand, and France do recommend low-dose aspirin for FGR prevention.[70–72]

UFH and LMWH are both attractive options for FGR prevention because they both suppress inflammation,[73] inhibit complement activation,[74] and promote angiogenesis in addition to their established role in thrombosis prevention.[75–79] The use of heparin to prevent placenta-mediated complications seemed promising after early studies reported reduction in preeclampsia and FGR.[80,81] These positive results were not consistently replicated, possibly due to varying trial quality or heterogeneity in populations included, outcomes assessed, or the formulation of LMWH used.[80–87] A study-level meta-analysis of 6 trials (N = 848 participants) found that LMWH reduced a composite outcome of placental insufficiency complications including SGA birthweight, but when the investigators repeated the meta-analysis using individual patient data with the addition of data from 3 new trials, they found no effect, including in a subanalysis of women with a prior SGA neonate.[88,89] When analyzing SGA alone (N = 873), LMWH was associated with reduced risk of SGA, but this effect was only present in single-center trials, suggesting bias introduced from lower trial quality.[89] Since the publication of this meta-analysis, data from 2 more trials has become available: the Enoxaparin for Preeclampsia and Intrauterine Growth Restriction (EPPI)[87] (N = 149) and the Heparin-Preeclampsia[84] (N = 257) trials. Neither found a difference in a variety of outcomes, including SGA less than 10th and fifth percentiles. Although it remains possible that UFH or LMWH have a role in preventing placenta-mediated complications in specific subpopulations or using specific formulations, the highest quality data available show no benefit, and so LMWH is not recommended for this purpose.

Phosphodiesterase-5 inhibitors such as sildenafil and tadalafil promote vasodilation by inhibiting the breakdown of intracellular cGMP by phosphodiesterase-5. Across multiple animal models of preeclampsia and FGR, sildenafil administration rescues abnormal pup growth and normalizes umbilical artery abnormalities,[90–93] although not all animal studies have shown benefit.[94,95] A meta-analysis of preclinical sildenafil trials that included 22 animal studies and 2 human trials found that sildenafil conferred a dose-responsive improvement in both fetal growth and maternal hypertension in pregnancies affected by preeclampsia or FGR but had no effect on fetal growth in uncomplicated controls.[96] A meta-analysis of human data that included 598 participants from 7 trials described an increase in birth weight (mean difference 228g, 95% CI 28–417) but did not find any difference in other outcomes, including mortality.[97] Subsequent human trials have derailed early optimism, however. The Sildenafil Therapy in Dismal Prognosis Early-Onset Intrauterine Growth Restriction (STRIDER) trials represent the effort of an international consortium that included 5 trials in the United Kingdom, Canada, Australia, New Zealand, and the Netherlands. These studies were planned as independent trials with coordinated outcomes designed to be compatible with meta-analysis. The Dutch STRIDER trial was halted early when a planned interim analysis found that sildenafil-exposed neonates had higher rates of

Table 2
Summary of pharmacologic interventions in clinical trials

Intervention	Drug Actions	Effect on SGA	Recommended for FGR Prevention by Professional Societies? (Year)
Aspirin	Platelets: • ↓ thromboxane A2 production • ↓ aggregation Endothelium: • ↑ NO availability • ↑ heme catabolism (suppresses inflammation, oxidative stress)	2019 Meta-analysis (50 trials, N = 35,761)[68]: • BW <10th percentile: RR SGA 0.86 (0.76–0.92) • BW <3rd percentile: RR 0.91 (0.69–1.19) ASPRE trial (N = 1620)[67]: • BW<10th percentile: OR 0.77 (0.56–1.06) • BW <3rd percentile: OR 0.92 (0.57–1.51)	SMFM[69]: no (2020) ACOG[26]: no (2019) PSANZ[71]: yes (2019) CNGOF[70]: yes (2016) RCOG[109]: no (2013) SOGC[72]: yes (2013)
Heparins	• ↓ inflammation • ↓ complement activation • ↑ angiogenesis • ↓ thrombosis	Meta-analysis (2016, 9 RCTs, N = 873)[89]: • Overall: decreased SGA (14 vs 22%, $P<.01$) • Single-center trials: decreased SGA, 8% vs 23%, $P<.01$ • Multicenter trials: no difference, 18% vs 21%, $P = .3$ EPPI trial (2017): no difference, 31.9% vs 29.9%, p = NS Heparin-Preeclampsia trial (2016)[84]: 21.3% vs 27.3%, p = NS	SMFM[69]: no (2020) ACOG[26]: n/a (2019) PSANZ[71]: n/a (2019) CNGOF[70]: no (2016) RCOG[109]: no (2013) SOGC[72]: no (2013)

(continued on next page)

Table 2
(continued)

Intervention	Drug Actions	Effect on SGA	Recommended for FGR Prevention by Professional Societies? (Year)
Sildenafil, Tadalafil	• ↑vasodilation • Rescues poor fetal growth in animal models	Meta-analysis (2019, 7 trials, N = 598)[97] • Increase BW 223g (28–417) • No difference in GA at birth, delivery for fetal distress, neonatal mortality. STRIDER trials: • Netherlands[98]: stopped early due to more pulmonary hypertension in treated group (N = 216; 18.8% vs 5.1%, P<.01). No difference in composite primary outcome. • UK[101]: completed enrolment (N = 135); No difference in primary outcome (time from randomization to delivery). No harm. • Aus/NZ[100]: completed enrolment (N = 122). No difference in primary outcome (increased growth velocity). No harm. • Canada: stopped early (N = 21).[99]	For investigational use only

Abbreviations: ACOG, American College of Obstetricians and Gynecologists; BW, birth weight; CNGOF, College National des Gynecologues et Obstetriciens Francais (French College of Gynaecologists and Obstetricians); FGR, fetal growth restriction; OR, odds ratio; PSANZ, Perinatal Society of Australia and New Zealand; RCOG, Royal College of Obstetricians and Gynaecologists; RR, relative risk; SGA, small for gestational age; SMFM, Society for Maternal Fetal Medicine; SOGC, Society of Obstetricians and Gynaecologists of Canada.

pulmonary hypertension after birth (18.8% vs 5.1%, $P = .008$) with no improvement in the primary outcome of perinatal death or major neonatal morbidity before discharge.[98] Reports from the Dutch trial led to the halting of the Canadian trial after recruiting 21 participants.[99] Reports from the UK and Australia/New Zealand trials reported no improvement in outcomes in sildenafil groups, although they did not find increased neonatal pulmonary hypertension or other signals of harm.[100,101] A planned individual patient data meta-analysis of STRIDER trial results is underway. It is unclear why sildenafil did not improve outcomes in the STRIDER trials after such promising early results. It may be that the STRIDER trial did not test the ideal dosing regimen or that STRIDER participants had such severe FGR that the disease was no longer reversible. For now, clinicians should not prescribe sildenafil for FGR except in the context of a clinical trial with institutional review board oversight and participant consent.

There are several additional therapies in preclinical or clinical stages of investigation. Some of these include repurposing of existing drugs classes, including statins, proton pump inhibitors, melatonin, creatine, and N-acetylcysteine. Additional therapeutics in development include the use of nanoparticles coated in peptide sequences selectively taken up by the placenta, allowing for targeted delivery of agents such as growth factors or antioxidants.[102–107] Maternal gene therapy to temporarily increase vascular endothelial growth factor expression in the uteroplacental circulation has been tested in animal models and shows promise.[108] The use of micro-RNAs, which regulate placental growth, and hydrogen sulfide, a vasodilator and angiogenesis promoter, for FGR is in early phases of preclinical development.[108] Because the ideal intervention is one that is both accessible and low cost, investigators and funding agencies should prioritize the repurposing of exiting drugs.

For now, the only therapeutic option available to clinicians caring for those with pregnancies complicated by FGR remains delivery before stillbirth based on close fetal surveillance to identify progressive fetal compromise and placental insufficiency. Risk stratification and surveillance strategies are beyond the scope of this review but are covered in more detail in Jessica M. Page and colleagues' article, "Fetal Growth and Stillbirth," in this issue. Pharmacologic interventions tested in pPhase III trials are summarized in **Table 2**.

SUMMARY

FGR is a condition of considerable public health importance. The recurrence of FGR characterized by fetal compromise is not well described, although the recurrence of SGA birthweight is consistently reported to be 20% to 30%. There are limited options for prevention, as low-dose aspirin and heparin are not recommended for FGR prevention without another indication. The most impactful modifiable risk factor is maternal tobacco smoking. Nutritional approaches that may be modestly beneficial include balanced energy and protein supplementation, daily fruit and vegetable intake, iron supplementation, and avoidance of excessive caffeine intake. For now, clinical management of subsequent pregnancies should include ultrasonographic fetal growth surveillance without nonstress or biophysical profile tests unless otherwise indicated. Once FGR is diagnosed, management is directed at close surveillance and carefully timed delivery before stillbirth occurs.

CLINICS CARE POINTS

- SGA recurs in 20% to 30% of subsequent pregnancies.
- Smoking cessation is a key modifiable risk factor for FGR, and cessation early in pregnancy attenuates the risks of SGA at birth.
- Low-dose aspirin is modestly effective to prevent FGR, whereas unfractionated or low-molecular weight heparins are not.
- Balanced energy and protein supplementation, daily fruit and vegetable intake, along with iron supplementation and avoidance of excess caffeine intake may reduce the risk of SGA.
- Subsequent pregnancy FGR surveillance should consist of ultrasound fetal growth surveillance, although the ideal regimen is not known.

DISCLOSURE

1. NICHD, grant number 2K12HD085816-06; 2. R Baby Foundation.

REFERENCES

1. McIntire DD, Bloom SL, Casey BM, et al. Birth weight in relation to morbidity and mortality among newborn infants. N Engl J Med 1999;340(16):1234–8.
2. Jarvis S, Glinianaia SV, Torrioli M-G, et al. Cerebral palsy and intrauterine growth in single births: European collaborative study. Lancet. 2003;362(9390):1106–11.
3. Ludvigsson JF, Lu D, Hammarström L, et al. Small for gestational age and risk of childhood mortality: A Swedish population study. PLOS Med 2018;15(12): e1002717.
4. Broere-Brown ZA, Schalekamp-Timmermans S, Jaddoe VWV, et al. Deceleration of fetal growth rate as alternative predictor for childhood outcomes: a birth cohort study. BMC Pregnancy Childbirth 2019;19(1):216.
5. Crispi F, Miranda J, Gratacós E. Long-term cardiovascular consequences of fetal growth restriction: biology, clinical implications, and opportunities for prevention of adult disease. Am J Obstet Gynecol 2018;218(2):S869–79.
6. Lee AC, Katz J, Blencowe H, et al. National and regional estimates of term and preterm babies born small for gestational age in 138 low-income and middle-income countries in 2010. Lancet Glob Health 2013;1(1):e26–36.
7. Sheen K, Slade P. Examining the content and moderators of women's fears for giving birth: A meta-synthesis. J Clin Nurs 2018;27(13–14):2523–35.
8. Voskamp BJ, Kazemier BM, Ravelli ACJ, et al. Recurrence of small-for-gestational-age pregnancy: analysis of first and subsequent singleton pregnancies in The Netherlands. Am J Obstet Gynecol 2013;208(5):374.e1-6.
9. Ananth CV, Kaminsky L, Getahun D, et al. Recurrence of fetal growth restriction in singleton and twin gestations. J Maternal-Fetal Neonatal Med 2009;22(8): 654–61.
10. Hinkle S, Albert P, Mendola P, et al. Differences in risk factors for incident and recurrent small-for-gestational-age birthweight: a hospital-based cohort study. BJOG 2014;121(9):1080–9.
11. Okah FA, Cai J, Dew PC, et al. Risk factors for recurrent small-for-gestational-age birth. Am J Perinatol 2010;27(1):1–7.
12. van Oostwaard MF, Langenveld J, Schuit E, et al. Recurrence of hypertensive disorders of pregnancy: an individual patient data metaanalysis. Am J Obstet Gynecol 2015;212(5):624.e1-7.
13. Rotshenker-Olshinka K, Michaeli J, Srebnik N, et al. Recurrent intrauterine growth restriction: characteristic placental histopathological features and association with prenatal vascular Doppler. Arch Gynecol Obstet 2019;300(6): 1583–9.
14. Khong TY, Mooney EE, Ariel I, et al. Sampling and definitions of placental lesions: amsterdam placental workshop group consensus statement. Arch Pathol Lab Med 2016;140(7):698–713.
15. Zur RL, Kingdom JC, Parks WT, et al. The placental basis of fetal growth restriction. Obstet Gynecol Clin North Am 2020;47(1):81–98.
16. Chen A, Roberts DJ. Placental pathologic lesions with a significant recurrence risk - what not to miss! APMIS 2018;126(7):589–601.
17. Odibo A, Nelson D, Stamilio D, et al. Advanced maternal age is an independent risk factor for intrauterine growth restriction. Am J Perinatol 2006;23(5):325–8.

18. Lean SC, Derricott H, Jones RL, et al. Advanced maternal age and adverse pregnancy outcomes: A systematic review and meta-analysis. PLoS One 2017;12(10):e0186287.

19. Manzanares S, Maroto-Martín MT, Naveiro M, et al. Risk of recurrence of small-for-gestational-age foetus after first pregnancy. J Obstet Gynaecol 2017;37(6):723–6.

20. Schummers L, Hutcheon JA, Hernandez-Diaz S, et al. Association of Short Inter-pregnancy Interval With Pregnancy Outcomes According to Maternal Age. JAMA Intern Med 2018;178(12):1661.

21. Class QA, Rickert ME, Oberg AS, et al. Within-family analysis of interpregnancy interval and adverse birth outcomes. Obstet Gynecol 2017;130(6):1304–11.

22. Hanley GE, Hutcheon JA, Kinniburgh BA, et al. Interpregnancy interval and adverse pregnancy outcomes: an analysis of successive pregnancies. Obstet Gynecol 2017;129(3):408–15.

23. Liauw J, Jacobsen GW, Larose TL, et al. Short interpregnancy interval and poor fetal growth: Evaluating the role of pregnancy intention. Paediatric Perinatal Epi-demiol 2019;33(1):O73–85.

24. Günther V, Alkatout I, Vollmer C, et al. Impact of nicotine and maternal BMI on fetal birth weight. BMC Pregnancy Childbirth 2021;21(1):127.

25. Xaverius PK, O'Reilly Z, Li A, et al. Smoking cessation and pregnancy: timing of cessation reduces or eliminates the effect on low birth weight. Matern Child Health J 2019;23(10):1434–41.

26. Fetal Growth Restriction: ACOG Practice Bulletin, Number 227. Obstet Gynecol 2021;137(2):e16–28.

27. Infante-Rivard C, Rivard G-E, Yotov WV, et al. Absence of association of throm-bophilia polymorphisms with intrauterine growth restriction. N Engl J Med 2002;347(1):19–25.

28. McCowan LME, Craigie S, Taylor RS, et al. Inherited thrombophilias are not increased in "idiopathic" small-for-gestational-age pregnancies. Am J Obstet Gynecol 2003;188(4):981–5.

29. Verspyck E, Le Cam-Duchez V, Goffinet F, et al. Thrombophilia and immunolog-ical disorders in pregnancies as risk factors for small for gestational age infants. BJOG 2002;109(1):28–33.

30. Liu L, Sun D. Pregnancy outcomes in patients with primary antiphospholipid syndrome: A systematic review and meta-analysis. Medicine (Baltimore). 2019;98(20):e15733.

31. Abou-Nassar K, Carrier M, Ramsay T, et al. The association between antiphos-pholipid antibodies and placenta mediated complications: A systematic review and meta-analysis. Thromb Res 2011;128(1):77–85.

32. Skeith L, Abou-Nassar K, Walker M, et al. Are Anti-β2 glycoprotein 1 antibodies associated with placenta-mediated pregnancy complications? a nested case–control study. Am J Perinatol 2018;35(11):1093–9.

33. Morikawa M, Kato-Hirayama E, Mayama M, et al. Glycemic control and fetal growth of women with diabetes mellitus and subsequent hypertensive disorders of pregnancy. PLoS One 2020;15(3):e0230488.

34. Glinianaia SV, Tennant PWG, Bilous RW, et al. HbA1c and birthweight in women with pre-conception type 1 and type 2 diabetes: a population-based cohort study. Diabetologia 2012;55(12):3193–203.

35. American College of Obstetricians and Gynecologists' Committee on Practice Bulletins—Obstetrics. ACOG Practice Bulletin No. 203: chronic hypertension in pregnancy. Obstet Gynecol 2019;133(1):e26–50.

36. Magee LA, von Dadelszen P, Rey E, et al. Less-tight versus tight control of hypertension in pregnancy. N Engl J Med 2015;372(5):407–17.
37. Akhter Z, Rankin J, Ceulemans D, et al. Pregnancy after bariatric surgery and adverse perinatal outcomes: A systematic review and meta-analysis. PLOS Med 2019;16(8):e1002866.
38. Heusschen L, Krabbendam I, Van Der Velde JM, et al. A matter of timing—pregnancy after bariatric surgery. Obes Surg 2021. https://doi.org/10.1007/s11695-020-05219-3.
39. ACOG practice bulletin no. 105: bariatric surgery and pregnancy. Obstet Gynecol 2009;113(6):1405–13.
40. Ota E, Mori R, Middleton P, et al. Zinc supplementation for improving pregnancy and infant outcome. Cochrane Database Syst Rev 2015;(2):CD000230.
41. Buppasiri P, Lumbiganon P, Thinkhamrop J, et al. Calcium supplementation (other than for preventing or treating hypertension) for improving pregnancy and infant outcomes. Cochrane Database Syst Rev 2015;(2):CD007079.
42. Makrides M, Crosby DD, Shepherd E, et al. Magnesium supplementation in pregnancy. Cochrane Database Syst Rev 2014;(4):CD000937.
43. Rumbold A, Ota E, Nagata C, et al. Vitamin C supplementation in pregnancy. Cochrane Database Syst Rev 2015;(9):Cd004072.
44. De-Regil LM, Palacios C, Lombardo LK, et al. Vitamin D supplementation for women during pregnancy. Cochrane Database Syst Rev 2016;(1):Cd008873.
45. Rumbold A, Ota E, Hori H, et al. Vitamin E supplementation in pregnancy. Cochrane Database Syst Rev 2015;(9):CD004069.
46. Saccone G, Berghella V, Maruotti GM, et al. Omega-3 supplementation during pregnancy to prevent recurrent intrauterine growth restriction: systematic review and meta-analysis of randomized controlled trials. Ultrasound Obstet Gynecol 2015;46(6):659–64.
47. Alwan NA, Cade JE, McArdle HJ, et al. Maternal iron status in early pregnancy and birth outcomes: insights from the Baby's Vascular health and Iron in Pregnancy study. Br J Nutr 2015;113(12):1985–92.
48. Peña-Rosas JP, De-Regil LM, Gomez Malave H, et al. Intermittent oral iron supplementation during pregnancy. Cochrane Database Syst Rev 2015;(10):CD009997.
49. Peña-Rosas JP, De-Regil LM, Garcia-Casal MN, et al. Daily oral iron supplementation during pregnancy. Cochrane Database Syst Rev 2015;(7):Cd004736.
50. Das JK, Hoodbhoy Z, Salam RA, et al. Lipid-based nutrient supplements for maternal, birth, and infant developmental outcomes. Cochrane Database Syst Rev 2018;(8):CD012610.
51. Haider BA, Bhutta ZA. Multiple-micronutrient supplementation for women during pregnancy. Cochrane Database Syst Rev 2017;(4):CD004905.
52. Cottrell E, Tropea T, Ormesher L, et al. Dietary interventions for fetal growth restriction - therapeutic potential of dietary nitrate supplementation in pregnancy. J Physiol 2017;595(15):5095–102.
53. Terstappen F, Tol AJC, Gremmels H, et al. Prenatal Amino Acid Supplementation to Improve Fetal Growth: A Systematic Review and Meta-Analysis. Nutrients. 2020;12(9):2535.
54. McCowan L, Roberts C, Dekker G, et al. Risk factors for small-for-gestational-age infants by customised birthweight centiles: data from an international prospective cohort study. BJOG 2010;117(13):1599–607.

55. Mikkelsen TB, Osler M, Orozova-Bekkevold I, et al. Association between fruit and vegetable consumption and birth weight: A prospective study among 43,585 Danish women. Scand J Public Health 2006;34(6):616–22.

56. Ramo NR, Ballester F, Iñlguez C, et al. Vegetable but not fruit intake during pregnancy is associated with newborn anthropometric measures. J Nutr 2009; 139(3):561–7.

57. Chen L-W, Aubert AM, Shivappa N, et al. Associations of maternal dietary inflammatory potential and quality with offspring birth outcomes: An individual participant data pooled analysis of 7 European cohorts in the ALPHABET consortium. PLOS Med 2021;18(1):e1003491.

58. Amezcua-Prieto C, Martínez-Galiano JM, Salcedo-Bellido I, et al. Maternal seafood intake and the risk of small for gestational age newborns: a case–control study in Spanish women. BMJ Open. 2018;8(8). e020424.

59. Emmett PM, Jones LR, Golding J. Pregnancy diet and associated outcomes in the Avon Longitudinal Study of Parents and Children. Nutr Rev 2015;73(Suppl 3):154–74.

60. Maternal caffeine intake during pregnancy and risk of fetal growth restriction: a large prospective observational study. BMJ 2008;337(nov03 2):a2332.

61. Bakker R, Steegers EA, Obradov A, et al. Maternal caffeine intake from coffee and tea, fetal growth, and the risks of adverse birth outcomes: the Generation R Study. Am J Clin Nutr 2010;91(6):1691–8.

62. Ota E, Hori H, Mori R, et al. Antenatal dietary education and supplementation to increase energy and protein intake. Cochrane Database Syst Rev 2015;(6):Cd000032.

63. Taubert D, Berkels R, Grosser N, et al. Aspirin induces nitric oxide release from vascular endothelium: a novel mechanism of action. Br J Pharmacol 2004; 143(1):159–65.

64. Grosser N, Abate A, Oberle S, et al. Heme oxygenase-1 induction may explain the antioxidant profile of aspirin. Biochem Biophys Res Commun 2003;308(4): 956–60.

65. Meher S, Duley L, Hunter K, et al. Antiplatelet therapy before or after 16 weeks' gestation for preventing preeclampsia: an individual participant data meta-analysis. Am J Obstet Gynecol 2017;216(2):121–8.e2.

66. Roberge S, Nicolaides K, Demers S, et al. The role of aspirin dose on the prevention of preeclampsia and fetal growth restriction: systematic review and meta-analysis. Am J Obstet Gynecol 2017;216(2):110–20.e6.

67. Rolnik DL, Wright D, Poon LC, et al. Aspirin versus Placebo in Pregnancies at High Risk for Preterm Preeclampsia. N Engl J Med 2017;377(7):613–22.

68. Duley L, Meher S, Hunter KE, et al. Antiplatelet agents for preventing preeclampsia and its complications. Cochrane Database Syst Rev 2019; 2019(10):CD004659.

69. Martins JG, Biggio JR, Abuhamad A. Society for Maternal-Fetal Medicine (SMFM) Consult Series #52: Diagnosis and Management of Fetal Growth Restriction. Am J Obstet Gynecol 2020;223(4):B2–17.

70. Vayssière C, Sentilhes L, Ego A, et al. Fetal growth restriction and intra-uterine growth restriction: guidelines for clinical practice from the French College of Gynaecologists and Obstetricians. Eur J Obstet Gynecol Reprod Biol 2015; 193:10–8.

71. Stillbirth PSoAaNZaCoRE. Position statement: detection and management of fetal growth restriction in singleton pregnancies. Brisbane, Australia: Centre of Research Excellence in Stillbirth; 2019.

72. Lausman A, Kingdom J, Gagnon R, et al. Intrauterine Growth Restriction: Screening, Diagnosis, and Management. J Obstet Gynaecol Can 2013;35(8): 741–8.

73. Mousavi S, Moradi M, Khorshidahmad T, et al. Anti-Inflammatory Effects of Heparin and Its Derivatives: A Systematic Review. Adv Pharmacol Sci 2015;2015: 507151.

74. Oberkersch R, Attorresi AI, Calabrese GC. Low-molecular-weight heparin inhibition in classical complement activaton pathway during pregnancy. Thromb Res 2010;125(5):e240–5.

75. Bose P, Black S, Kadyrov M, et al. Adverse effects of lupus anticoagulant positive blood sera on placental viability can be prevented by heparin in vitro. Am J Obstet Gynecol 2004;191(6):2125–31.

76. Bose P, Black S, Kadyrov M, et al. Heparin and aspirin attenuate placental apoptosis in vitro: Implications for early pregnancy failure. Am J Obstet Gynecol 2005;192(1):23–30.

77. McLaughlin K, Baczyk D, Potts A, et al. Low Molecular Weight Heparin Improves Endothelial Function in Pregnant Women at High Risk of Preeclampsia. Hypertension 2017;69(1):180–8.

78. Sobel ML, Kingdom J, Drewlo S. Angiogenic response of placental villi to heparin. Obstet Gynecol 2011;117(6):1375–83.

79. Yinon Y, Ben Meir E, Margolis L, et al. Low molecular weight heparin therapy during pregnancy is associated with elevated circulatory levels of placental growth factor. Placenta. 2015;36(2):121–4.

80. De Vries JIP, Van Pampus MG, Hague WM, et al. Low-molecular-weight heparin added to aspirin in the prevention of recurrent early-onset pre-eclampsia in women with inheritable thrombophilia: the FRUIT-RCT. J Thromb Haemost 2012;10(1):64–72.

81. Rey E, Garneau P, David M, et al. Dalteparin for the prevention of recurrence of placental-mediated complications of pregnancy in women without thrombophilia: a pilot randomized controlled trial. J Thromb Haemost 2009;7(1):58–64.

82. Rodger MA, Hague WM, Kingdom J, et al. Antepartum dalteparin versus no antepartum dalteparin for the prevention of pregnancy complications in pregnant women with thrombophilia (TIPPS): a multinational open-label randomised trial. Lancet. 2014;384(9955):1673–83.

83. Martinelli I, Ruggenenti P, Cetin I, et al. Heparin in pregnant women with previous placenta-mediated pregnancy complications: a prospective, randomized, multicenter, controlled clinical trial. Blood. 2012;119(14):3269–75.

84. Haddad B, Winer N, Chitrit Y, et al. Enoxaparin and Aspirin Compared With Aspirin Alone to Prevent Placenta-Mediated Pregnancy Complications: A Randomized Controlled Trial. Obstet Gynecol 2016;128(5):1053–63.

85. Visser J, Ulander V-M, Helmerhorst F, et al. Thromboprophylaxis for recurrent miscarriage in women with or without thrombophilia. Thromb Haemost 2011; 105(02):295–301.

86. Kaandorp SP, Goddijn M, Van Der Post JAM, et al. Aspirin plus Heparin or Aspirin Alone in Women with Recurrent Miscarriage. N Engl J Med 2010; 362(17):1586–96.

87. Groom KM, McCowan LM, Mackay LK, et al. Enoxaparin for the prevention of preeclampsia and intrauterine growth restriction in women with a history: a randomized trial. Am J Obstet Gynecol 2017;216(3):296.e1-e4.

88. Rodger MA, Carrier M, Le Gal G, et al. Meta-analysis of low-molecular-weight heparin to prevent recurrent placenta-mediated pregnancy complications. Blood. 2014;123(6):822–8.

89. Rodger MA, Gris J-C, De Vries JIP, et al. Low-molecular-weight heparin and recurrent placenta-mediated pregnancy complications: a meta-analysis of individual patient data from randomised controlled trials. Lancet. 2016;388(10060): 2629–41.

90. Kanasaki K, Palmsten K, Sugimoto H, et al. Deficiency in catechol-O-methyltransferase and 2-methoxyoestradiol is associated with pre-eclampsia. Nature 2008;453(7198):1117–21.

91. Stanley JL, Andersson IJ, Poudel R, et al. Sildenafil Citrate Rescues Fetal Growth in the Catechol- O -methyl transferase knockout mouse model. Hypertension 2012;59(5):1021–8.

92. Dilworth MR, Andersson I, Renshall LJ, et al. Sildenafil citrate increases fetal weight in a mouse model of fetal growth restriction with a normal vascular phenotype. PLoS One 2013;8(10):e77748.

93. Oyston C, Stanley JL, Oliver MH, et al. Maternal administration of sildenafil citrate alters fetal and placental growth and fetal–placental vascular resistance in the growth-restricted ovine fetus. Hypertension 2016;68(3):760–7.

94. Miller SL, Loose JM, Jenkin G, et al. The effects of sildenafil citrate (Viagra) on uterine blood flow and well being in the intrauterine growth-restricted fetus. Am J Obstet Gynecol 2009;200(1):102.e1-7.

95. Nassar A, Masrouha K, Itani H, et al. Effects of Sildenafil in Nω-Nitro-l-Arginine Methyl Ester-Induced Intrauterine Growth Restriction in a Rat Model. Am J Perinatol 2012;29(06):429–34.

96. Paauw ND, Terstappen F, Ganzevoort W, et al. Sildenafil During Pregnancy. Hypertension 2017;70(5):998–1006.

97. Ferreira RDDS, Negrini R, Bernardo WM, et al. The effects of sildenafil in maternal and fetal outcomes in pregnancy: A systematic review and meta-analysis. PLoS One 2019;14(7). e0219732.

98. Pels A, Derks J, Elvan-Taspinar A, et al. Maternal sildenafil vs placebo in pregnant women with severe early-onset fetal growth restriction. JAMA Netw Open 2020;3(6):e205323.

99. STRIDER CANADA. PREgnancy Evidence, Monitoring, Partnerships and Treatment (Pre-empt) Consortium. 2021. Available at: https://pre-empt.obgyn.ubc.ca/evidence/strider-canada. Accessed February 17, 2021.

100. Groom K, McCowan L, Mackay L, et al. STRIDER NZAus: a multicentre randomised controlled trial of sildenafil therapy in early-onset fetal growth restriction. BJOG 2019;126(8):997–1006.

101. Sharp A, Cornforth C, Jackson R, et al. Maternal sildenafil for severe fetal growth restriction (STRIDER): a multicentre, randomised, placebo-controlled, double-blind trial. Lancet Child Adolesc Health 2018;2(2):93–102.

102. Harris LK. Could peptide-decorated nanoparticles provide an improved approach for treating pregnancy complications? Nanomedicine (Lond) 2016; 11(17):2235–8.

103. Constância M, Hemberger M, Hughes J, et al. Placental-specific IGF-II is a major modulator of placental and fetal growth. Nature 2002;417(6892):945–8.

104. King A, Ndifon C, Lui S, et al. Tumor-homing peptides as tools for targeted delivery of payloads to the placenta. Sci Adv 2016;2(5):e1600349.

105. van der Heijden OW, Essers YP, Fazzi G, et al. Uterine artery remodeling and reproductive performance are impaired in endothelial nitric oxide synthase-deficient mice. Biol Reprod 2005;72(5):1161–8.

106. Phillips TJ, Scott H, Menassa DA, et al. Treating the placenta to prevent adverse effects of gestational hypoxia on fetal brain development. Sci Rep 2017;7(1): 9079.

107. Cureton N, Korotkova I, Baker B, et al. Selective Targeting of a Novel Vasodilator to the Uterine Vasculature to Treat Impaired Uteroplacental Perfusion in Pregnancy. Theranostics. 2017;7(15):3715–31.

108. Groom KM, David AL. The role of aspirin, heparin, and other interventions in the prevention and treatment of fetal growth restriction. Am J Obstet Gynecol 2018; 218(2):S829–40.

109. Gynaecologists RCoOa. The Investigation and Management of the Small for Gestational Age Fetus2013. Located at: Green-top Guideline.